Roshan Lall Gupta's
Recent Advances in
SURGERY

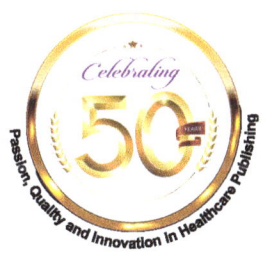

Roshan Lall Gupta's
Recent Advances in
SURGERY

Volume 16

Editor

Puneet
MS DNB (Surg) MNAMS FACS
Professor
Department of Surgery
Institute of Medical Sciences
Banaras Hindu University
Varanasi, Uttar Pradesh, India

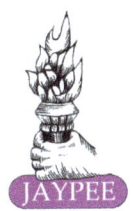

JAYPEE BROTHERS MEDICAL PUBLISHERS
The Health Sciences Publisher
New Delhi | London | Panama

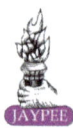 **Jaypee Brothers Medical Publishers (P) Ltd**

Headquarters
Jaypee Brothers Medical Publishers (P) Ltd.
4838/24, Ansari Road, Daryaganj
New Delhi 110 002, India
Phone: +91-11-43574357
Fax: +91-11-43574314
E-mail: jaypee@jaypeebrothers.com

Overseas Offices

JP Medical Ltd.
83, Victoria Street, London
SW1H 0HW (UK)
Phone: +44-20 3170 8910
Fax: +44(0)20 3008 6180
E-mail: info@jpmedpub.com

Jaypee-Highlights Medical Publishers Inc.
City of Knowledge, Bld. 235, Clayton
Panama City, Panama
Phone: +1 507-301-0496
Fax: +1 507-301-0499
E-mail: cservice@jphmedical.com

Jaypee Brothers Medical Publishers (P) Ltd.
Bhotahity, Kathmandu, Nepal
Phone: +977-9741283608
E-mail: kathmandu@jaypeebrothers.com

Website: www.jaypeebrothers.com
Website: www.jaypeedigital.com

© 2019, Jaypee Brothers Medical Publishers

The views and opinions expressed in this book are solely those of the original contributor(s)/author(s) and do not necessarily represent those of editor(s) of the book.

All rights reserved. No part of this publication may be reproduced, stored or transmitted in any form or by any means, electronic, mechanical, photocopying, recording or otherwise, without the prior permission in writing of the publishers.

All brand names and product names used in this book are trade names, service marks, trademarks or registered trademarks of their respective owners. The publisher is not associated with any product or vendor mentioned in this book.

Medical knowledge and practice change constantly. This book is designed to provide accurate, authoritative information about the subject matter in question. However, readers are advised to check the most current information available on procedures included and check information from the manufacturer of each product to be administered, to verify the recommended dose, formula, method and duration of administration, adverse effects and contraindications. It is the responsibility of the practitioner to take all appropriate safety precautions. Neither the publisher nor the author(s)/editor(s) assume any liability for any injury and/or damage to persons or property arising from or related to use of material in this book.

This book is sold on the understanding that the publisher is not engaged in providing professional medical services. If such advice or services are required, the services of a competent medical professional should be sought.

Every effort has been made where necessary to contact holders of copyright to obtain permission to reproduce copyright material. If any have been inadvertently overlooked, the publisher will be pleased to make the necessary arrangements at the first opportunity. The **CD/DVD-ROM** (if any) provided in the sealed envelope with this book is complimentary and free of cost. **Not meant for sale.**

Inquiries for bulk sales may be solicited at: jaypee@jaypeebrothers.com

Roshan Lall Gupta's Recent Advances in Surgery (Volume 16)

First Edition: **2019**

ISBN: 978-93-5270-828-4

Dedicated to
My wife, Ritu Ragini
son, Akshat and daughter, Aanya

Contributors

Aditya Kumar
Senior Resident
Minimal Access Surgery
Department of Surgical Disciplines
All India Institute of Medical Sciences
New Delhi, India

Ajay K Khanna
Professor
Department of Surgery
Institute of Medical Sciences
Banaras Hindu University
Varanasi, Uttar Pradesh, India

Arunima Verma
Consultant Surgeon
Tata Main Hospital
Jamshedpur, Jharkhand, India

Arvind Kumar
Senior Consultant and Chairman
Department of Thoracic Surgery
Director
Institute of Robotic Surgery
Sir Ganga Ram Hospital
New Delhi, India

Belal Bin Asaf
Consultant
Department of Thoracic Surgery
Institute of Robotic Surgery
Sir Ganga Ram Hospital
New Delhi, India

Gaurav Agarwal
Professor
Department of Endocrine and
Breast Surgery
Sanjay Gandhi Postgraduate
Institute of Medical Sciences
Lucknow, Uttar Pradesh, India

Gaurav Joshi
Senior Resident
Minimal Access Surgery
Department of Surgical Disciplines
All India Institute of Medical Sciences
New Delhi, India

Harsh Vardhan Puri
Associate Consultant
Department of Thoracic Surgery
Institute of Robotic Surgery
Sir Ganga Ram Hospital
New Delhi, India

Jaya Ghosh
Professor
Department of Medical Oncology
Tata Memorial Hospital
Homi Bhabha National Institute
Mumbai, Maharashtra, India

Manish Pandey
Senior Resident
Department of Urology
Institute of Medical Sciences
Banaras Hindu University
Varanasi, Uttar Pradesh, India

Manish S Bhandare
Assistant Professor and Consultant
Surgeon
Department of Gastrointestinal and
Hepato-Pancreatico-Biliary Surgery
Tata Memorial Hospital
Mumbai, Maharashtra, India

N Ananthakrishnan
Professor
Department of Surgery
Mahatma Gandhi Medical College
and Research Institute
Sri Balaji Vidyapeeth Deemed University
Puducherry, India

PK Sasmal
Associate Professor
Department of General Surgery
All India Institute of Medical Sciences
Bhubaneswar, Odisha, India

Puneet
Professor
Department of Surgery
Institute of Medical Sciences
Banaras Hindu University
Varanasi, Uttar Pradesh, India

R Kalayarasan
Associate Professor of Surgical Gastroenterology
Jawaharlal Institute of Postgraduate Medical Education and Research
Puducherry, India

Rahul
Assistant Professor
Department of Surgical Gastroenterology
Sanjay Gandhi Postgraduate Institute of Medical Sciences
Lucknow, Uttar Pradesh, India

Rahul Khanna
Professor
Department of Surgery
Institute of Medical Sciences
Banaras Hindu University
Varanasi, Uttar Pradesh, India

Rajeev Sinha
Professor
Department of Surgery
Maharani Laxmi Bai Medical College
Jhansi, Uttar Pradesh, India

Rajinder Parshad
Professor of Surgery
Department of Surgical Disciplines
All India Institute of Medical Sciences
New Delhi, India

Ramya VC
Senior Resident
Department of Endocrine and Breast Surgery
Sanjay Gandhi Postgraduate Institute of Medical Sciences
Lucknow, Uttar Pradesh, India

Richa Sinha
Assistant Professor
Department of Microbiology
Indira Gandhi Institute of Medical Sciences
Patna, Bihar, India

RN Meena
Assistant Professor
Department of Surgery
Institute of Medical Sciences
Banaras Hindu University
Varanasi, Uttar Pradesh, India

S Suresh Kumar
Additional Professor
Department of Surgery
Jawaharlal Institute of Postgraduate Medical Education and Research
Puducherry, India

Sajal Rai
Consultant Laparoscopic and Colorectal Surgeon
Stepping Hill Hospital
Stockport, Manchester, UK

Sameer Trivedi
Professor
Department of Urology
Institute of Medical Sciences
Banaras Hindu University
Varanasi, Uttar Pradesh, India

Satyendra K Tiwary
Associate Professor
Department of Surgery
Institute of Medical Sciences
Banaras Hindu University
Varanasi, Uttar Pradesh, India

Seema Khanna
Professor
Department of Surgery
Institute of Medical Sciences
Banaras Hindu University
Varanasi, Uttar Pradesh, India

Shaifali Goel
Attending Consultant
Department of Gastrointestinal and Hepato-Pancreatico-Biliary Oncosurgery
Rajiv Gandhi Cancer Institute and Research Center
New Delhi, India

Shailesh V Shrikhande
Professor and Head
Division of Cancer Surgery
Chief
Department of Gastrointestinal and Hepato-Pancreatico-Biliary Surgery
Deputy Director
Tata Memorial Hospital
Mumbai, Maharashtra, India

Shaleen Agarwal
Senior Consultant
Department of Liver Transplant and Hepato-Pancreatico-Biliary Surgery
Center for Liver and Biliary Sciences
Max Superspecialty Hospital
New Delhi, India

Shivendra Singh
Senior Consultant and Chief
Department of GI and Hepato-Pancreatico-Biliary Oncosurgery
Rajiv Gandhi Cancer Institute and Research Center
New Delhi, India

Sujith Kumar M
Specialist Registrar
Department of Medical Oncology
Tata Memorial Hospital
Homi Bhabha National University
Mumbai, Maharashtra, India

Sunil Kumar
Professor and Head
Consultant Surgery
Tata Main Hospital
Jamshedpur, Jharkhand, India

Vikram Chaudhari
Assistant Professor and Consultant Surgeon
Department of Gastrointestinal and Hepato-Pancreatico-Biliary Surgery
Tata Memorial Hospital
Mumbai, Maharashtra, India

Vikram Kate
Professor
Department of General and Gastrointestinal Surgery
Jawaharlal Institute of Postgraduate Medical Education and Research
Puducherry, India

VK Kapoor
Professor
Department of Surgical Gastroenterology
Sanjay Gandhi Postgraduate Institute of Medical Sciences
Lucknow, Uttar Pradesh, India

Preface

This edition of *Roshan Lall Gupta's Recent Advances in Surgery (Vol. 16)* is a compilation of evidence-based knowledge for postgraduate and young practicing surgeons and will update them with the latest developments in the field of surgery. The chapters are concise and not only discuss the surgical techniques and management, but also the detail preoperative evaluation, postoperative management and follow-ups of surgical patients. This book will also help to postgraduate students and young surgeons in preparation of various examinations.

This book has contributions from eminent surgeons in their respective specialties. They have compiled best of their knowledge in clinical practice with evidence. In the present era, evidence-based practice has taken precedence and is to be strictly followed. In this fast-changing world, it is also imperative to keep abreast with the latest developments in the field of imaging, evaluation and management of surgical problems. In surgical practice, it is important to have knowledge of newer imaging modalities for not only accurate diagnosis and but also for planning of surgical procedure.

Puneet

Acknowledgments

I thank all the authors for their contribution to this edition. The text is in simple language and student-friendly for easy understanding, and appropriate for young surgeons to adapt in clinical practice. I am quite hopeful that this edition will be informative. I am thankful to M/s Jaypee Brothers Medical Publishers (P) Ltd, New Delhi, India, for publishing this book.

Contents

1. Energy Sources in Surgical Practice 1
   Rajeev Sinha

2. Management of Colorectal Liver Metastases 27
   Shaleen Agarwal

3. Complications of Acute Pancreatitis 43
   PK Sasmal, VK Kapoor

4. Management of Colon Cancer: Changing Trends,
   Recent Advances and Current Practices 62
   *Vikram Kate, R Kalayarasan, S Suresh Kumar, Sajal Rai,
   N Ananthakrishnan*

5. Management of Intestinal Obstruction 89
   Sunil Kumar, Arunima Verma

6. Barrett's Esophagus 108
   Rajinder Parshad, Aditya Kumar, Gaurav Joshi

7. Borderline Resectable and Locally Advanced
   Pancreatic Cancer 129
   Manish S Bhandare, VikramChaudhari, Shailesh V Shrikhande

8. Minimally Invasive Thoracic Surgery 146
   Belal Bin Asaf, Harsh Vardhan Puri, Arvind Kumar

9. Abdominal Tuberculosis 165
   Rahul, Richa Sinha, Puneet

10. Recent Advances in Renal Cell Carcinoma 190
    Sameer Trivedi, Manish Pandey

11. Peritoneal Carcinomatosis 219
    Shaifali Goel, Shivendra Singh

12. Drug Resistance in Cancer 239
    Sujith Kumar M, Jaya Ghosh

13. Vascular Malformations 249
    Satyendra K Tiwary, Ajay K Khanna

14. Triple-negative Breast Cancer 268
    Seema Khanna, RN Meena, Rahul Khanna

15. Hormone Therapy for Breast Cancer 280
    Ramya VC, Gaurav Agarwal

Index *297*

Chapter 1

Energy Sources in Surgical Practice

Rajeev Sinha

INTRODUCTION

The present day surgeon has a number of energy sources at his disposal, to help him to cut and coagulate tissues. These energy sources include electrical, laser, ultrasonic, and mechanical. Each of these has unique properties that determine its effectiveness and limitations when used during any kind of surgery, including minimally invasive surgery. The surgeon must realize that learning the use of a specific energy source, does not in itself practically lessen the chance of a complication. A complete understanding of the equipment, physics of the energy source, its potential hazards and limitations is essential, if energy source-related complications are to be reduced.

THERMAL TISSUE EFFECTS

Hyperthermia-induced tissue changes, start at, as early as 44°C in the form of tissue necrosis. Between 50°C and 80°C protein coagulation and collagen is converted to glucose. Between 80°C and 100°C, total desiccation of tissue occurs, and beyond 100°C, tissue is vaporized. With fulguration, when the temperature climbs to 200°C and above, carbonization starts and a visible black eschar can be seen (Fig. 1). The various energy sources utilized clinically, achieve varying degrees of hyperthermia. The ultrasonic wave achieves 80°C, the laser works at 200°C, and electrosurgery can achieve temperatures as high as 400°C. The final temperature acheived, however, also depends on the time that the energy source is applied to the tissue.

Hypothermia to –40°C and below, results in tissue freezing and in the postthaw period, there is vascular endothelial damage leading to thrombosis and cell membrane dysfunction. With temperature decreasing to –195°C below zero, there is intracellular and extracellular ice formation, leading to cell dehydration and shrinkage. With thawing, the melted extracellular water rushes inside the cell and the cell bursts.

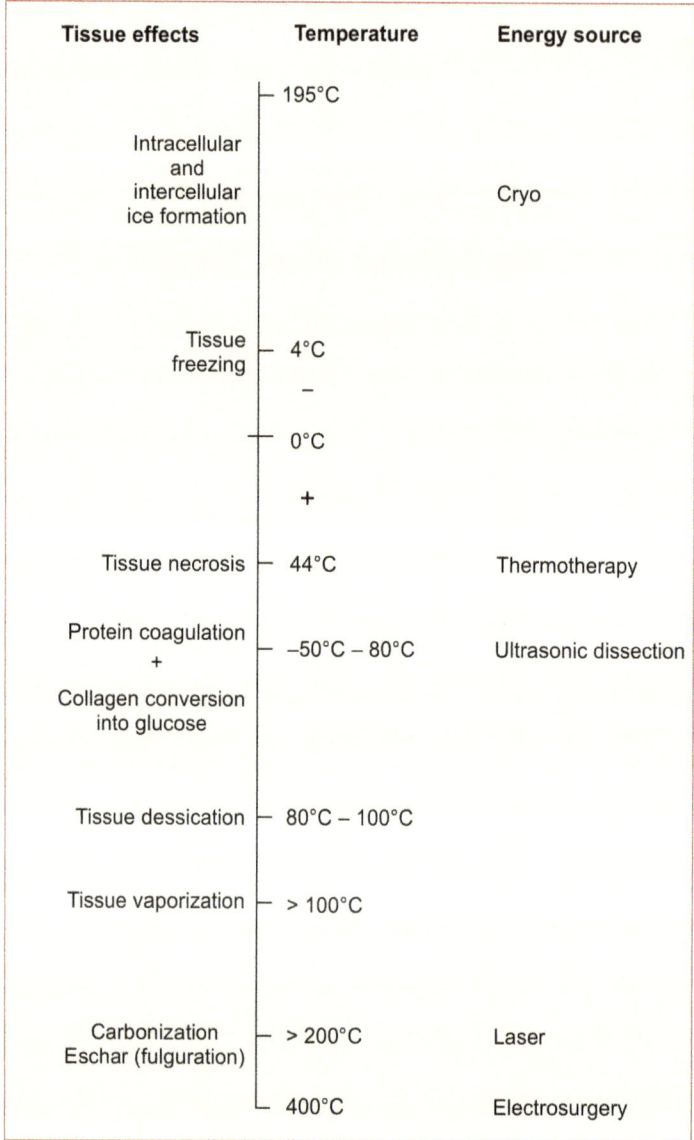

Fig. 1: Temperature determined tissue changes.

Electrosurgery

Physics

- Electrosurgery uses an alternating radiofrequency current in the frequency range of 500,000 to 2 million Hz per second. The rapid reversal of this very high frequency alternating current means that ion positions across cellular membranes do not change. As a result, neuromuscular membranes do not depolarize, and there is no danger of muscle contraction or cardiac defibrillation at these high frequencies. On the other hand, household current, with its low frequency of 60 Hz can produce ventricular fibrillation and gives the typical shock.[1,2]

- The terms *electrocautery* and *electrosurgery* are often used interchangeably in modern surgical practice. However, these terms define two distinctly different electrical applications.[3,4] Electrocautery is the use of electricity to heat a metallic object which then transfers the heat to the tissue helping to coagulate or burn, but, there is no current flow through the object being cauterized. In electrosurgery, the electrical current flows through the tissue and heats the tissue by the excitation of cellular ions.[5,6]
- There are 3 types of electrical currents in clinical usage:
    1. *Direct current*, which is unidirectional, is also known as galvanic current and is used in acupuncture and endothermy but not for electrosurgery.
    2. *AC or alternating current* where the flow changes in a sinusoidal fashion and is used in electrosurgery.
    3. *Pulsed current* where a high amount of electrical energy is discharged in a very short time. It is used for electromyography and nerve stimulation.
- Current flowing through the body takes the path of least resistance which in the human body means tissues with maximal water or in other words, the electrical resistance is in inverse proportion to water content of tissues. Thus blood is most conductive followed by nerve, muscle, adipose tissue and finally, least conductive is the bone. The path of the current in body tissues is not always a straight one. As soon as the current passes through a tissue it dries or it desiccates it, thus increasing its resistance and making it nonconductive. The current then takes the path through adjacent tissues which are still hydrated and thus have lesser resistance. Hence, the flow pattern of current through live tissue can never be predicted. Also this changing resistance of body tissues during the current flow requires that electrosurgical generators must deliver current at increasing voltages that should match the expected increase in tissue resistance of the human body, otherwise, current flow can be too low to produce the desired effect or too great, resulting in injury.
- The current density is an important variable determining the biological effect of the current and can be defined as amperes/area or amp/cm^2. This explains why the pinpoint tip of an electrosurgical pencil works more effectively than a spatula. The less the area of contact, the more the density of the current at the point of contact and thus greater would be the effect (Fig. 2). Current flowing through the tissue raises the temperature of

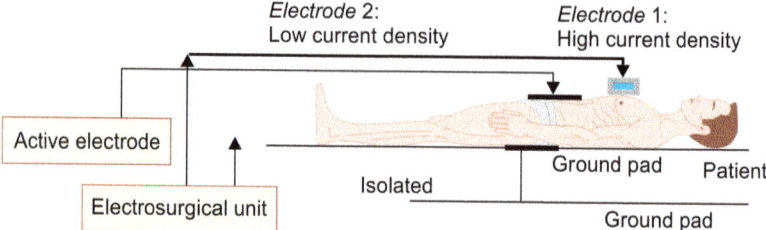

Fig. 2: Current density. Electrode 1 with a smaller surface area, generates current density more than under electrode 2, similarly the area of the ground pad, would determine the current density at its site of attachment. Larger surface areas for the ground pad are obviously better.

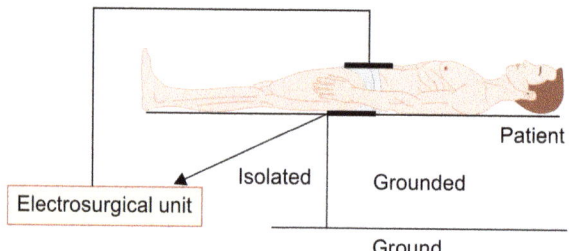

Fig. 3: Isolated and grounded generator system. In the grounded generator, the current returns to the earth while in the isolated generator, the current goes back into the electrosurgical unit. All present day ESUs are isolated types.

the tissue and generates heat. The amount of heat thus released is directly proportional to the resistance of the tissues.

- The electrical current in electrosurgery can be delivered through two kinds of circuits. In the unipolar circuit, the ground pad (which is incorrectly called earth plate) takes the current back to the machine after traveling through the body.[3,7] Thus it should be the aim to minimize the distance between the operating electrode and the ground pad. In the bipolar circuit, because both the positive and negative electrodes are near to each other, the current flow inside the body is minimal and is thus less damaging.

- Electrosurgical generator units (ESU) are essentially of two types: grounded and isolated (Fig. 3). The newer isolated generators eliminate the possibility of an alternate site burn by requiring the current to return to the generator.[5,8] In the early grounded generators the current returned to earth via any contact point and thus caused inadvertent alternate site burns.

- Both the unipolar and bipolar circuits can further be modified as open and closed circuit. Open circuit is typically formed when the electrode does not make contact with the tissues or the tissue in contact with the electrode is already desiccated. In the circuit the resistance increases and generator increases the voltage to close the circuit and the waveform also becomes erratic. The current in closed circuit is safe and delivers lesser voltage.

Biophysics

The electrosurgical effect on the tissue results in three definable effects:[9,10]
1. Cutting
2. Coagulation and/or fulguration
3. Desiccation.

1. *Cutting:* True electrosurgical cutting is a *noncontact* activity in which the electrosurgical instrument must be a short distance from the tissue to be cut. If there is contact, desiccation leading to mechanical cutting rather than pure-cutting ensues. True-cutting requires the generation of sparks between the electrode and the tissue, which generates extreme heat which leads to cell explosion.

2. *Fulguration:* In this mode also, there is a *no contact* between the electrosurgical delivery device and the tissue. In contrast to cutting, fulguration requires short bursts of high voltage only 10% of the time to produce sparks but a low power to produce coagulation. Coagulation and fulguration thus utilize higher voltage than cutting but the pause between current flows is more (maximum pause in fulguration). Both cause coagulative necrosis of tissues and fluid.

3. *Desiccation:* Is the process by which the tissue is heated and the water in the cell boils to steam, resulting in a drying out of the cell. Desiccation can be achieved with either the cutting or the coagulation current by *contact* of the electrosurgical device with the tissue because no sparks are generated. Therefore, desiccation is a low power form of coagulation without sparking, and *it is the most common mode used by the surgeon.*

- *The blend current*: The pure-cutting current will cut the tissue but will provide poor hemostasis. The coagulation current will provide excellent coagulation but minimal cutting. The blend current is an intermediate current between the cutting and the coagulation current, as one might expect. In actuality, it is a cutting current–the duty cycle or time that the current is actually lowing during activation of the electrosurgical delivery device is decreased from 100% of the time to 80–50% (Fig. 4).[11,12] It is important to note that setting the generator to blend mode does nothing to alter the coagulation current that is provided. Only the cutting current is altered so that the duty cycle is reduced to provide more hemostasis.

- *Use in laparoscopic surgery*: It was initially believed that the use of electrosurgery in laparoscopic surgery would have unique problems. The low heat capacity of the insufflating gas would result in instruments not cooling as rapidly as in the open environment. In addition the high-water content of the insufflated gas would increase the conductive capacity of the medium. But evidence does not substantiate these beliefs. However, laparoscopic application of electrosurgery has other problems, giving rise to unique complications.[3,13]

Complications

Injudicious use of the ESU in open and laparoscopic surgery can be associated with:
- Grounding failures
- Alternate site injuries
- Demodulated currents
- Insulation failure
- Tissue injury at a distal site
- Sparking
- Direct coupling
- Capacitive coupling
- Surgical glove injury
- Explosion.

Ground pad failures: The large surface area of contact of the return electrode with the body and prevents injury by dispersing the current over a larger surface area. Lack of uniform contact, however, can result in significant current concentration and damage, and any conductive low resistance object

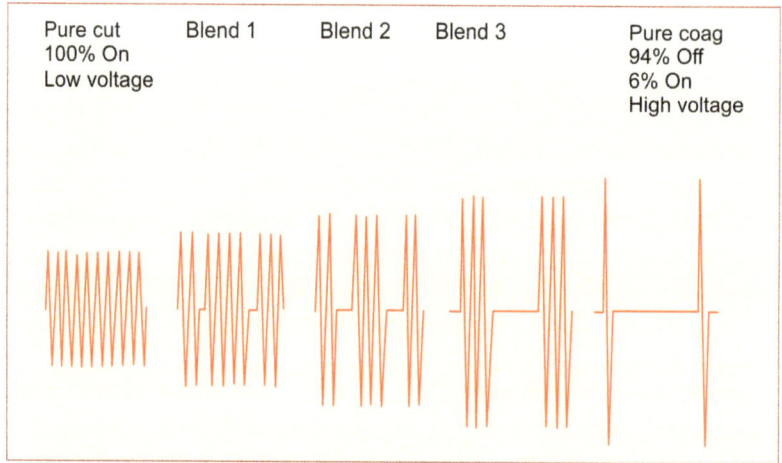

Fig. 4: Difference between pure cut and pure coagulation current. Pure cut is a low voltage continuous current, while a coagulation current is of very high voltage in very short bursts. Blend mode—only the cutting current is altered so that the duty cycle is reduced (i.e. time off becomes more than on) to provide more hemostasis.

can then serve as the alternate conduit. Exit of current at these alternate sites can produce injury because of the high current density.

The application of the ground pad to a body surface which is uneven results in inadequate contact and causes tissue injury. Thus the pad is best not kept under the scapulas, heels or other bony structures such as the skull. It is always safe to keep it under the buttocks or thighs or the calf muscles.

Demodulated currents: Modern generators have filters that remove demodulated currents so that only electrical current of 250–2,000 kHz is delivered. Demodulated currents occur most commonly when an electrosurgical instrument is activated off metal and then touched to the metal, such as the common practice of "buzzing a hemostat." Demodulated currents produce neuromuscular activity that is usually of no significance unless directly coupled to the heart through a catheter or during a cardiothoracic surgical procedure. Another example of demodulated current is muscle fasciculation at the site of application during the use of electrosurgery.

Insulation failure: Insulation failure is thought to be the most common reason for electrosurgical injury during laparoscopic procedures and more commonly seen with high voltage coagulation currents. The key factor that determines the magnitude of injury from insulation failure resides in the size of the break in the insulation.[5,14] Paradoxically, the smaller the break, the more the chances of it being missed and greater the likelihood of injury on contact with tissue.[5,15]

This is related to the concept of power density. Protection against insulation failure is provided by the active electrode monitoring system, available in many machines and which switches the current off, if there is an insulation failure.[5,16]

Tissue injury: Current passing through structures of small cross-sectional area may have current concentrated there, with resultant unintentional thermal injury. For example, if the testicle and cord are skeletonized and mobilized from the scrotum, application of energy to the testicle can result in damage to the cord, because the current must return to the indifferent electrode (ground pad) through the small diameter cord before it is dissipated in the body through numerous pathways. Another example is of cutting an adhesive band from the gallbladder to the duodenum with electrosurgery. If the adhesion is wider near the gallbladder than on the duodenum, the current density will be greater on the duodenum injuring the duodenum (Fig. 5).

Another inadvertent method of tissue injury may occur as follows. Reapplication of current near anal ready desiccated or fulgurated tissue may create an unwanted exit route through a small contact area, which builds up a high current density. The typical example is during electrosurgical distal tubal cauterization. Initial cauterization of the tube near the isthmus produces an

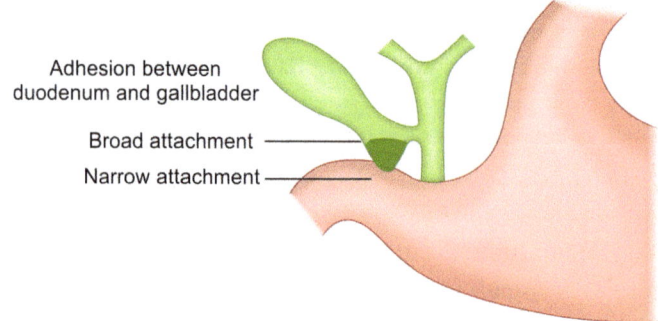

Fig. 5: Tissue injury during adhesionolysis. The attachment of the adhesion has a narrower duodenal attachment as compared to the gallbladder end; hence there is greater current density at the duodenal end of the adhesion. This translates into greater chances of duodenal injury.

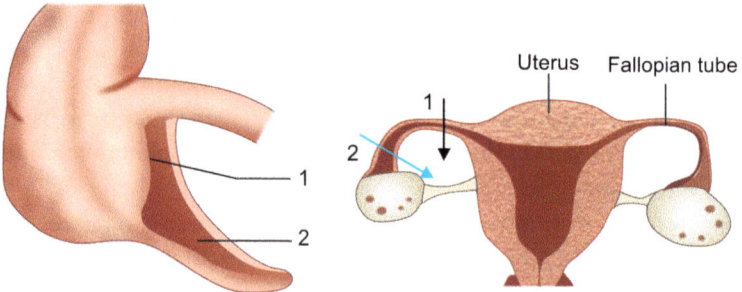

Fig. 6: Tissue injury at distal site. Because the first application 1 desiccates the tissue and makes it nonconductive, thus the second cauterization site denoted as 2 can only disseminate current through the tip of the appendix or the terminal end of the tubes. This would damage the adjacent structure to these sites and would present as delayed cautery burns and if the current passes to an intestinal segment in the vicinity, then usually perforation results. So after cauterization at site 1 further cauterization should not be done at site 2.

electrical nonconductive tissue. If further application is done toward the uterine side, the current exits through the uterus and out of the body. But if the current is reapplied towards the tubal side, the current can only flow out toward the ground plate through the fimbrial end and if the fimbrial end is in contact with a bowel loop it sets up a thermal injury (Fig. 6).

The tissue injury can also occur with other freely mobile or small area structures near to vital structures, such as infundibulopelvic, uterosacral, ovarian ligaments and the appendix.

Direct tissue injury is easy to recognize and repair. Indirect gastrointestinal tract (GIT) injuries are usually missed at the time when they occur only to manifest 72 hours later when coagulative necrosis is complete. Thus the clinical presentation is always delayed and the patient then presents with peritonitis.

- *Sparking and arcing:* Jumping of sparks from the electrode to tissues is the mechanism for fulguration and true electrosurgical cutting. However, it can also occur in an unintended fashion such that injury results, especially in laparoscopic surgery. Current can jump from any place on the uninsulated end of the electrode or an area of insulation break and not necessarily only from the tip. In addition, build up of eschar, or desiccated tissue sticking on the electrosurgical instrument may promote arcing from the shaft instead of the tip of the electrode leading to sparking to a secondary site. However fortunately, sparking with monopolar electric current is small because, under normal operating conditions at 30–35 W, 50% of the time, the spark jumps only 2–3 mm, and this is not enough to allow significant air or CO_2 gaps to bebridged. However, the tip of the laparoscopic instrument should always be kept clean.
- *Direct coupling:* Direct coupling occurs when an electrosurgical device is in contact with a conductive instrument which then conducts electricity.[9,17] Direct coupling can be reduced by using only insulated instruments and careful attention to avoid contact with any metallic object in the operative field and activating the electrosurgical electrode only inside the visual field and never near another metal object such as a clip, staple, laparoscope, or metal instrument (Fig. 7).
- *Capacitive coupling:* Capacitance is stored electrical charge that occurs between two conductors which are separated by an insulator

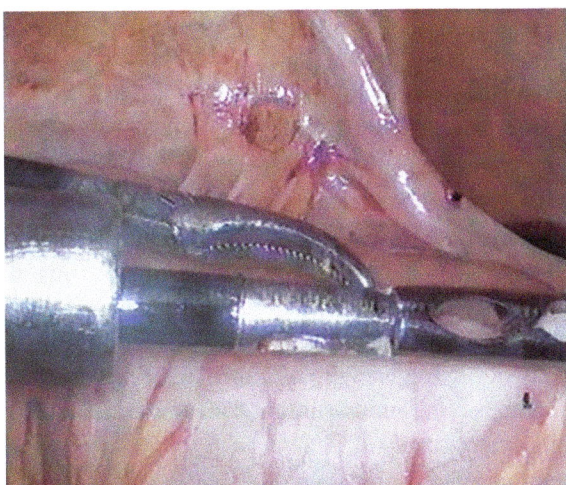

Fig. 7: Direct coupling. Accidental direct contact between the cautery connected Maryland dissector and 2nd instrument.

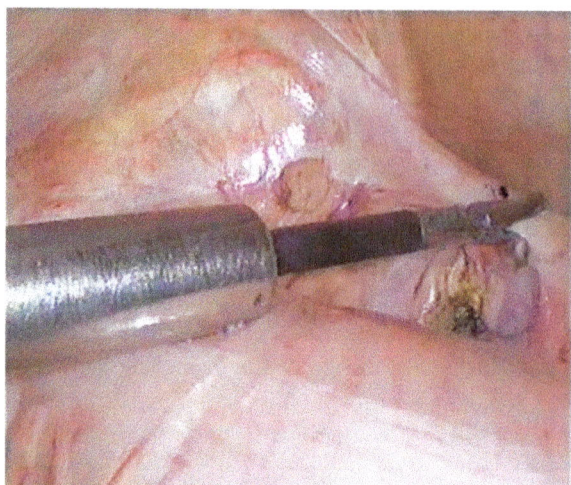

Fig. 8: Capacitive coupling. Current generated in the outer metal trocar sheath, containing the cautery connected instrument, in accidental contact with the large intestine causes bowel injury.

(Fig. 8)[3,18]. The capacitively coupled current wants to complete the circuit by finding a pathway to the patient's return electrode. The charge is stored in the capacitor until either the generator is deactivated or a pathway to complete the circuit is achieved. Capacitive coupling is greatest in the coagulation mode when there is no load on the circuit (open circuit). Capacitive coupling is considerably greater through a 5 mm cannula than through an 11 mm cannula and greater through a longer cannula. Every object in the room, the surgeon, the patient, the operating table, all have a small but finite capacitance to earth. In context to laparoscopic application it must be remembered that compound cannulas (metal with plastic sheath) should never be used. Because when capacitative current is set up in a metal cannula it must logically exit through the abdominal wall but if the plastic sheath is in place it separates the cannula from the abdominal wall and the current can only exit when the cannula tip comes in contact with any intra-abdominal structure causing unrecognized injury. Hence, the cannulas should either be only metal or only plastic, where no capacitive current is built up. Another example of capacitance can be seen with excessive length of the cautery cord lying on the table and the surgeons hand or instrument comes in contact leading to minor shock to the surgeon (Fig. 9).

A large number of the above complications can be reduced by using the electroshield system which shuts off the generator in the event of an insulation failure, or if capacitative coupled current has been generated.

Energy Sources in Surgical Practice

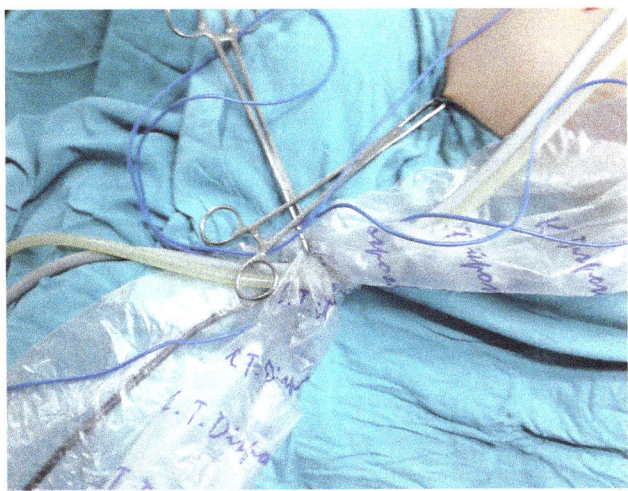

Fig. 9: Capacitive current because of extra length of ESU cord, which generates electrical field on the adjacent instruments.

Bipolar Electrosurgery

The principal tissue effect achieved with bipolar electrosurgery is tissue coagulation through the process of desiccation. Bipolar electrosurgery can coagulate vessels up to 7 mm diameter%.[5,19]

In contrast to unipolar circuits, bipolar shows a 50% reduction in the overall amount of tissue damage, but requires more time. With the bipolar mode, there is reduced depth of penetration, less smoke is generated and the risk of perforation is less also decreased lateral spread.[5,20] Another obvious advantage of bipolar over monopolar electrosurgery is the absence of a return electrode on the patient which eliminates the possibility of ground pad or alternate site burns, and capacitive coupling.[3,21] In addition, it almost eliminates the risk of insulation failure. Finally, direct coupling can occur only if metal is grasped or placed between the electrodes in a bipolar circuit or extremely close to the electrodes. But the bipolar, too, has its share of problems. The visual appearance of surface coagulation may not correspond to actual full-thickness desiccation and thus there are chances that there may be over desiccation or under desiccation, both of which are problematic. As the outer layers of tissue desiccates, the resistance to current flow increases which results in lateral spread of current almost 3-4 mm and tissue heating over an additional 2-3 mm, in all directions, because of steam dispersion through tissue (Fig. 10).

With under desiccation the coagulation may cease before it is completed. This can result in bleeding. Inadequate coagulation canal so explain, in part, the occasional high rates of pregnancy following bipolar sterilization, where

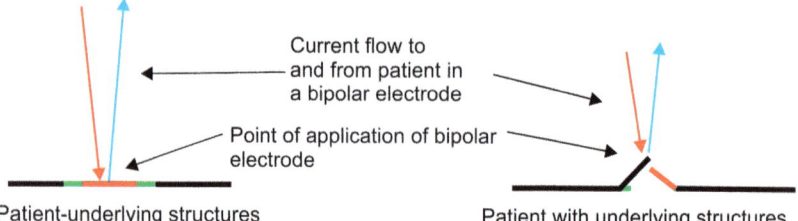

Fig. 10: Bipolar current effects red area–extent of current flow (usual 3–4 mm), green area denotes extent of thermal effect (up to 3–5 mm). Lifting the tissues before current is switched on minimizes the thermal damage to underlying structures.

the tubes may be incompletely blocked. It canal so result inside wall injury of vessels both because of current and thermal effect. Thus retraction and lifting up of tissue from vital structures is essential. A significant problem with bipolar electrodes is tissue sticking. This can be reduced or eliminated by irrigation of the bipolar electrodes at the time of activation. The irrigant not only cools the electrodes but also the tissue, thereby minimizing conducted thermal injury. Nonelectrolytic solutions such as glycine or weakly electrolytic solutions work best.

This problem can be overcome by the use of an attached ammeter which denotes optimal desiccation indirectly by showing a cessation of current flow through that tissue. Under desiccation leads to obvious failure to achieve the desired effect.

Electrosurgery in patients with metal implants or pacemaker has to be used with care. Preferable mode to be used should be bipolar mode. In unipolar mode the ground plate should be as near to the site of surgery, as away from the implant or pacemaker, minimum time of activation and under electrocardiogram (ECG) monitoring, and care should be taken that the unit should be stopped on the slightest change in cardiac rhythm.

Do's and Don'ts

- Inspect insulation carefully
- Use lowest possible power setting
- Use a low voltage waveform (cut)
- Use brief intermittent activation versus prolonged activation
- Do not activate in open circuit
- Do not activate in close proximity or direct contact with another instrument
- Use bipolar electrosurgery when appropriate
- Select an all metal cannula system as the safest choice. Do not use hybrid cannula systems that mix metal with plastic.

- Utilize available technology, such as a tissue response generator to reduce capacitive coupling or an active electrode monitoring system, to eliminate concerns about insulation failure and capacitive coupling
- Maximum contact between body and ground plate preferably under gluteus, thigh or leg
- Do not use under bony structures such as scapula, heel or head.

Use of Electrosurgery in Laparoscopic Applications

A few safety precautions would be helpful:
- Use up to 30 W of power.
- Choose a smaller contact patch to achieve cutting and a larger contact patch to achieve coagulation.
- Use the thin wire electrodes to cut and the tissue has to be placed on tension to achieve cutting and for precise bloodless dissection.
- The foot switch or hand switch should be activated for short periods only. If the current is on long, the chance of remote site electrical injury is increased (in the event, there is an unrecognized insulation failure).
- If the surgeon observes blanching of tissue, a precursor of charring, too much power is being used. Charring should be avoided. In the liver bed, this will result in the liver tissue adhering to the electrode and, when the electrode is moved, it will tear the liver tissue.

Recent Technological Advances in Electrosurgery

With the development of newer generators and innovative instrumentation, better delivery of the appropriate amount of energy resulting in better sealing of vessels, can now be achieved by a number of methods.

Argon Beam Coagulator

Argon gas is an inert, noncombustible and easily ionized gas that is used in conjunction with monopolar electrosurgery to produce fulguration. Essentially, the electrical current ionizes the argon gas, thereby making a more efficient pathway for the current to flow because the gas is more conductive than air, therefore providing an efficient bridge between the tissue and the electrode. The plasma beam is conducted to the area of lowest resistance during fulguration. Thus, when it is used, rising resistance in desiccated tissue, beam will move to an adjoining area of relatively lower resistance result in more limited and uniform area of eschar formation. This eschar formed with ABC is more stable and depth of 2–3 mm coagulation is achieved depending on the power- and gas-flow settings.[22,23] Since ABC is non-contact in nature, it ensures that the eschar created is not pulled away which normally occur with conventional diathermy. Also less smoke is produced with the argon beam coagulator. Despite these advantages, the argon beam coagulator suffers from on every significant drawback in laparoscopic surgery, namely, high flow infusion of argon gas into the abdominal cavity which not only increases the intra-abdominal pressure to potentially dangerous levels, but can also result in fatal gas embolism. The effect is obviously not seen in open surgery, where it is extensively utilized in hepatic resection or for hemostasis in any solid organ.[22,23]

Vapor Pulse Coagulation

A unique technology called vapor pulse coagulation (VPC) produces faster, more uniform results with pulsed energy instantly delivered in a controlled manner. The energy delivery device generates up to 200 W of radiofrequency output. The energy curve is sinusoidal, with variable amplitude between 320 kHz and 450 kHz. VPCs pulse-off periods allow tissue to cool and moisture to return to the targeted area, greatly reducing hotspots and coagulum formation. This technology also results in evenly coagulated target tissue, minimal thermal spread, less sticking, and enhanced hemostasis. This technology is only available in the *Gyrus PK Tissue Management System* with its own innovative generator, which works in tandem with the *Gyrus PK* instruments. The delivery device has several settings for different applications. For the current usage, it is set up for coagulation with an adjustable setting for maximum energy delivery. In addition, energy delivery has an integral pulse-off, making delivery intermittent and thereby allowing for tissue cooling and preventing desiccation. This, in addition to a bipolar mode, enhances its safety due to minimal lateral spread of energy.[24]

Smart Electrode Technology

The *Surg Rx EnSeal System* incorporates *Smart Electrode Technology*. The *EnSeal* instruments adjust dose energy simultaneously to various tissue types in a tissue bundle each with its own impedance characteristics. This electrode consists of millions of nanometer-sized conductive particles embedded in a temperature-sensitive material. Each particle acts like a discrete thermostatic switch to regulate the amount of current that passes into the tissue region with which it is in contact, thereby generating heat within it. To keep temperature from rising to potentially damaging levels, each conductive nanoparticle interrupts current flow to a specific tissue region engaged by the electrode region. When temperature dips below the optimal fusion level, the individual particle switches back on, reinstating current flow and heat deposition. The process continues until the entire tissue segment is uniformly fused without charring or sticking. Less heat is required to accomplish fusion, as the tissue volume is minimized through compression energy, is focused on the captured segment and the vessel walls are fused through compression, protein denaturation, and then renaturation.[25]

Modified Bipolar Electrosurgery

The *Ligasure System* or LVSS (Ligasure vessel sealing system) utilizes a new bipolar technology for vascular sealing with a higher current and lower voltage (180 V) than conventional electrosurgery. It uses a unique combination of pressure and energy to create vessel fusion. This fusion is accomplished by melting the collagen and elastin in the vessel wall and reforming it into a permanent, plastic-like seal. It does not rely on a proximal thrombus as the classic bipolar electrocautery. A feedback-controlled response system automatically discontinues energy delivery when the seal cycle is complete, eliminating guess work and minimizing thermal spread to approximately 2 mm for most *LigaSure* instruments. This unique energy output results in virtually no sticking or charring, and the seals can withstand 3 times normal systolic blood pressure seals vessels up to 7 mm.[26,27] This system also requires a designated generator that works with several different specific instruments designed by the company.

Ultrasonic Energy

Today virtually all laparoscopic procedures and many open surgical procedures can be performed safely and efficiently without the use of electrosurgery by utilizing ultrasound. Furthermore, ultrasonic surgery has also replaced mechanical surgical clips and scissors in many laparoscopic procedures.[28]

Physics of Ultrasound

- Audible sound waves are confined to the frequency range of 20 cycle per second (Hz) to about 20,000 cycles per second. A longitudinal wave, whose frequency is above the audible range is an ultrasonic wave. When ultrasonic waves are applied at low power levels, no tissue effect occurs, as is the case for diagnostic ultrasound imaging. However, higher power levels and power densities can be harnessed to produce surgical cutting, coagulation, and dissection of tissues. This involves mechanical propagation of sound (pressure) waves from an energy source through a solid, liquid, or gaseous medium to an active blade element (longitudinal mechanical waves).
- Ultrasonic dissectors are of two types—*low power* which cleaves water-containing tissues by cavitations leaving organized structures with low-water content intact, e.g. blood vessels, bile ducts, etc. It does not coagulate vessels and is used as cavitational aspirators for liver surgery

and neurosurgery (Cusa, Selector) and *high power systems* which cleave loose areolar tissues by frictional heating and thus cut and coagulate the edges at the same time. High power systems (Autosonix, Ultracision) are used extensively, especially in advanced laparoscopic surgery. The harmonic scalpel and the AutoSonix system operate at a frequency of 55.5 kHz.
- Therapeutic ultrasurgical devices are composed of a generator, hand piece, and blade. The handpiece houses the ultrasonic transducer, as tack of piezoelectric crystals sandwiched under pressure between metal cylinders. The transducer is attached to amount, which is then attached to the blade extender and blade. The harmonic scalpel cools the hand piece with air while AutoSonix and Sonosurg systems rely principally on large diameter hand piece made of heat dissipating materials to remove the heat and prevent heat buildup.[28,29]

Ultrasonic Cutting, Coagulation and Cavitation

- The basic mechanism for *coagulation* of bleeding vessels ultrasonically is similar to that of electrosurgery or lasers. The difference is that with ultrasonic probes vessels are sealed by tamponading and coapting with a denatured protein coagulum by mechanical energy of the vibrating probe as opposed to thermal injury.
- Ultrasurgical hook, or spatula blade can coagulate blood vessels in the 2 mm diameter range without difficulty and the scissors can coagulate vessels up to 5 mm in diameter. Heat generated with the use of dissector is limited to temperature below 80°C. The overall temperatures achieved by the dissector, even after prolonged use, remains well below the 250–400°C achieved with electrosurgery and laser surgery. This results in reduced tissue charring and desiccation and also minimizes the zone of thermal injury. Skin incisions made with the ultrasonically activated scalpel or cold steel scalpel heal almost identically and are superior to electrosurgically made incisions. The minimal tissue damage may explain the marked reduction in postoperative adhesions to the liver bed following laparoscopic cholecystectomy with the ultrasonically activated scalpel, when compared with electrosurgery or laser surgery.
- Although coagulation produced by ultrasonic surgery is slower than that observed with either electrosurgery or laser surgery, nonetheless, it is as effective or even more effective, because despite the slower rate of tissue coagulation, the entire process of tissue coagulation combined with transection, the ultimate goal of surgery, is faster with the ultrasonic scalpel than with other energy modalities. However, greater depth of thermal injury can result with ultrasonic dissection ultrasurgery, as compared to electrosurgery, if activation of the probe persists for more than 10 seconds.

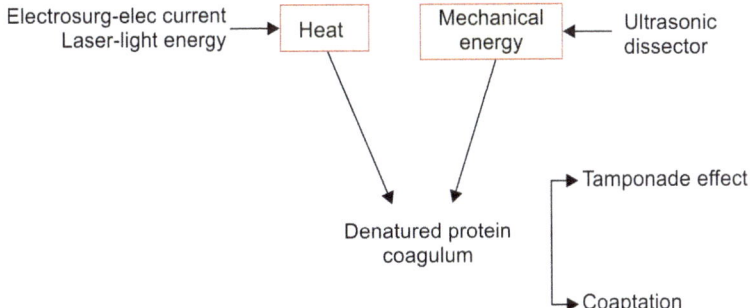

Fig. 11: Different energy sources all ultimately result in protein denaturation.

- The mechanisms of coagulation also offer an advantage for ultrasonic surgery over electrosurgery with regards to the sidewall of a blood vessel. Blood vessels are usually not coapted significantly by electrosurgery because of the concomitant reduction in power density. Furthermore, the blood within the vessels has a high heat capacity and acts as a heat sink, which allows one side to coagulate prior to the other, with resultant bleeding from a hole in the wall of the vessel that was in contact with the electrosurgical device. But with the ultrasonic shears the blood vessel can be gripped and then coagulated (Fig. 11).
- Absence of coagulated tissue sticking to the active element, because of the vibration of the active blade, is another unique feature of ultrasurgical coagulation compared with other energy modalities. In addition, the grasper blade allows unsupported tissue to be grasped and coagulated without difficulty, or cut and coagulated as with scissors.
- The *cutting mechanism* for the ultrasonically activated scalpel is also different from that observed with electrosurgery or laser surgery. At least two mechanisms exist. The first is *cavitational fragmentation* in which cells are disrupted. This occurs primarily in low protein density areas such as liver. This mechanism is utilized by the cavitational ultrasonic aspirating device (CUSA). The device is composed of an ultrasonic generator that vibrates at 23,000 Hz. When coupled with powerful aspiration device, the ultrasonic aspirator fragments cells and aspirates the resulting cellular debris and water. This action leaves collagen rich tissues such as blood vessels, nerves, and lymphatic intact. Thus, there is no cutting or coagulation with the ultrasonic aspirator. In marked contrast, the ultrasonically activated scalpel not only coagulates and cavitates, it also cuts high protein density areas such as collagen or muscle rich tissues. This occurs via the second cutting mechanism, which is the actual *"power cutting"* offered by a relatively sharp blade vibrating 55,500 times per second over a distance of 80 µm.

- A major advantage of the ultrasonically activated scalpel's coagulation ability is the absence of melting and charring of tissues. This allows the tissue planes to be clearly and sharply visualized at all times. The ultrasonically activated scalpel can also be used as a blunt dissector to aid in identifying tissue planes. However, the high power ultrasonic dissection systems may cause collateral damage by excessive heating and this is well documented in clinical practice. Ultrasonic surgical dissection allows coagulation and cutting with less instrument traffic (reduction in operating time), less smoke and no electrical current.[28-30]

Laser

(LASER: Light Amplification through Stimulated Emission of Radiation)

The laser beam is generated in a cavity (Fig. 12). By using a foot pedal, the surgeon has three options as to how the laser beam can be released from the cavity. The first mode is known as the continuous wave (CW) where the beam continues to be emitted at a steady rate. In the *pulse mode (PW)*, the pulse is released for a limited period of time at a higher peak power and the *Q switched mode* where the energy is released in exceedingly narrow pulses in very high peak power. This type of laser is used frequently in ophthalmologic procedures and the power in these lasers tends to be measured in milliwatts. High power and short pulse duration are the hallmark of ophthalmologic lasers (Fig. 13).

Unique Properties of the Lasers (Table 1)

- First the light is *monochromatic*. The laser emits light over a very narrow, well-defined wavelength.
- Second, the light is *coherent*. Because of the properties of stimulated emission, laser light is perfectly in phase; that is each peak and valley of the sine wave curves align exactly.

Finally laser beam is virtually *nondivergent* (up to 1° of divergence), giving a highly focused beam.

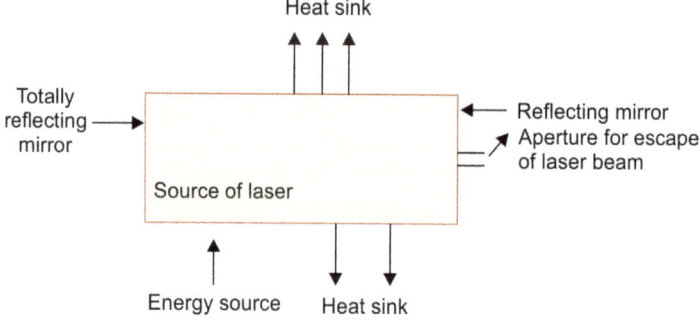

Fig. 12: Method of laser generation.

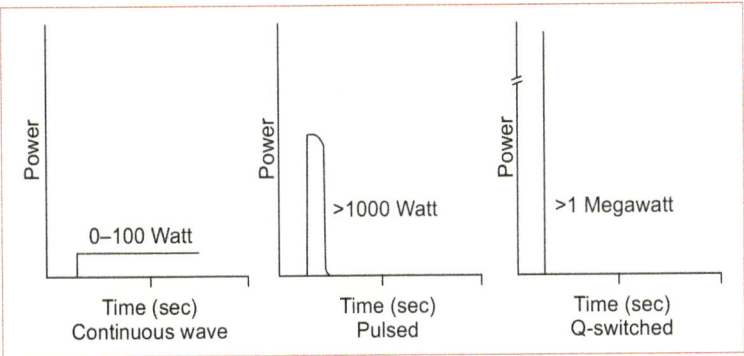

Fig. 13: Methods of release of laser beam.

Table 1: Properties of commonly used lasers.

Properties	Nd:YAG	CO_2	Argon	Holmium:YAG
Wavelength	within near 1,064 nm	Far infrared region 10,600 nm	Infrared region 450–528 mm	2,010 mm
Energy reflected (Back scatter)	30–40% So cannot act effectively	<10%	55%	
Effective depth of penetration and coagulation	3–4 mm	0.1 mm	1.0 mm	1.3 mm good cut good coagulation
Transmission through fibers	+ can – coagulate/cuts – endoscopic use	Poor transmission through fibers requires mirrors	Fibers transmission ++	Glass fiber ++
Transmission through liquids	+	Heavily absorbed by water vaporizes and cuts	Heavily absorbed by hemoglobin or melanin pigments	+
Clinical use	Good coagulation	Superficial skin lesions ENT Good cutting		BEP excellent cut Blood vessel coagulates Stone fragmentation

Biophysical Principles of Lasers

The biophysical effects can be described as:
- *Electromechanical:* Dielectric breakdown in tissue caused by shock wave-plasma expansion resulting in localized mechanical rupture.
- *Photoablative*: Photo-dissociation or breaking of molecular bonds in tissue.

- *Photothermal*: Laser light generates heat which heats and vaporizes tissues.
- *Photochemical*: Target cells are induced by laser light to chemical reactions.
- *Holmium laser* vaporizes water inside the stone causing thermal expansion and calculus disintegration.

There are a number of types of laser available. The major types of medical lasers available commercially today, are all named after the medium in the laser cavity.

Laser Tissue Interaction

It depends upon:
- Wavelength
- Power density
- Exposure time (3 types available) Q-switched, pulsed and cautious wave
- Absorption and scatter.

Depth of penetration denotes extinction length or the tissue thickness at which 90% of laser beam has been absorbed. The effect generated:
- Is directly proportional to the time of application more than the power rating.
- Is inversely proportional to distance from tissue.
- Some cooling at the surface of application results in lesser vaporization at surface and deeper penetration (blooming effect).

Specific properties:
- Nd:YAG, CO_2 and argon lasers.
- All three of the above lasers work fundamentally by thermal action. When tissue is heated by any of these lasers up to 60°C, there is no permanent or visible damage to the tissue. By 65°C, denaturation of protein occurs. The tissue will visibly turn white or gray and will disintegrate approximately 4–7 days later. This is the temperature range in which the Nd:YAG laser works. Once tissue has been heated to 90–100°C, there is tissue drying, some shrinkage, and permanent damage due to dehydration. Over 100°C, carbonization or blackening of tissue occurs. As the temperature rise continues, there is evolution of gas with tissue vaporization. This is the temperature in which the CO_2 and argon laser works.
- *Argon-pumped dye laser*: The only laser system that does not work by the thermal cavity is combined with hematoporphyrin derivative. In this laser system, hematoporphyrin derivative is administered intravenously 48 hours prior to therapy. The hematoporphyrin derivative is concentrated within the tumor cells in preference to the normal cells in certain organ system of the body including the bladder. When exposed to the red light, the hematoporphyrin derivative is excited and cleaves oxygen to from

singlet oxygen within the mitochondria, leading to cell death. This is a nonthermal effect.
- Holmium:YAG laser is based on a mixture of helium and neon gas is visible as red light. It is used as a guiding medium for nonvisible lasers and also for stone disintegration by vaporization of the water inside calculus causing thermal expansion and calculus disintegration.[31,32]
- Excimer laser uses rare gas halides as the medium. It lies in the ultraviolet spectrum. Maximum usage in ophthalmology and laser angioplasty.
- KTP/YAG laser (wavelength 532 nm) is the green light laser. Potassium-titanyl-phosphate which is used to guide the beam of Nd:YAG laser is visible as green light. It is used in prostatectomy, and skin lesions.[33]

Visible and Invisible Lasers

- Visible lasers are located in the wavelength between 400–700 nm. Best examples are argon and KTP laser.
- Invisible lasers are located in the range of 700 nm or more. The best examples are Nd:YAG laser, carbon dioxide laser.

Common Complications

- Skin related—skin burn.
- Photokeratitis, skin malignancy
- Eye—thermal retinal damage, corneal burn and cataract.

High-Velocity Water Jet Dissection or Hydro-dissection

Pulsatile high-velocity high-pressure water or crystalloid jet dissection involves the use of relatively simple device, produces clean cutting of reproducible depth. In hydrojet technology very thin water jet produced which acts almost like a cutting knife. It requires a special hydrojet generator and produces high-pressure jet of between 20 BAR and 60 BAR. Water stream under high pressure (hydrojet) is used to facilitate tissue dissection and release adhesions. Other advantages are the cleansing of the operating field by the turbulent flow zone and the small amount of water required to complete dissection. A relatively hemostatic method which exposes the blood vessels or biliary channels, once parenchymal dissection has occurred, which can then be dealt with appropriately.[34,35] Specific problems were identified with the use of this modality. The "hail storm" effect results in excessive misting which obscures vision. This has been solved to some extent by incorporating a hood over the nozzle. Difficulty in gauging distance and thus poor control of the depth of the cut are drawbacks. The spraying of tissue fragments also renders the procedure oncologically unsound. The present use of water-jet dissection is limited to dissection and resection of parenchymal organs, including liver, gallbladder, brain, kidney, prostate, lymphadenectomy and pleurectomy in thoracoscopic surgery and to cleaning wounds.[34,35] Other uses include, in orthopedic surgery for cutting and endoprosthesis and bone, in dental use for cutting and grinding of dental materials, in plastic surgery for cleaning skin graft, removal of tattoos, and liposuction and for dermatological lesions. The fluid used can be combined with an anesthetic agent or an antibiotic to reduce the pain and prevent infection. Microwave water jet scalpel is another application of the water flow. It is used for minimally invasive removal or resection of tumors. It is a combination of a microwave scalpel and a jet system.

Radiofrequency Ablation

Radiofrequency (RF) ablation is a minimally invasive method that uses thermal energy to destroy tumor cells in organs such as the lung, liver, kidney, benign bone tumors, pancreatic cancer and also biliary cancer. The tumor is located by a computed tomogram or an ultrasound scan. Energy is then delivered through a metal tube (probe) inserted into tumors or other tissues, under ultrasound guidance. When the probe is in place, metal prongs open out to extend the reach of the therapy. RF energy causes atoms in the cells to vibrate and create friction. This generates heat (50–100°C) and leads to the death of the cells. However, temperature controlled RFA can also be used. The efficacy of treatment is assessed by CT scan one month following treatment. Retreatments are often necessary. Risks of the procedure include bleeding, although this is extremely rare. It also finds use in heart tissue to destroy abnormal electrical pathways that are contributing to a cardiac arrhythmia. Thus it is used in recurrent atrial flutter (Afl), atrial fibrillation (AF), supraventricular tachycardia (SVT), atrial tachycardia, multifocal atrial tachycardia (MAT) and some types of ventricular arrhythmias.

Recent advances in treatment of varicose veins include varicose vein ablation by RF delivered with the help of a thin catheter. So also nerve ablation can be done to reduce the chronic pain of arthritis or lower back pain. Chronic lower back pain (CLBP) is also an area amenable to RF. The causes of CLBP tend to be multifactorial. Arthropathy of the lumbar facet joints is thought to be a common etiology (15–45%). RFA of the medial branch nerve of the facet joint is a well-established treatment modality used to decrease facet joint pains. A wide range of temperature is being used (70–90°C) but the optimal temperature that provides the best patient outcomes with the least side effects is not well established in the pain management literature.[36,37]

Microwave Ablation

An alternative means of producing thermal coagulation of tissue involves the use of microwaves (MW) to induce an ultra-high-speed (2,450 MHz) alternating electric field, causing the rotation of water molecules. Although the use of MV for tissue ablation is not new, the majority of the clinical experience with technique is with ablation of liver tumors. Percutaneous microwave ablation (PCMWA) was first used as an adjunct to liver biopsy in 1986, but it has since been used for hepatic tumor ablation. As with RFA, MWA involves placement of a needle electrode directly into the target tumor, typically under US guidance. MW energy spectrum ranges from 300 MHz to 300 GHz to produce tissue-heating effects. Each ablation also produces a hyperechoic region around the needle, similar to that observed with RFA. Unlike RFA, however, no retractable prongs are used, and the resulting ablation tends to be much more elliptical. For isolated, nonmetastatic lung tumors, surgical resection remains the treatment of choice. However, many patients are precluded from surgery due to poor cardiopulmonary function, advanced age, or extensive disease burden. For these patients, minimally invasive therapeutic options such as RFA, MWA, and cryoablation have emerged as possible alternatives. Tumor ablation of thoracic malignancies should be considered a viable treatment option for patients with early stage, primary or secondary lung cancers who are not surgical candidates or for patients in whom palliation of tumor-related symptoms is the intent. MWA is regarded as a particularly efficient option for the treatment of lung tumors since unlike RFA it does not rely on impedance to generate heat, rather electromagnetic microwave waves heat matter by agitating water molecules in the surrounding tissue, producing friction and heat.[38,39]

Cryotherapy

Cryotherapy uses the principle of rapid freezing and slow thawing of the tissue in multiple cycles. These temperature changes affect several intra- and extracellular mechanisms leading to cell membrane disruption and thrombi formation in the blood vessels inducing apoptosis and ischemia.[40] Delayed effects include loss of microcirculation leading to anoxia and stimulation of cytotoxic T cells.[41] The cryogens used are liquid nitrogen, nitrous oxide and liquid carbon dioxide. Liquid nitrogen has became the most popular cryogen as it is easily available, lack explosive potential, freeze tissue up to −197°C and predictable effect. The application is carried out through 3 mm or less probes. The application of ultracold liquid causes damage to the treated tissue due to intracellular ice formation. The osmotic gradient created by these crystals facilitates cell destruction by drawing water out of the cells. In addition, the cell membrane composed of lipid bilayer is also sensitive to hypothermia. During the cooling process, the membrane becomes highly permeable and allows mass transfers of ion, resulting in destructive changes in the ionic composition of the cell. The thawing process is the final step when the crystals dissolve due to increased temperatures, creating a reverse osmotic gradient.

Water reenters the cells, causing swelling and rupture. Furthermore, it has also been hypothesized that freezing results in vascular injury by causing stasis in blood flow. The resulting ischemia causes cell death by necrosis. The degree of damage depends upon the minimum temperature achieved and the rate of cooling. The gas is then switched off once the desired temperature is achieved. The tissue is allowed to thaw which leads to the cell destruction by hemorrhagic infarction. The cycle of freezing and thawing may then be repeated, a process known as "double freezing."

The uses of cryotherapy are esophageal premalignant lesion, bone tumors, hepatocellular carcinomas, precancerous condition of cervix, nephron-sparing kidney cancers prostate cancer, retinoblastoma and in the palliation of hepatocellular carcinoma (HCC) and liver metastsis.[40-42] It is also widely used in various skin conditions such as skin cancer, actinic keratosis, warts, moles, skin tags, and solar keratosis. The application of cryotherapy can be in both by open and, laparoscopic surgery. Cryotherapy can also be applied as ice-pack therapy, cold spray anesthetics and whole body cryotherapy.

CONCLUSION

In present era, wide range of energy devices are available, which are appealing and also safe alternative for cutting, coagulation and dissection. Its use in surgical practice has increased the versatility of the surgical procedure and decreases operating time. The use of energy devices in surgical practice depends on the task, surgeon experience, availability and cost. Monopolar and conventional bipolar electrosurgery are used freely, as it has wide range of dissection capability and cost effective. Because among the most commonly used sources, there is no major difference among their results. The only reason to select one over the other would be the site of application and the requirement.

REFERENCES

1. Taheri A, Mansoori P, Sandoval LF, et al. Electrosurgery: part I. Basics and principles. J Am Acad Dermatol. 2014;70(4):591.e1-4.
2. Harrell AG, Kercher KW, Heniford BT. Energy sources in laparoscopy. Semin Laparosc Surg. 2004;11(3):201-9.
3. Brill AI. Electrosurgery: principles and practice to reduce risk and maximize efficacy. Obstet Gynecol Clin North Am. 2011;38(4):687-702.
4. Wu MP, Ou CS, Chen SL, et al. Complications and recommended practices for electrosurgery in laparoscopy. Am J Surg. 2000;179(1):67-73.
5. Law KS, Abbott JA, Lyons SD, et al. Energy sources for gynecologic laparoscopic surgery: a review of the literature. Obstet Gynecol Surv. 2014;69(12):763-76.
6. Sutton C, Abbott J. History of power sources in endoscopic surgery. J Minim Invasive Gynecol. 2013;20(3):271-8.

7. Brill AI, Feste JR, Hamilton TL, et al. Patient safety during laparoscopic monopolar electrosurgery: principles and guidelines. JSLS. 1998; 2(3):221-5.
8. Lipscomb GH, Givens VM. Preventing electrosurgical energy-related injuries. Obstet Gynecol Clin North Am. 2010;37(3):369-77.
9. Advincula AP, Wang K. The evolutionary state of electrosurgery: where are we now? Curr Opin Obstet Gynecol. 2008,20(4):353-8.
10. Wicker P. Electrosurgery-part 2: the principles of electrosurgery. NATNEWS. 1990;27(9):6-7;10.
11. Suchanek S, Grega T, Zavoral M. The role of equipment in endoscopic complications. Best Pract Res Clin Gastroenterol. 2016;30(5):667-78.
12. Morris ML, Tucker RD, Baron TH, et al. Electrosurgery in gastrointestinal endoscopy: principles to practice. Am J Gastroenterol. 2009;104(6):1563-74.
13. Brill AI. Energy systems in laparoscopy. In: A Practical Manual of Laparoscopy and Minimally Invasive Gynecology. Florida: CRC Press; 2007. pp. 86-9.
14. Yazdani A, Krause H. Laparoscopic instrument insulation failure: the hidden hazard. J Minim Invasive Gynecol. 2007;14(2):228-32.
15. Montero PN, Robinson TN, Weaver JS, et al. Insulation failure in laparoscopic instruments. Surg Endosc. 2010;24(2):462-5.
16. Vancaillie TG. Active electrode monitoring: how to prevent unintentional thermal injury associated with monopolar electrosurgery at laparoscopy. Surg Endosc. 1998;12(8):1009-12.
17. Association of Surgeons in Training. (1999). Principles of electrosurgery. [online] Available from https://www.asit.org/assets/documents/Prinicpals_in_electrosurgery.pdf/.
18. Wu MP, Ou CS, Chen SL, et al. Complications and recommended practices for electrosurgery in laparoscopy. Am J Surg. 2000;179:67-73.
19. Newcomb WL, Hope WW, Schmelzer TM, et al. Comparison of blood vessel sealing among new electrosurgical and ultrasonic devices. Surg Endosc. 2009;23(1):90-6.
20. Sutton PA, Awad S, Perkins AC, et al. Comparison of lateral thermal spread using monopolar and bipolar diathermy: the Harmonic Scalpel and the LigaSure. Br J Surg Mar. 2010;97(3):428-33.
21. Brill AI. Bipolar electrosurgery: convention and innovation. Clin Obstet Gynecol. 2008;51(1):153-8.
22. Farin G, Grund KE. Technology of argon plasma coagulation with particular regard to endoscopic applications. Endosc Surg Allied Technol. 1994;2(1):71-7.
23. Aoki T, Kato T, Yasuda D, et al. Cyst wall resection and ablation by hand-assisted laparoscopic surgery combined with argonplasma coagulator for huge hepatic cysts. Int Surg. 2007;92(6):361-6.
24. Abouljoud MS, Arenas J, Yoshida A, et al. New application of the bipolar vapor plasma coagulation system for laparoscopic major liver resections. Surg Endosc. 2008;22(2):426-9.
25. Jaiswal A, Huang KG. Energy devices in gynecological laparoscopy: archaic to modern era. Gynecol Minim Invasive Ther. 2017;6(4):147-51.

26. Kim FJ, Chammas Jr MF, Gewehr E, et al. Temperature safety profile of laparoscopic devices: harmonic ACE (ACE), Ligasure V (LV), and plasma trisector (PT). Surg Endosc. 2008;22(6):1464-9.
27. Carbonell AM, Joels CS, Kercher KW, et al. A comparison of laparoscopic bipolar vessel sealing devices in the hemostasis of small-, medium-, and large-sized arteries. J Laparoendosc Adv Surg Tech. 2003;13(6):377-80.
28. Emam TA, Cuschieri A. How safe is high-power ultrasonic dissection? Ann Surg. 2003;237(2):186-91.
29. Sankaranarayanan G, Resapu RR, Jones DB, et al. Common uses and cited complications of energy in surgery. Surg Endosc. 2013;27(9):3056-72.
30. Obonna G, Mishra R. Differences between Thunderbeat, LigaSure and Harmonic scalpel energy system in minimally invasive surgery. World J Lap Surg. 2014;7(1):41-4.
31. Kronenberg P, Somani B. Advances in Lasers for the Treatment of Stones: a systematic review. Curr Urol Rep. 2018;19(6):45.
32. Kronenberg P, Traxer O. Update on lasers in urology 2014: current assessment on holmium:yttrium-aluminum-garnet (Ho:YAG) laser lithotripter settings and laser fibers. World J Urol. 2015;33(4):463-9.
33. Marks AJ, Teichman JM. Lasers in clinical urology: state-of-the art and new horizons. World J Urol. 2007;25(3):227-33.
34. Durai R, Ng PC. Multistream saline-jet dissection using simple irrigation system defines difficult tissue planes. JSLS. 2010;14(1):53-9.
35. Shekarriz B. Hydro-Jet technology in urologic surgery. Expert Rev Med Devices. 2005;2(3):287-91.
36. Larghi A, Rimbaş M, Tringali A, et al. Endoscopic radiofrequency biliary ablation treatment: a comprehensive review. Dig Endosc. 2018;16.
37. Chua NH, Vissers KC, Sluijter ME. Pulsed radiofrequency treatment in interventional pain management: mechanisms and potential indications: a review. Acta Neurochir (Wien). 2011;153(4):763-71.
38. Vogl TJ, Nour-Eldin NA, Hammerstingl RM, et al. Microwave Ablation (MWA): Basics, Technique and Results in Primary and Metastatic Liver Neoplasms–Review Article. Rofo. 2017;189(11):1055-66.
39. Huo YR, Eslick GD. Microwave ablation compared to radiofrequency ablation for hepatic lesions: a meta-analysis. J Vasc Interv Radiol. 2015; 26(8):1139-46.
40. Baust JG, Gage AA, Clarke D, et al. Cryosurgery: a putative approach to molecular-based optimization. Cryobiology. 2004;48(2):190-204.
41. Johnson JP. Immunologic aspects of cryosurgery: potential modulation of immune recognition and effector cell maturation. Clin Dermatol. 1990;8(1):39-47.
42. Lal P, Thota PN. Cryotherapy in the management of premalignant and malignant conditions of the esophagus. World J Gastroenterol. 2018;24(43):4862-9.

Chapter 2

Management of Colorectal Liver Metastases

Shaleen Agarwal

INTRODUCTION

Colorectal cancer is a major global health problem. It is the most common malignancy of the gastrointestinal tract and third most common globally diagnosed cancer.[1,2] About 20–25% patients with colorectal cancer have liver metastases at the time of diagnosis and nearly 50% patients will develop metastases during the course of their disease; mostly to the liver. The natural history of metastatic colorectal cancer (mCRC) is variable, however, untreated mCRC has a poor prognosis with median survival rates of less than 8 months. Unfortunately, only 15–20% of the liver metastases are amenable to curative resection, however, those undergoing a curative resection can expect an overall 5-year survival of 50–60% and 10-year overall survival of 25%.[3]

DEFINITION: SYNCHRONOUS VERSUS METACHRONOUS LIVER METASTASES

There are different definitions of synchronous liver metastases but most studies define synchronous metastases as those diagnosed before or at the time of diagnosis or surgery for primary tumor. Any metastases discovered after the surgery/treatment of primary tumor are termed as metachronous. There are some studies which consider metastases discovered up to 6 months after the treatment of primary tumor as synchronous.

DIAGNOSIS AND WORKUP

Majority of colorectal liver metastases (CRLM) are asymptomatic and are typically diagnosed on imaging studies either at diagnosis or during follow-up after treatment of the primary tumor. During the workup of the primary tumor it is essential to look for metastatic disease, since it has bearing on the overall management and outcome. For the purposes of detection and surveillance, the National Comprehensive Cancer Network (NCCN) guidelines recommend contrast-enhanced computed tomography (CECT) of abdomen and pelvis.[4] Carcinoembryonic antigen (CEA) is a useful tumor marker that helps in prognostication and assessing the response to treatment. Molecular studies for determining the RAS mutations have a bearing on deciding treatment with biological agents in advanced cases. In those cases where metachronous CRLM is found, a colonoscopy within a year of the diagnosis is considered standard.

Once liver metastases are detected cross-sectional imaging is required for further staging and treatment planning. A high resolution chest computed tomography (CT) would suffice for imaging of the chest. For abdomen and pelvis either a CECT or a contrast-enhanced magnetic resonance imaging (MRI) should be performed.

Colorectal liver metastases lesions on CT are hypovascular and are usually visualized as hypodense lesions on the portovenous phase. Contrast-enhanced CT and MRI have comparable sensitivity and specificity for detecting liver metastases; 73% and 96% for CECT versus 82% and 92% for contrast-enhanced MRI. MRI is particularly helpful in a steatotic liver or for evaluation of response to chemotherapy and radioembolization. Representative CT and MRI pictures of liver metastases from colorectal cancer are shown in Figures 1 and 2.

Till recently there was no consensus on the role of positron emission tomography/computed tomography (PET/CT) in the evaluation of CRLM. A French study published in 2005 found that PET/CT was more cost-effective than CT alone.[5] However, a randomized trial of PET/CT versus CT in patients

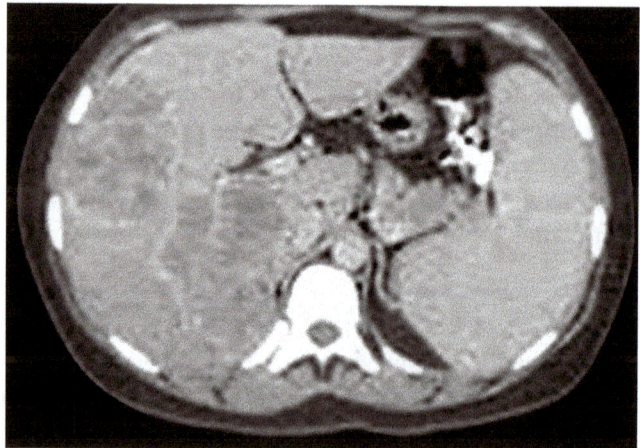

Fig. 1: Venous phase contrast-enhanced computed tomography (CECT) image of large metastatic deposit in right lobe of liver.

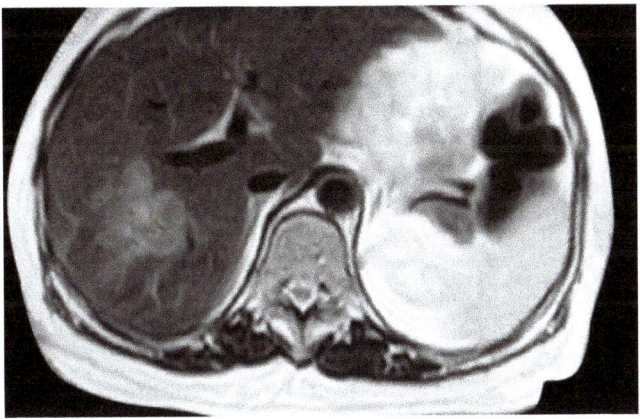

Fig. 2: Noncontrast magnetic resonance image (MRI) of right lobe colorectal liver metastasis.

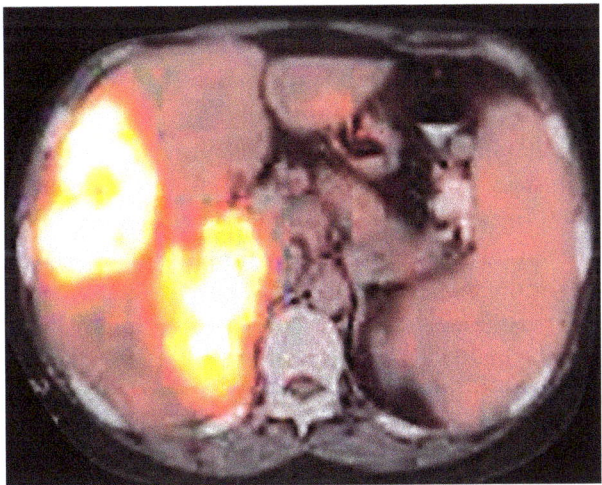

Fig. 3: Fluorodeoxyglucose (FDG) avid liver metastases from rectal cancer.

with potentially resectable CRLM did not show any significant advantage of PET/CT in surgical planning. This trial provides definitive evidence that the routine use of PET does not significantly affect outcomes among patients with potentially resectable CRLM.[6] NCCN guidelines for localized colon cancer do not recommend routine PET/CT for surveillance or for monitoring therapeutic progress for mCRC.[7] According to the guidelines laid down by American College of Radiology PET/CT is not routinely indicated but may be useful in cases of advanced bilobar disease for ruling out extrahepatic disease and nodal metastases.[8] PET image of right lobe colorectal metastases is shown in Figure 3.

FACTORS INFLUENCING THE TREATMENT STRATEGY

Several factors that should be taken into account when planning a treatment strategy; these include age, performance status (PS), and the comorbidities of the patient, the extent of disease, surgical intervention to remove the primary tumor, the location of the tumor, the status of biomarkers, and the disease heterogeneity inherent to colorectal cancer.

SURGICAL MANAGEMENT OF COLORECTAL LIVER METASTASES

Surgery for liver metastases has evolved markedly during the last few decades. Currently surgery is considered the standard of care for the management of CRLM. Surgery should be performed in all cases where complete disease extirpation is considered safe and feasible.[9] Even patients with multiple bilobar nodules or synchronous extrahepatic disease are commonly considered for resection.[10] Excellent results in terms of safety (mortality risk less than 2%) and efficacy (5-year actual survival rates of about 50%) have strongly encouraged these broader indications.

With the availability of high quality imaging and advances is surgical technique, liver surgery has become safe but the risk of postresection liver failure is always present when major hepatic resections are considered, particularly, when the patient has already received chemotherapy for the primary tumor or the metastatic disease. Modern chemotherapy regimens and new targeted therapies have contributed to improved survival for mCRC patients.[9] This favorable scenario has led clinicians to adopt an aggressive multidisciplinary approach to colorectal liver metastases (CLM), including nonsurgical treatments, to maximize disease control and patient survival.

DEFINING RESECTABILITY

In the context of CRLM resection, resectability is defined as the probability of achieving a negative (R0) resection margin and at the same time ensuring a sufficient functional liver remnant. It is well-known that a margin of 10 mm or more is associated with a favorable outcome, however, negative margins regardless of the width are associated with a positive outcome.[10] However, in the overall context, R0 resection is just one part of the entire paradigm of patient outcomes in metastatic colorectal cancer. Tumor biology, disease burden, performance status of the patient, and risk of recurrence have a very significant bearing on the outcome. The technical aspects of resectability have been summarized by the Americas Hepato-Pancreato-Biliary Association (AHPBA) as:[11]

- *Ability to obtain R0 resection*: No tumor present at margin
- *Adequate postoperative liver volume and function*:
  - At least 20% of total liver volume with normal function
  - At least 30% if any chemotherapy-associated liver injury
  - At least 40% if any hepatic fibrosis or cirrhosis from other causes
  - At least two functional contiguous segments with intact portal and arterial inflow, venous outflow, and biliary drainage
- Limited extrahepatic disease that is resectable
- No portal lymphadenopathy or multiple metastatic sites
- Limited progression if received preoperative chemotherapy
- No development of new hepatic lesions
- Medically fit to undergo a major operation.

APPROACH TO A PATIENT WITH SYNCHRONOUS LIVER METASTASES

The treatment strategy for a patient with synchronously detected liver metastases is determined by:
- Location and extent of primary tumor
- Whether the primary tumor is symptomatic
- Burden of liver metastases
- Extent of liver resection required
- Presence of extrahepatic disease
- Performance status of the patient
- Available surgical expertise.

Three main strategies have been described for dealing with synchronously detected liver metastases:

1. *Classical approach*: Involves surgery of the primary tumor as first stage surgery followed by adjuvant chemotherapy and liver resection as second surgery. This approach is recommended when the primary tumor is symptomatic and when a major hepatectomy is required for removal of liver metastases. Classical approach is safe when the patient is not in a condition to undergo two major surgical procedures in the same sitting. However, this approach carries the drawback of leaving behind the metastatic disease which may progress during the waiting period.

2. *Simultaneous approach*: As the name suggests, this approach involves simultaneous resection of the primary tumor and liver metastases (Figs. 4 and 5). This technique has the advantage of dealing with the primary tumor and liver metastases during a single surgery, thus, avoiding the trauma of a second surgery and preventing disease progression during the waiting period, as is the case with classical approach. Simultaneous resection shortens the length of overall hospital stay, length of gap between treatments, and is especially advantageous if operations are

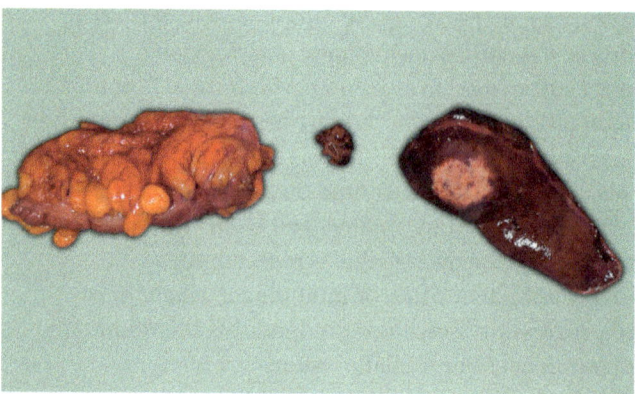

Fig. 4: Photograph showing specimen of sigmoid colectomy and left lateral sectionectomy along with metastatectomy in segment VII (in middle) done as simultaneous resection.

done with a minimally invasive approach. The major drawback with this approach is that it is not suitable when there is large disease burden in the liver and when the patient's performance status is not adequate for undergoing to major surgical procedures.

3. *Liver-first approach*: This strategy is based on the logic that since the metastatic disease is the primary determinant of long-term patient outcome, it should be treated first. "Liver-first" approach involves systemic chemotherapy followed by liver resection. Chemotherapy is continued after liver resection and primary tumor is dealt with at a second surgery. This approach cannot be used when the primary tumor is symptomatic and needs urgent attention such as in cases of bleeding and obstructing tumors. A treatment algorithm based on the recommendations of the expert group on oncosurgery management of liver metastases is presented in Flowchart 1.[12]

TECHNICAL ASPECTS OF HEPATIC RESECTION

Two factors need to be considered while planning for liver resection of CRLM, namely anatomic distribution of disease and the future liver remnant (FLR).

A hepatic parenchyma-sparing partial hepatectomy is feasible in 30–50% of cases.[13] It is not mandatory to do a formal lobectomy for achieving good long-term outcomes. Type of liver resection is determined by the distribution of disease. Moreover, parenchyma sparing nonanatomical resections are associated with lower morbidity (34% versus 25%) and postoperative liver failure (2% versus 7%).[14] Additionally, major liver resections are associated with much higher risk of mortality (8.3% versus 1.4%).[15] Sparing of hepatic parenchyma also increases salvage options for patients who recur in the liver after initial resection.

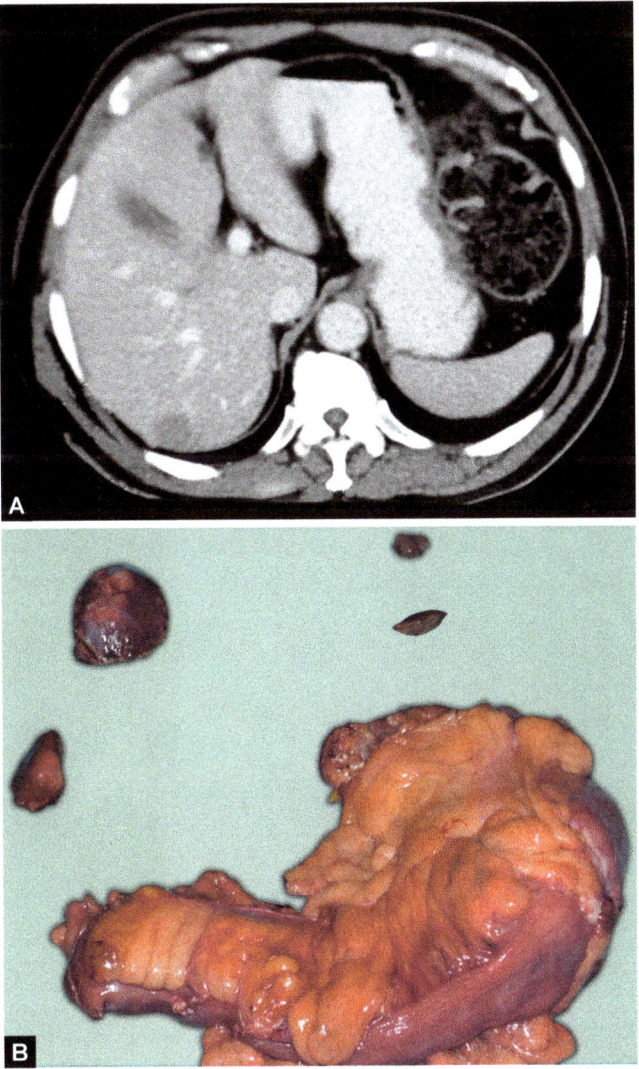

Figs. 5A and B: Contrast-enhanced computed tomography (CECT) showing mildly enhancing lesion in segment VI of right lobe of liver representing colorectal metastases. (B) Photograph following synchronous resection of sigmoid lesion and multiple liver metastases.

Two-stage hepatectomy is a useful option when dealing with large tumor volume or bilobar distribution of metastatic disease and the FLR is likely to be inadequate if a single stage operation is performed. In two-stage hepatectomy, the future liver remnant, usually the left lobe is cleared of the disease by small nonanatomical resections. In the same sitting, the right portal vein is ligated or embolized postoperatively, allowing for the hypertrophy of FLR. Interval CECT, usually performed after 4–6 weeks of the first surgery is used to document the

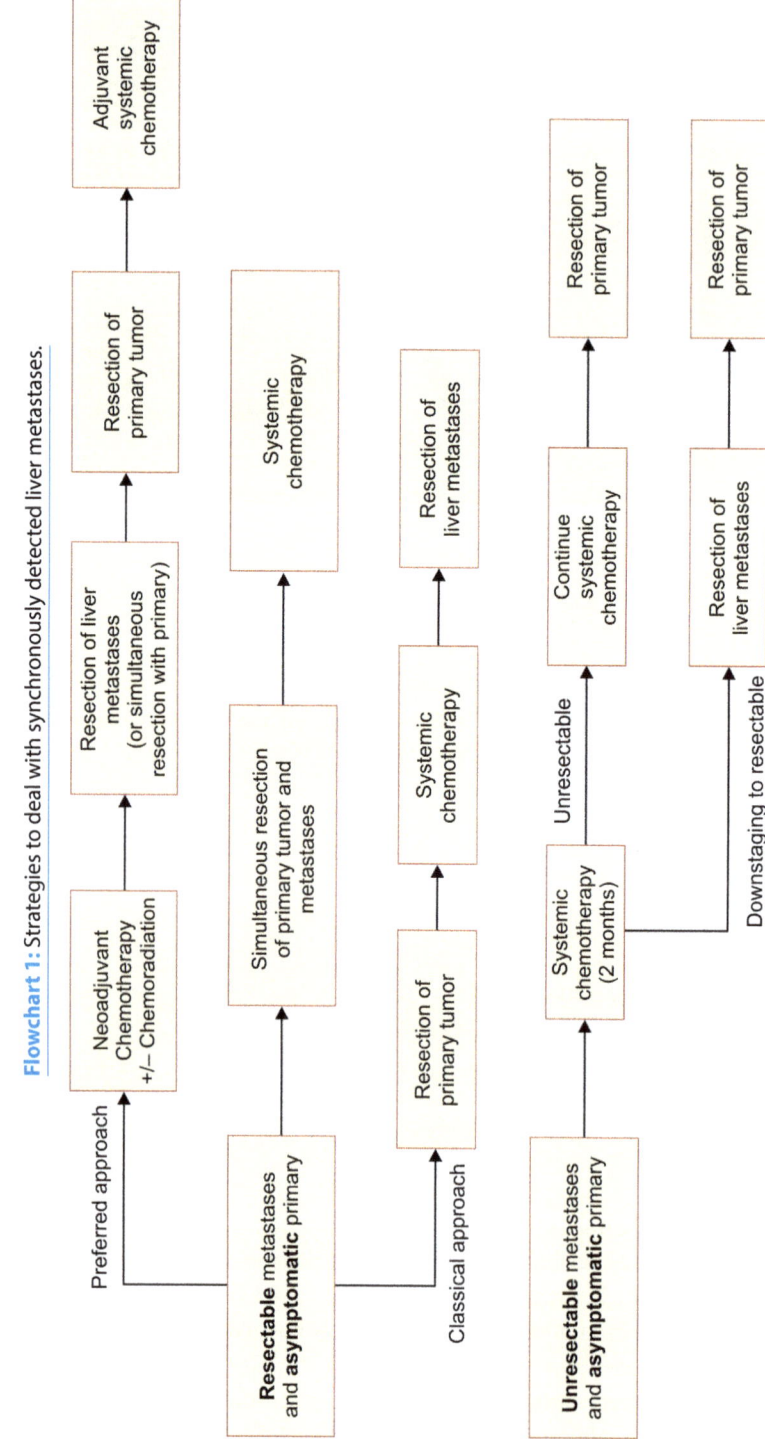

Flowchart 1: Strategies to deal with synchronously detected liver metastases.

hypertrophy of the FLR. Growth rate of greater than 2% per week is associated with low rates of liver failure after the second stage of resection. In the second stage, an extended (usually right) hepatectomy is done to remove all remaining tumors. Dropout after the first stage because of tumor progression occurs in up to 35% of patients. Prognostic factors for dropout include CEA greater than 30, tumor size greater than 4 cm, greater than 12 cycles of chemotherapy, or progression during first-line treatment. Completion of the second stage has a distinct survival advantage of median 37 months compared with 16 months for those who only complete the first stage.[16]

As a result of increasing experience with minimally invasive surgical techniques, laparoscopic liver resections are being performed with greater frequency at experienced hepatobiliary centers. Besides the benefits of avoiding a large laparotomy incision, laparoscopic approach is associated with reduced intraoperative blood loss due to the tamponade effect of pneumoperitoneum. This amounts to faster postoperative recovery, lesser analgesic requirement and reduced length of hospital stay; without compromising the oncologic outcomes.[17,18] It has been suggested that laparoscopic liver resection techniques require advanced training and a learning curve of 60 major hepatectomies before decreasing morbidity and mortality to acceptable rates of 17.2% and 3.4%.[19]

As part of multimodality management of CRLM, preoperative chemotherapy is being increasingly used, especially in patients with large tumor burden. This strategy has led to a unique finding of so-called "disappearing metastases". About 10–38% of CRLM disappear after neoadjuvant chemotherapy especially those less than 2 cm in size.[20] However, it has been clearly shown that disappearance on cross-sectional imaging is not synonymous with complete pathological response. Residual tumor is found in up to 80% of such cases on pathological examination. Contrast MRI is a better imaging modality in such a scenario. It is recommended that such disappearing lesions should be aggressively searched for during surgery and resected. Pathologic complete response occurs in 9% of tumors and is an excellent prognostic factor with 5-year survival of 75%.[21]

Neoadjuvant chemotherapy is a boon for patients having unresectable disease at initial presentation. Conversion to resectable disease has been reported in 17–40% in these cases with 5-year survival rates of up to 30% in those where negative resection margins are achieved. However, disease recurrence rates are higher in these patients.[22] Recurrence rates after hepatectomy for CRLM range from 60% to 70%. Fortunately, for patients who present with recurrence confined to the liver repeat resection may be feasible in up to 27%. Major morbidity and mortality rates are similar to the primary hepatectomy. Repeat resections are associated with up to 50% 5-year survival rates.[23]

PROGNOSTIC FACTORS

In an attempt to improve outcomes in patients with CRLM, studies have looked into the prognostic factors that have a bearing on long-term outcomes. The most important prognostic factors associated with worse outcome are: increasing number and size of tumors, shorter disease free interval, synchronous metastases, node positive primary disease, positive resection margins, and bulky extrahepatic disease. Using data from 1,001 patients treated for CRLM at Memorial Sloan Kettering Cancer Center (MSKCC), Fong et al. combined these prognostic factors to develop a clinical risk score (CRS) that predicts survival in patients with CRLM undergoing hepatic resection.[24] According to CRS, poor prognostic factors are node-positive primary, disease-free interval less than 12 months, more than one tumor, largest tumor greater than 5 cm, and CEA greater than 200 ng/mL. There are other scoring systems besides CRS but none of these systems is specific enough and therefore even patients with poor prognostic score should not be denied treatment because some of these patients will still have good long-term survival despite the poor risk scores. Nomograms have also been developed in order to help predict outcomes. Using data on 1477 CRLM patients, a nomogram was developed incorporating several of the CRS elements, resection characteristics, and colon or rectal origin to predict 96 month disease specific survival.[25] In another work, a Japanese group developed both a preoperative and postoperative nomogram in 578 CRLM patients to predict 5-year disease-specific survival (DSS) using six clinical variables.[26] Nomograms are potentially useful tools because they are dynamic and can adapt readily to clinical, pathologic, and genomic information, and provide a more precise assessment of individual risk.

CHEMOTHERAPY

Over the last few years it has become amply clear that the key to improving survival in patients with CRLM, a multimodality approach to treatment has to be adopted. Chemotherapy, either neoadjuvant or adjuvant or palliative has become a very important component of the multimodality approach. Moreover, it has been seen that many patients with initially unresectable disease can be staged down to resectable disease with chemotherapy, aptly called "conversion chemotherapy". Standard regimens comprising 5-fluorouracil (FU)/folinic acid plus either irinotecan (FOLFIRI) or oxaliplatin (FOLFOX) can facilitate resection in 7–40% of patients.[27] In 1999, Giacchetti et al. reported that 5-FU/leucovorin (LV) plus oxaliplatin treatment could reduce the size of liver metastases by more than 50% in 59% of the patients with unresectable CRLM; giving a complete resection rate of up to 38%.[28]

A phase II randomized trial comparing intensified chemotherapy regimens including high dose FOLFIRI, FOLFIRINOX with standard regimens showed greater activity of intensified regimens in cases with initially unresectable disease. Conversion rates of up to 67% and median overall survival of more than 48 months were achieved with the intensified regimens.[29]

Recurrence has been reported in 50–70% of patients undergoing liver resection for CRLM. Perioperative chemotherapy has therefore become an important tool for increasing the disease-free survival in patients with initially resectable disease. A randomized, phase III trial, European Organisation for Research and Treatment of Cancer (EORTC) 40983, comparing perioperative (both neoadjuvant and adjuvant) FOLFOX-4 chemotherapy with surgery alone in 364 patients with resectable CRLM, has shown a significant increment of progression free survival in favor of perioperative treatment but no significant differences in long-term overall survival between the two treatment arms.[30, 31] However, postoperative morbidity was found to be higher in the chemotherapy plus surgery arm.

TARGETED BIOLOGICAL TREATMENT

Greater understanding of the molecular pathways involved in cancer progression has led to the development of biologic therapies targeting two different mechanisms, epidermal growth factor receptors inhibitors (EGFRs) (cetuximab and panitumumab) and angiogenesis (bevacizumab).[32] Inhibitors of EGFR have been found to be active both when used alone or in combination with standard chemotherapy regimes in CRLM that are RAS wild type.[33] The Outcomes following Vaginal Prolapse Repair and Mid Urethral Sling (OPUS) trial showed that the association of FOLFOX-4 plus cetuximab nearly doubled R0 resection rates (4.7%).[34] The Cetuximab Combined with Irinotecan in First-line Therapy for Metastatic Colorectal Cancer (CRYSTAL) study showed that combination of FOLFIRI plus cetuximab increased the R0 resection rate from 3.7% to 7.0%.[35] The cetuximab in a multidisciplinary concept (CELIM) trial reported that neoadjuvant treatment with FOLFIRI plus cetuximab or FOLFOX-6 resulted in 34% of R0 resections.[36] Overall response rate is in the range 60–79%, however, resection rates after chemotherapy/cetuximab are very variable. Addition of bevacizumab to first and second-line chemotherapy for mCRC improves progression-free survival and in some studies overall survival.[37,38] However, data on the role of bevacizumab added to chemotherapy in the perioperative setting is limited. It can be stated with confidence that "biologically directed" chemotherapy reduces the number and size of unresectable lesions and allows rescue of 15–35% of patients, bringing them to surgery. These therapies are being increasingly used worldwide.

ADJUNCTS TO RESECTION

Ablation techniques such as radiofrequency ablation (RFA) and microwave ablation (MWA) are another component of multimodality approach to treatment of CRLM. They have a role to play in patients with poor performance status and in situations where there are small centrally located tumors that will require removal of large volume of healthy liver parenchyma at resection, risking the patient to postoperative liver failure.[39] Another role for ablation therapies is in the palliative setting in combination with systemic chemotherapy. The use of RFA with systemic chemotherapy in the setting of unresectable disease is associated with higher progression-free survival at 3 years (27.6%) compared with systemic chemotherapy alone (10.6%) and better 5-year overall survival (43.1% versus 30.3%).[40] A relative contraindication to ablation is use for central tumors near major biliary structures. Hepatic arterial infusion pump for regional liver chemotherapy is another adjuvant treatment modality that can be combined with liver resection.[41]

SUMMARY OF TREATMENT OPTIONS FOR UNRESECTABLE LIVER METASTASIS AS CONVERSION OR PALLIATIVE THERAPIES

- *Systemic chemotherapy*: FOLFOX, FOLFIRI, capecitabine plus oxaliplatin (CAPE-OX), FOLFOXIRI ± Bevacizumab or panitumumab/cetuximab [Kirsten rat sarcoma wild-type (KRAS WT)].
- *Ablation therapies*: RFA, microwave, irreversible electroporation.
- *Stereotactic body radiotherapy (SBRT)*: Highly focused locoregional therapy using 34–75 Gy delivered in 3–6 fractions.
- *Yttrium-90 selective internal radiotherapy (Y-90 SIRT) (Radioembolization)*: Locoregional therapy using glass or resin beads with Y-90 delivered through the hepatic artery in doses of 100–3000 Gy. Advantage of delivering high doses to the tumor without causing damage to surrounding healthy liver parenchyma due to limited penetration.
- Isolated hepatic artery perfusion
- *Drug-eluting beads preloaded with irinotecan [Transarterial Chemoembolization (TACE)-DEBIRI]*: Locoregional therapy of drug-eluting beads delivered through the hepatic artery.

CONCLUSION

The surgical management of CRLM is complex. Factors such as accurate preoperative staging, role of tumor biology, need and timing of chemotherapy, and appropriate surgical plan have to be considered before embarking on the treatment of patients with CRLM. Therefore, treatment has to be multimodality in order to achieve the best possible outcome. Treatment has to be individualized for each patient and discussed in a multidisciplinary meeting. Surgical resection clearly has a central role in the entire treatment paradigm because this is one treatment modality that can lead to long-term survival. R0 resection is the goal and not the type of resection. Limited non-anatomical resections are safer, with results nearly equal to those of major lobar resections. Overall mortality after hepatic resection for CRLM at major centers is less than 1%, likely resulting from improved operative technique and patient selection.

Systemic chemotherapy in different settings and formats has become an indispensable part of the treatment algorithm despite the fact that randomized trials have not shown any major improvement in outcomes in the perioperative setting. Predictors of survival include size and number of tumors, short disease-free interval, node-positive primary tumor, positive margins, and the presence of bulky extrahepatic disease. However, neither the individual risk factors nor the risk scores developed on the basis of these factors are very specific, and therefore do not preclude the possibility of long-term survival even in patients with poor prognostic factors. Molecular and immunologic markers have acquired an important role and help in selection of patients appropriate for targeted biological agents.

REFERENCES

1. World Health Organization; International Agency for Research in Cancer. (2012) Globocan 2012: estimated cancer incidence, mortality and prevalence worldwide 2012. [online] Available from http://publications.iarc.fr/Databases/Iarc-Cancerbases/GLOBOCAN-2012-Estimated-Cancer-Incidence-Mortality-And-Prevalence-Worldwide-In-2012-V1.0-2012.
2. Zhang YL, Zhang ZS, Wu BP, et al. Early diagnosis for colorectal cancer in China. World J Gastroenterol. 2002;8:21-5.
3. Tzeng CW, Aloia TA. Colorectal liver metastases. J Gastrointest Surg. 2013;17(1):195-201.
4. Benson AB 3rd, Bekaii-Saab T, Chan E, et al. Metastatic colon cancer, version 3.2013: featured updates to the NCCN Guidelines. J Natl Compr Canc Netw. 2013;11(2):141-52.
5. Lejeune C, Bismuth MJ, Conroy T, et al. Use of a decision analysis model to assess the cost-effectiveness of 18F-FDG PET in the management of metachronous liver metastases of colorectal cancer. J Nucl Med. 2005;46(12):2020-8.
6. Moulton CA, Gu CS, Law CH, et al. Effect of PET before liver resection on surgical management for colorectal adenocarcinoma metastases: a randomized clinical trial. JAMA. 2014;311(18):1863-9.
7. Benson AB 3rd, Bekaii-Saab T, Chan E, et al. Localized colon cancer, version 3.2013: featured updates to the NCCN Guidelines. J Natl Compr Canc Netw. 2013;11(5):519-28.

8. Fowler KJ, Kaur H, Cash BD, et al. Expert Panel on Gastrointestinal Imaging. ACR Appropriateness Criteria® Pretreatment Staging of Colorectal Cancer. J Am Coll Radiol. 2017;14(5S):S234-244.
9. Adam R, De Gramont A, Figueras J, et al. Jean-NicolasVauthey of the EGOSLIM (Expert Group on Onco Surgery management of LIver Metastases) group: The oncosurgery approach to managing liver metastases from colorectal cancer: a multidisciplinary international consensus. Oncologist. 2012;17(10):1225-39.
10. Are C, Gonen M, Zazzali K, et al. The impact of margins on outcome after hepatic resection for colorectal metastasis. Ann Surg. 2007;246(2):295-300.
11. Adams RB, Aloia TA, Loyer E, et al. Selection for hepatic resection of colorectal liver metastases: expert consensus statement. HPB (Oxford). 2013;15(2): 91-103.
12. Adam R, de Gramont A, Figueras J, et al. Managing synchronous liver metastases from colorectal cancer: a multidisciplinary international consensus. Cancer Treat Rev. 2015;41(9):729-41.
13. de Jong MC, Pulitano C, Ribero D, et al. Rates and patterns of recurrence following curative intent surgery for colorectal liver metastasis: an international multi-institutional analysis of 1669 patients. Ann Surg. 2009;250(3):440-8.
14. Memeo R, de Blasi V, Adam R, et al. Parenchymal-sparing hepatectomies (PSH) for bilobar colorectal liver metastases are associated with a lower morbidity and similar oncological results: a propensity score matching analysis. HPB (Oxford). 2016;18(9):781-90.
15. Reddy SK, Pawlik TM, Zorzi D, et al. Simultaneous resections of colorectal cancer and synchronous liver metastases: a multi-institutional analysis. Ann Surg Oncol. 2007;14(12):3481-91.
16. Imai K, Benitez CC, Allard MA, et al. Failure to achieve a 2-stage hepatectomy for colorectal liver metastases: how to prevent it? Ann Surg. 2015;262(5):772-8.
17. Allard MA, Cunha AS, Gayet B, et al. Early and long-term oncological outcomes after laparoscopic resection for colorectal liver metastases: a propensity score based analysis. Ann Surg. 2015;262(5):794-802.
18. Martinez-Cecilia D, Cipriani F, Vishal S, et al. Laparoscopic versus open liver resection for colorectal metastases in elderly and octogenarian patients: a multicentre propensity score based analysis of short- and long-term outcomes. Ann Surg. 2017;265(6):1192-200.
19. Vigano L, Laurent A, Tayar C, et al. The learning curve in laparoscopic liver resection: improved feasibility and reproducibility. Ann Surg. 2009;250(5):772-82.
20. Bischof DA, Clary BM, Maithel SK, et al. Surgical management of disappearing colorectal liver metastases. Br J Surg. 2013;100(11):1414-20.
21. Blazer DG, Kishi Y, Maru DM, et al. Pathologic response to preoperative chemotherapy: a new outcome end point after resection of hepatic colorectal metastases. J Clin Oncol. 2008;26(33):5344-51.
22. Devaud N, Kanji ZS, Dhani N, et al. Liver resection after chemotherapy and tumour downsizing in patients with initially unresectable colorectal cancer liver metastases. HPB (Oxford). 2014;16(5):475-80.

23. Wicherts DA, de Haas RJ, Salloum C, et al. Repeat hepatectomy for recurrent colorectal metastases. Br J Surg. 2013;100(6):808-18.
24. Fong Y, Fortner J, Sun RL, et al. Clinical score for predicting recurrence after hepatic resection for metastatic colorectal cancer: analysis of 1001 consecutive cases. Ann Surg. 1999;230(3):309-18.
25. Kattan MW, Gonen M, Jarnagin WR, et al. A nomogram for predicting disease specific survival after hepatic resection for metastatic colorectal cancer. Ann Surg. 2008;247(2):282-7.
26. Takakura Y, Okajima M, Kanemitsu Y, et al. External validation of two nomograms for predicting patient survival after hepatic resection for metastatic colorectal cancer. World J Surg. 2011;35(10):2275-82.
27. Van Cutsem E, Nordlinger B, Cervantes A. Advanced colorectal cancer: ESMO Clinical Practice Guidelines for treatment. Ann Oncol. 2010;21 Suppl 5:v93-7.
28. Giacchetti S, Itzhaki M, Gruia G, et al. Long-term survival of patients with unresectable colorectal cancer liver metastases following infusional chemotherapy with 5-fluorouracil, leucovorin, oxaliplatin and surgery. Ann Oncol. 1999;10:663-9.
29. Ychou M, Rivoire M, Thezenas S, et al. A randomized phase II trial of three intensified chemotherapy regimens in first-line treatment of colorectal cancer patients with initially unresectable or not optimally resectable liver metastases. The METHEP trial. Ann Surg Oncol. 2013;20:4289-97.
30. House MG, Ito H, Gönen M, et al. Survival after hepatic resection for metastatic colorectal cancer: trends in outcomes for 1,600 patients during two decades at a single institution. J Am Coll Surg. 2010;210:744-52, 752-5.
31. Nordlinger B, Sorbye H, Glimelius B, et al. Perioperative FOLFOX4 chemotherapy and surgery versus surgery alone for resectable liver metastases from colorectal cancer (EORTC 40983): long-term results of a randomised, controlled, phase 3 trial. Lancet Oncol. 2013;14:1208-15.
32. Peeters M, Price T. Biologic therapies in the metastatic colorectal cancer treatment continuum—applying current evidence to clinical practice. Cancer Treat Rev. 2012;38:397-406.
33. Fausto N. Growth factors in liver development, regeneration and carcinogenesis. Prog Growth Factor Res. 1991;3:219-34.
34. Fausto N, Webber EM. Mechanisms of growth regulation in liver regeneration and hepatic carcinogenesis. Prog Liver Dis. 1993;11: 115-37
35. Mangnall D, Smith K, Bird NC, et al. Early increases in plasminogen activator activity following partial hepatectomy in humans. Comp Hepatol. 2004;3(1):11.
36. Van den Eynde M, Hendlisz A. Treatment of colorectal liver metastases: a review. Rev Recent Clin Trials. 2009;4(1):56-62.
37. Hurwitz H, Fehrenbacher L, Novotny W, et al. Bevacizumab plus irinotecan, fluorouracil, and leucovorin for metastatic colorectal cancer. N Engl J Med. 2004;350(23):2335-42.
38. Saltz LB, Clarke S, Díaz-Rubio E, et al. Bevacizumab in combination with oxaliplatin-based chemotherapy as first-line therapy in metastatic colorectal cancer: a randomized phase III study. J Clin Oncol. 2008;26(12):2013-9.

39. Eltawil KM, Boame N, Mimeault R, et al. Patterns of recurrence following selective intraoperative radiofrequency ablation as an adjunct to hepatic resection for colorectal liver metastases. J Surg Oncol. 2014;110(6):734-8.
40. Ruers T, Van Coevorden F, Punt CJ, et al. Local treatment of unresectable colorectal liver metastases: results of a randomized phase II trial. J Natl Cancer Inst. 2017;109(9).
41. Lewis HL, Bloomston M. Hepatic artery infusional chemotherapy. Surg Clin North Am. 2016;96(2):341-55.

3
Chapter

Complications of Acute Pancreatitis

PK Sasmal, VK Kapoor

INTRODUCTION

Acute pancreatitis (AP) is one of the most common gastrointestinal (GI) disorders worldwide, despite improvements in intensive care, imaging, and interventional techniques it continues to be a major cause of morbidity and mortality. The autoactivation of the pancreatic enzymes inside the acinar cells, due to various causes like gallstones or alcohol, leads to damage to the gland itself along with adjacent tissues and other organs. The diagnosis of AP is made upon the presence of two of the following three features: (1) acute onset severe upper abdominal pain, often radiating to the back; (2) raised serum amylase and/or lipase more than and equal to three times the upper limit of normal; and (3) radiological findings suggestive of pancreatitis on transabdominal ultrasonography (USG), contrast-enhanced computed tomography (CECT) or less commonly magnetic resonance imaging (MRI).[1]

The early assessment of severity of pancreatitis aids in the successful management of this dreadful disease. A range of predictive scoring systems are commonly used in clinical practice, that includes Ranson's criteria, Acute Physiologic Assessment and Chronic Health Evaluation II (APACHE II), and the Bedside Index for Severity in Acute Pancreatitis (BISAP) score.[2] As suggested by the revised Atlanta classification 2012, AP has two phases—early (first 1 or 2 weeks) and late (weeks or months).[3] The revised classification system is targeted to correlate the detailed imaging findings and appropriate interpretation of the severity and complications of the disease process, which will ultimately assist the treating clinician in efficient and timely management of the patient.

TYPES OF ACUTE PANCREATITIS

There are two different morphological forms of AP: (1) interstitial edematous pancreatitis and (2) necrotizing pancreatitis (terms emphysematous pancreatitis and pancreatic phlegmon are no longer used). Majority of the patients have edematous pancreatitis with a mild course and recover without sequelae, but 10-20% will have a severe and more complicated clinical course with higher risks of morbidity and mortality.[4]

SEVERITY CLASSIFICATION

Severity of the disease is categorized into three levels: mild, moderately severe, and severe.

The complications of AP depend upon the disease severity which is stratified by organ failure, local complications (fluid collections and necrosis), and systemic complications (Table 1).[5]

About 5-10% of individuals with severe acute pancreatitis (SAP) develop necrosis which affects the pancreatic parenchyma in 5%, peripancreatic tissue in 20% and both of them in 70% of cases, respectively.[6,7] The increased morbidity and mortality of patients with SAP are due to development of infection in the pancreatic and peripancreatic necrosis and subsequent multiple organ failure (MOF). The presence of pancreatic parenchymal necrosis indicates a more severe disease compared with peripancreatic necrosis alone.[8] Based on the radiological changes and extent of necrosis present, the estimation of the severity of the disease process was done by the CT severity index (CTSI) of Balthazar in 1990. But after the framing of revised Atlanta classification in 2012, it is most commonly used to assess the severity of the disease and predict mortality. The natural history of pancreatic and peripancreatic necrosis is variable because it may remain solid or liquefy, remain sterile or become infected and persist, or disappear over time.[5] Patients who develop persistent organ failure within the first few days of the disease have a mortality rate as high as 30-50%.[9] The classification of AP and associated collections as per the revised Atlanta classification 2012, are described by Zhao et al (Flowchart 1).[10]

Table 1: Severity grades of acute pancreatitis with mortality.

	Mortality
Mild acute pancreatitis • No organ failure • No local or systemic complications	**Rare (1–2%)**
Moderately severe acute pancreatitis • Organ failure that resolves within 48 hour (transient organ failure) and/or • Local or systemic complications without persistent organ failure	**Low (2–5%)**

Severe acute pancreatitis
• Persistent organ failure (>48 hour)
  – Single organ failure
  – Multiple organ failure
	High (20–30%)

Flowchart 1: Classification of acute pancreatitis and its associated collections (Revised Atlanta Classification, 2012).

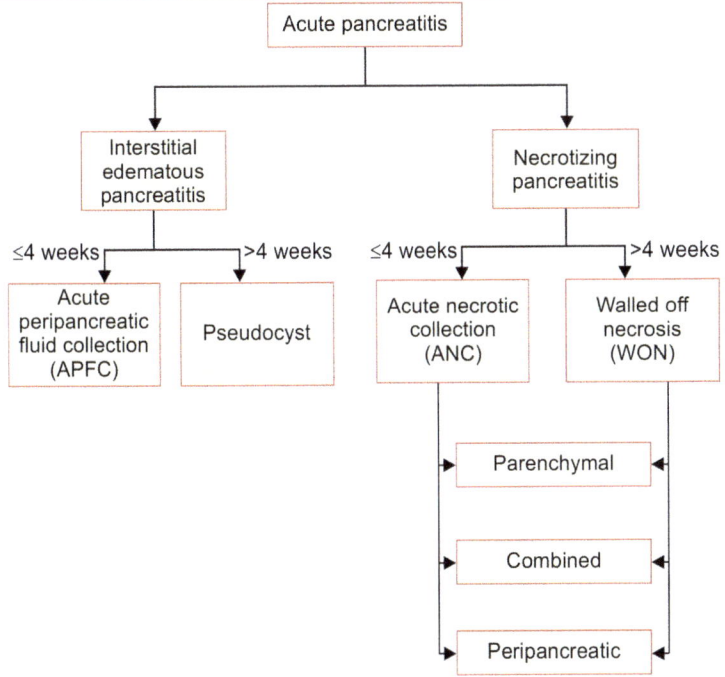

PHASES OF ACUTE PANCREATITIS

Acute pancreatitis has two overlapping phases of presentation with two peaks of mortality: early and late.[11,12] The early phase, which usually lasts for the first 1–2 weeks, is followed by a second later phase, which can run a protracted course from weeks to months. Mortality in the early phase is usually due to MOF and in the late phase due to sepsis caused by infection (bacterial and fungal) of necrosis.

Early Phase

During this phase, the systemic manifestations result from host response to local pancreatic injury. This early phase is usually over by the end of the first week, but may extend into the second week. Pancreatic insult due to any etiology leads to release of proinflammatory mediators, such as zymogens, cytokines, and vasoactive factors. Cytokine cascades are activated by the pancreatic inflammation which manifests clinically as the systemic inflammatory response syndrome (SIRS) (Box 1).[13,14] These mediators cause endothelial cell activation leading to arteriolar vasoconstriction, increased permeability, and circulatory stasis, thereby inducing ischemia.[15] The

> **Box 1:** Systemic inflammatory response syndrome.
>
> Response to a variety of severe clinical insults, manifested by two or more of the following:
> - Temperature > 38° C or < 36° C
> - Heart rate > 90 beats/min
> - Respiratory rate > 20/min or $PaCO_2$ < 32 mm Hg
> - White blood cell (WBC) count > 12,000 cells/mm^3, < 4,000 cells/mm^3 or > 10% immature (band) forms

($PaCO_2$: partial pressure of carbon dioxide)

presence of SIRS particularly when three or more criteria are present, or when it persists for 48 hours or more after admission, identifies patients at risk of multiple organ dysfunction syndrome (MODS).

The severity of this dynamic disease is based on the presence and duration of organ failure. The organ failure may resolve within 48 hours *"transient organ failure"* or may persist beyond 48 hours *"persistent organ failure"*. If the organ failure affects more than one organ system, it is termed as MOF. Although local complications may be identified during the early phase, they are not the predominant determinants of severity,[16] and it is the presence and duration of organ failure which determines the severity of AP. During the early phase, the severity of AP needs to be reassessed on a daily basis while the pancreatitis is still evolving. Convenient time points to re-evaluate are 24 hours, 48 hours, and 7 days after admission to hospital.

Late Phase

This phase is characterized by the persistence of systemic signs of inflammation or by the presence of local complications of AP. During this phase, it is important to distinguish the different morphologic characteristics of the local complications by radiologic imaging, for deciding the further course of management. Persistent organ failure, however, remains the main determinant of severity; hence characterization of AP in the late phase requires both clinical and morphologic criteria.

The SIRS of the early phase may be followed by a compensatory anti-inflammatory response syndrome (CARS) in the late phase that may contribute to an increased risk of infection; however, these events are complex and poorly understood.[17]

COMPLICATIONS OF ACUTE PANCREATITIS

The complications of AP are broadly classified into systemic or local and regional (Table 2).

Table 2: Complications of acute pancreatitis.

Systemic	Local and regional
• SIRS • MODS • Respiratory • Renal • CVS • Metabolic • Encephalopathy	• Acute peripancreatic fluid collections • Pseudocyst • Acute necrotic collection • Walled off pancreatic necrosis • Pancreatic abscess • Hemorrhage • Portal vein/splenic thrombosis • Gastrointestinal obstruction • Obstruction of extraintestinal structures • Pancreatic ascites and pleural effusions • Abdominal compartment syndrome

(CVS: cyclic vomiting syndrome; MODS: multiple organ dysfunction syndrome; SIRS: systemic inflammatory response syndrome)

Systemic Complications of Acute Pancreatitis

The systemic complications in the form of SIRS and MODS are most commonly seen during the early phase of the dynamic disease. The local and regional complications usually become clinically apparent in the late phase of the disease process. Hence, it is prudent to discuss the systemic complications first along with the pathophysiology of the inflammatory disease.

Organ Failure (Persistent or Transient)

The most reliable marker for disease severity in AP is organ failure that persists for longer than 48 hours.[18] The universally applicable modified Marshall scoring system stratifies organ dysfunction easily and objectively.[5,9,14] The system evaluates the three organ systems most commonly affected by SAP: respiratory (tachypnea, rhonchi, crepitation, and bilateral hilar fluffy infiltrates on chest X-ray), renal [acute renal failure (ARF)], cardiovascular [hypotension, disseminated intravascular coagulation (DIC) platelets < 100,000, and fibrinogen < 1 g/L, fibrin degradation product (FDP) > 80 mg/mL], neurological (disorientation, drowsiness, and altered sensorium), and GI (gastroparesis and paralytic ileus) system. Organ failure is defined as a score of 2 or more for one of these three organ systems. The modified Marshall scoring system (Table 3) has the advantage of being simple to use hence used globally to stratify disease severity objectively.[5]

Serial evaluation of organ dysfunction by sequential organ failure assessment (SOFA) has been evaluated and shown to be reliable in intensive care unit (ICU) practice as it takes into account the use of inotropic and respiratory support.[19] Of the multiple factor scoring systems, APACHE II of 8 or higher at baseline or in the first 72 hours is suggestive of SAP, provides the best prediction of mortality, but requires repeated careful clinical observation.[20]

Table 3: Modified Marshall scoring system for organ dysfunction.[5]

Organ system	Score				
	0	1	2	3	4
Respiratory (PaO$_2$/FiO$_2$)	>400	301–400	201–300	101–200	≤101
Renal* (serum creatinine, mg/dL)	<1.4	1.4–1.8	1.9–3.6	3.6–4.9	>4.9
Cardiovascular (systolic blood pressure, mm Hg)†	>90	<90, fluid responsive	<90, not fluid responsive	<90, pH < 7.3	<90, pH < 7.2

A score of 2 or more in any system defines the presence of organ failure.
* A score for patients with pre-existing chronic renal failure depends on the extent of further deterioration of baseline renal function. No formal correction exists for a baseline serum creatinine ≥1.4 mg/dL.
† Off inotropic support.
(FiO$_2$: fraction of inspired oxygen; PaO$_2$: partial pressure of arterial oxygen)

The diagnosis of SAP should be made if the patient has a serum C-reactive protein (CRP) more than and equal to 150 mg/dL at baseline or in the first 72 hours; APACHE II score more than and equal to 8 at baseline or in the first 72 hours; or exhibits signs of persistent organ failure for more than 48 hours despite adequate intravenous fluid resuscitation and organ support.[21] There are various other scoring systems [Ranson, BISAP (**B**UN, **I**mpaired mental status, **S**IRS, **A**ge, **P**leural effusion), etc.] that help stratify the severity of AP.

Metabolic Complications

Severe acute pancreatitis is associated with SIRS and a hypercatabolic state.[22] The adverse consequences of this include protein calorie malnutrition, expansion of the extracellular fluid compartment, and immune suppression. Other metabolic derangements in AP are hyperglycemia and hypocalcemia. AP results in a severe catabolic response causing malnutrition.

Local and Regional Complications

In the revised Atlanta classification 2012, an important distinction is made between collections that are composed of fluid alone versus those that arise from necrosis and contain a solid component (also contain varying amounts of fluid).[10]

Acute Peripancreatic Fluid Collection

Fluid collections usually develop in the early phase of interstitial edematous pancreatitis, with no associated peripancreatic necrosis.[22] This term applies only to homogeneous peripancreatic fluid collection seen within the first

4 weeks after onset of interstitial edematous pancreatitis without a discrete wall of fibrous or granulation tissue and confined to normal anatomical planes. On CECT, acute peripancreatic fluid collections (APFCs) are homogeneous collection (solitary or multiple) of fluid adjacent to pancreas in the setting of interstitial edematous pancreatitis, without a definable wall and are confined by normal fascial planes in the retroperitoneum. Collections can be seen remote from the pancreas also.

Most acute fluid collections remain sterile and usually resolve spontaneously without intervention.[23] The fluid collection lack true communication with the pancreatic duct. When a localized APFC persists beyond 4 weeks it is likely to develop into a pancreatic pseudocyst, this is although rare in AP. APFCs which resolve or remain asymptomatic do not require treatment and do not by themselves constitute SAP.

Pancreatic Pseudocyst

An encapsulated collection of fluid with high pancreatic enzyme concentrations in the peripancreatic tissues, with a well-defined inflammatory wall of fibrous or granulation tissues devoid of epithelial lining, with minimal or no necrosis. At times the pseudocyst may be partly or completely intrapancreatic. Pseudocyst not only arises as a result of AP but also from chronic pancreatitis, pancreatic trauma or obstruction of the pancreatic duct by a neoplasm. This entity usually forms at least 4 weeks after onset of interstitial edematous pancreatitis. A pancreatic pseudocyst is assumed to arise from disruption of the main pancreatic duct or its branches without any recognizable pancreatic parenchymal necrosis. The consequent extravasation of pancreatic juice results in a persistent localized fluid collection, persisting beyond 4 weeks. Initially the wall of the cyst is thin fibrous tissue, which progressively thickens over time with maturation. The revised Atlanta classification 2012,[10] classifies the peripancreatic collections in interstitial edematous pancreatitis as pseudocyst only if it persists after 4 weeks of the onset of the AP. However, the development of a pancreatic pseudocyst is rare in the setting of AP.

Imaging modality like CECT is most commonly used to describe pseudocysts, but MRI or USG may be required to confirm the absence of solid content in the collection which will change the nomenclature to walled-off pancreatic necrosis. The CECT findings in a pseudocyst are well circumscribed usually round or oval peripancreatic fluid collection with homogeneous fluid density but without necrotic content (Fig. 1). It has a well-defined wall; it is, completely encapsulated and takes more than 4 weeks to mature. Pseudocysts occur more frequently in chronic pancreatitis (20–40%) as compared to AP (10–20%).[24] Half of them occur in or around the head of the pancreas, whereas the rest are evenly located in the body and tail of the gland.

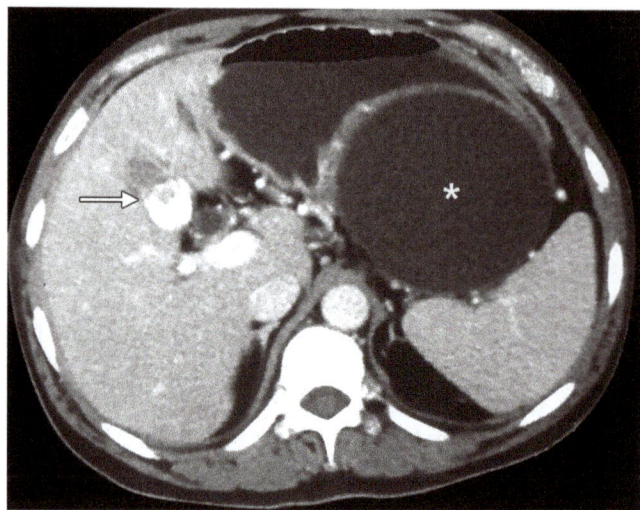

Fig. 1: Axial contrast-enhanced computed tomography (CECT) showing a large pancreatic pseudocyst (asterisk) compressing the stomach anteriorly and presence of a large gallstone (arrow).

Expectant management is important in the first 6–12 weeks of existence of pseudocysts that have arisen during an acute attack of AP. Spontaneous resolution of the pseudocyst does occur in up to 40% of cases requiring no treatment. Persistence of a pseudocyst usually occurs due to communication with the pancreatic ductal system.

Pseudocysts can be complicated in up to 40% of cases with infection, rupture (5%), hemorrhage or compression or obstruction of adjacent structures.[25] The principal indications for treatment are to relieve symptoms and to prevent complications. Larger the size of the cyst, more are the chances for intervention required.

Treatment options include internal drainage (preferred method of treatment), which can be either a Roux-en-Y cystojejunostomy, cystogastrostomy, or cystoduodenostomy, excision of the cyst, or external drainage (surgical or percutaneous). Endoscopic transgastric and transduodenal drainage are gaining popularity as treatment options due to a reported decrease in complication and mortality rates.[26]

Acute Necrotic Collection

In necrotizing pancreatitis, during the first 4 weeks, a collection containing variable amounts of fluid and necrotic tissue is termed as acute necrotic collection (ANC). The necrosis can involve the pancreatic parenchyma and/or the peripancreatic tissues. ANC is different from APFC as the former occurs only in the setting of acute necrotic pancreatitis and contains necrotic material in addition to fluid. An ANC may be associated with disruption of

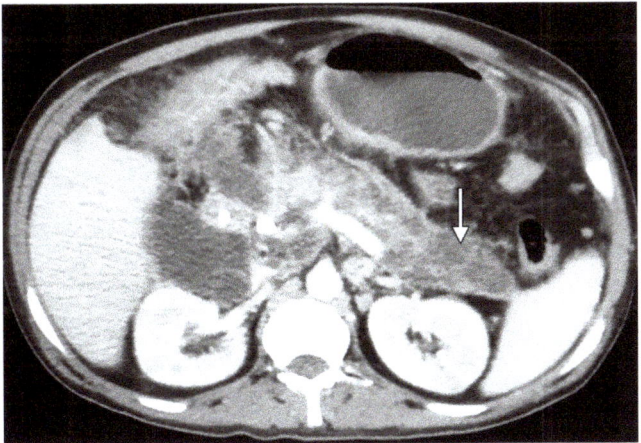

Fig. 2: Axial contrast-enhanced computed tomography (CECT) showing pancreatic necrosis (arrow) with nonenhancing parenchyma.

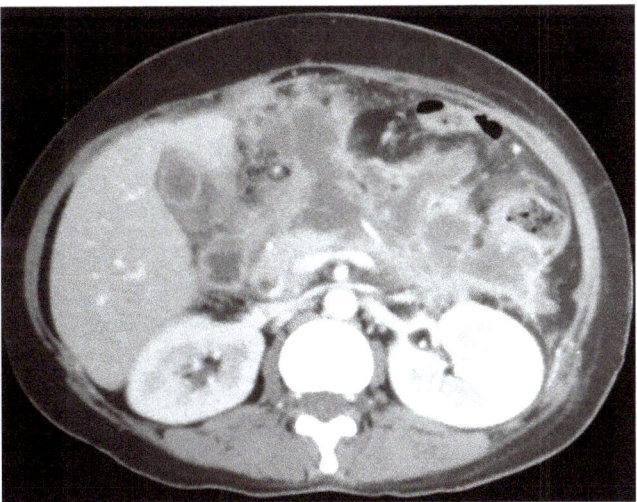

Fig. 3: Axial contrast-enhanced computed tomography (CECT) in second week of acute necrotizing pancreatitis, showing acute necrotic collection (ANC) with absence of a well-defined wall involving the pancreatic and peripancreatic region.

the main pancreatic duct within the zone of parenchymal necrosis and it can become infected.

On CECT, acute pancreatic (Fig. 2) or peripancreatic necrotic collections contain varying amounts of solid necrotic material and fluid, may be loculated or multiple with no definable wall encapsulating the collection (Fig. 3). Radiological imaging may not be able to differentiate ANC from APFC within the first week. The highest risk of local and systemic complications is seen in patients with necrosis more than and equal to 50% of the pancreas on CECT or MRI.[27]

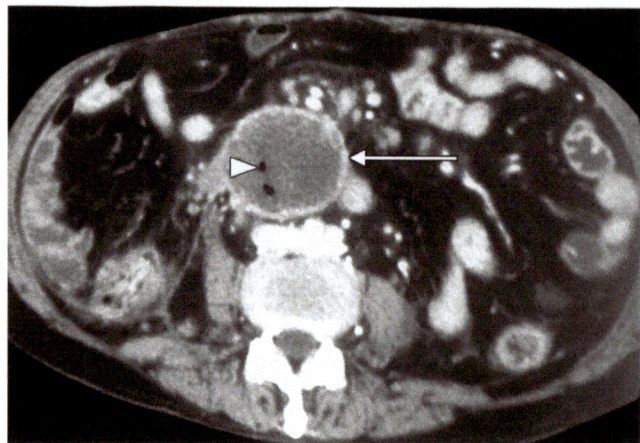

Fig. 4: Axial contrast-enhanced computed tomography (CECT) showing thick-enhancing wall (arrow) around a walled-off necrotic collection with air foci (arrowhead).

Walled-off Necrosis

Walled-off necrosis (WON) is the mature, encapsulated collection of pancreatic and/or peripancreatic necrosis with fluid surrounded by a well-defined inflammatory wall. The process of maturation occurs more than and equal to 4 weeks after onset of necrotizing pancreatitis. WON may be loculated or multiple, infected, and may be present at sites distant from the pancreas. It may be stressed that the presence of necrosis does not necessarily mean that it is infected. CECT may not readily distinguish solid from liquid content and ANC may be interpreted erroneously as pseudocyst (Fig. 4). In this setting, MRI, transabdominal USG or endoscopic ultrasonography (EUS) may be required to make the distinction.

Infected Necrosis/Pancreatic Abscess

The term pancreatic abscess is not mentioned separately in the revised Atlanta classification as it evolves from infection of APFC or pseudocyst or liquefaction of ANC. It is well localized, has a mature wall, and contains mainly pus with some solid necrotic debris. The diagnosis of infection [infected pancreatic necrosis (IPN)] of an ANC or of WON or pseudocyst can be suspected from the patient's systemic signs or by the presence of gas within the collection seen on CECT (Fig. 4). To distinguish pancreatic inflammation from secondary infection, Gram staining, and culture must be performed after image-guided aspiration.[28] Contents of some pseudocysts show evidence of bacteria on Gram stain and culture, but the fluid from these pseudocysts is not purulent and patients do not have clinical signs of infection.

When aspiration of the contents of the pseudocysts or WON reveals purulent fluid, it is termed as pancreatic abscess. It is one clinical condition in which percutaneous catheter drainage (PCD) is clearly the treatment of choice.[29] If PCD is not possible or successful, operative external drainage should be performed. The bacteriological analysis of an infected necrosis or pancreatic abscess reveals mostly intestinal gram-negative microbes like *Escherichia coli* most commonly followed by *Enterococcus* and *Klebsiella*.[30] However in recent years, a shift of the bacterial pattern has been found towards more gram-positive bacteria like *Staphylococcus aureus* and *Enterobacteriaceae*[31] and *Candida* species.[32]

The most common (up to 70%) cause of mortality in patients with AP, who survive the early phase, is infected pancreatic necrosis, although it is present in 5% cases only.[33] The principle of management of infected necrotizing pancreatitis has undergone sea change from aggressive surgical debridement or necrosectomy to more conservative staged multidisciplinary "step up" approach.[34]

Management in early phase: In the first week of admission, management mostly comprises of supportive care with adequate analgesia, hydration, nutrition, and frequent clinical evaluation. In the absence of clinical improvement in a week, CECT or MRI abdomen is indicated to evaluate for pancreatic or peripancreatic necrosis or extrapancreatic fluid collections. Any surgical interventions either elective early debridement or emergency procedures for bleeding/perforated viscus is associated with increased mortality rates of 40–80%.[35] Endoscopic retrograde cholangiopancreatography (ERCP) is indicated in early phase in the presence of choledocholithiasis with cholangitis.

Pharmacologic strategy (antibiotics): The prophylactic use of antibiotics or probiotics in patients with AP to prevent infection has always been a contentious issue. The recent systematic review and meta-analysis of 14 randomized control trials (RCTs) in 2011, including 841 patients diagnosed with SAP concluded no statistically significant reduction in mortality, incidence of infected pancreatic necrosis, incidence of nonpancreatic infections, and need of surgical interventions.[36] However, the usage of antibiotics/antifungals is recommended as per the antibiogram, if there is documentation of infection via blood culture and fine needle aspirations (FNA) of pancreatic necrosis.

Management in Intermediate phase (2–3 weeks): Imaging studies like CECT or MRI will assist in the diagnosis of pancreatic necrosis and peripancreatic collections. The evidence of retroperitoneal gas bubbles inside pancreatic fluid collections is pathognomonic of IPN. Fine-needle aspiration and culture of the necrotic material is not routinely advised. It is done only if the result will direct the treatment plan in patients who are not settling with conservative approaches.

It is now well established that avoiding early surgical intervention results in better outcome. The "step up" protocol for IPN recommends PCD and appropriate antibiotics. The PANTER trial recommends the "step up" approach over that of conventional open necrosectomy in terms of reduced major complications.[37] Also it was found that up to 30% of the patients of IPN with PCD did not require additional surgical interventions.

Management in late phase (≥4 weeks): The patients with IPN on PCDs, if clinically deteriorating or not showing signs of improvement despite adequate drainage are indicated for endoscopic transluminal drainage/ necrosectomy or minimally invasive drainage techniques like video-assisted retroperitoneal debridement (VARD),[38] minimal access retroperitoneal pancreatic necrosectomy (MARPN)[39] and laparoscopic necrosectomy. Open necrosectomy is indicated, if available expertise in the minimal access technique is not available.

Hemorrhage

Arterial hemorrhage may occur in up to 10% of patients with pancreatic pseudocysts.[40] Arterial bleeding mostly follows pseudoaneurysm formation due to weakening of the vessel wall by the pancreatic enzymes and eventual rupture. The most common source of pseudoaneurysm-associated bleeding is the splenic artery (up to 50%), followed by gastroduodenal and pancreaticoduodenal arteries.[41] Other uncommon sites of bleeding are from the portal, superior mesenteric, or splenic veins causing a retroperitoneal hematoma.

Contrast-enhanced CT is the best imaging study for evaluating vascular complications with conventional angiography done for arterial abnormalities (pseudoaneurysm) (Fig. 5).

Management of vascular bleeding is often successfully done by angioembolization.[42] Arterial bleeding can occur in pseudocyst or WON, into the GI tract or the peritoneal cavity, retroperitoneum, usually leading to acute hemorrhagic shock.[43] Operative interventions are rarely required. Control of arterial bleeding may require associated pancreatic resection (distal pancreatectomy pancreaticoduodenectomy) as ligation or over sewing of the bleeding vessels in the setting of inflammation and enzymatic erosion associated with pseudocysts is often unsuccessful. GI bleed may occur due to rupture of a pseudocyst into adjacent viscera.

Portal/Splenic Vein Thrombosis

Ongoing pancreatic inflammation may cause irritation and inflammation of the portal vein and/or splenic vein. The splenic vein is the most commonly affected vessel because of its extensive contact with the pancreatic gland.

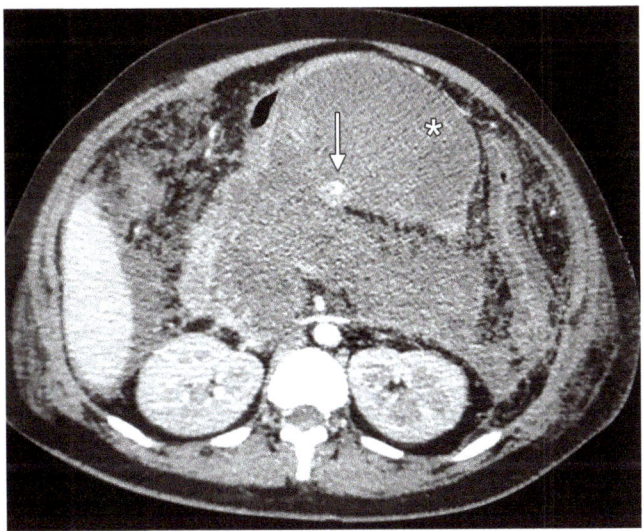

Fig. 5: Axial contrast-enhanced computed tomography (CECT) in arterial phase showing brightly enhancing vascular structure (pseudoaneurysm) marked by white arrow, in peripancreatic collection (asterisk).

Inflammation may lead to intrinsic damage to the venous intima or extrinsic compression secondary to edema or mass lesions. The stasis of blood flow may eventually lead to splenic vein thrombosis and manifest with left-sided portal hypertension and esophagogastric varices and GI bleeding.[44] Treatment of patients with bleeding gastroesophageal varices secondary to splenic vein thrombosis is splenectomy or splenic artery embolization in selected cases.

Gastrointestinal Obstruction

Acute pancreatitis can result in paralytic ileus as a result of dehydration, electrolyte abnormalities, or adjacent bowel inflammation. Later on with the disease progression, emergence of pseudocysts or abscess may result with compression effect on adjacent structures giving rise to GI tract obstruction. Although duodenal/jejunal obstruction is the most common site of mechanical obstruction, obstruction of the stomach, esophagus, and colon are also reported.[45,46] Adjacent duodenum, jejunum or colon may be involved in necrosis—causing thrombosis of vessels resulting in ischemia, gangrene, perforation, and fistula.

Obstruction of Extraintestinal Structures

Pseudocysts in/around the head of pancreas can cause biliary obstruction leading to cholangitis. Pseudocysts have been reported to obstruct retroperitoneal structures like inferior vena cava and the ureters.[47,48] Also there are reports of pseudocysts with mediastinal and pleural extension impeding cardiac performance secondary to obstruction of preload or increased afterload[49] and also causing congestive heart failure secondary to cardiac compression.[50]

Pancreatic Ascites and Pleural Effusion

The diagnostic criteria for pancreatic ascites and pleural effusion were initially proposed by Cameron et al. in 1967.[51] Fluid analysis to confirm the entity requires elevated amylase levels relative to serum values in all patients and fluid albumin levels elevated to 3 g/100 mL or more.

The pathogenesis of both pancreatic pleural effusion and ascites involves a disruption of the pancreatic duct and creation of an internal fistula into the retroperitoneum, which further tracks posteriorly into the pleural space or anteriorly into the peritoneal cavity.[52] The fluid is most often clear or straw colored but it may appear thick, chylous or even bloody. Clinically most patients with pancreatic ascites or effusions have an indolent illness that may not suggest pancreatic disease. The treatment options include intermittent paracentesis or thoracentesis to empty the pleural or peritoneal cavity. If conservative management (including nil by mouth, parenteral nutrition, and octreotide) for at least 3 weeks fails,[53] the pancreatic anatomy needs to be clearly defined by CECT or MRI/magnetic resonance cholangiopancreatography (MRCP). Pancreatic duct stents bridging the ductal disruption have shown promising results to heal internal pancreatic fistulas.[54] At times, e.g. for disconnected duct syndrome, surgical intervention may be addressed by distal pancreatectomy or drainage procedure of pseudocysts.

Abdominal Compartment Syndrome

Abdominal compartment syndrome (ACS) is defined as a sustained intra-abdominal pressure (IAP) more than 20 mm Hg (>27 cm H_2O) associated with new organ dysfunction/failure. SAP is frequently associated with intra-abdominal hypertension (IAH), defined as a sustained or repeated elevation of IAP more than 12 mm Hg (>16 cm H_2O).[55] The incidence of IAH in SAP, is approximately 60% whereas ACS is found in 30%.[55] In severe AP, IAH is partially related to the effects of the inflammatory process causing retroperitoneal, bowel and parietal edema, collections, ascites and ileus, and it partially results from medical intervention, especially aggressive fluid resuscitation.[55] Sustained IAP more than 20 mm Hg (>27 cm H_2O) can affect several intra-abdominal and extra-abdominal organs with frequent involvement of the cardiovascular system (decreased venous return and cardiac output), lungs (restricted ventilation due to elevation of domes of diaphragm), kidneys (impaired renal perfusion and function), splanchnic vessels (reduced blood flow to the bowel causing bacterial translocation from the lumen into the peritoneal cavity and retroperitoneum), and central nervous system.[56] ACS is associated with increased mortality in patients with severe AP. IAP can be measured directly using a peritoneal catheter or indirectly measuring intravesicular pressure using a bladder catheter.[56]

Other Rare Complications

Acute pancreatitis may rarely cause Purtscher's retinopathy resulting in varying degrees of visual impairment, due to systemic circulation of pancreatic proteases in pancreatitis. The entity was first described by Inkeles and Walsh in 1975.[57]

Acute Recurrent Pancreatitis

It is defined as more than one attack of AP. The etiology in majority of the cases is well recognized. Some of the common causes of acute recurrent pancreatitis (ARP) includes common bile duct stones (or sludge and crystals—microliths), chronic alcohol consumption, sphincter of Oddi dysfunction, anatomical ductal variants including anomalous pancreaticobiliary ductal junction (APBDJ) and pancreas divisum interfering with pancreatic juice outflow or obstruction of the main pancreatic duct.

In about 70% of cases, routine diagnostic tests such as blood chemistry, transabdominal ultrasound, MRCP, and CT scan generally detect the cause of ARP. However, despite advancement in radiologic and other diagnostic technologies, the etiology of ARP still remains unknown and "idiopathic" in up to 30% of cases.[58] In "idiopathic" recurrent pancreatitis advanced diagnostic modalities including specific pancreatic tests, genetic testing for *CFTR* or *SPINK1/PRSS1* gene mutations and immunoglobulin G4 (IgG4), MRCP with secretin stimulation, sphincter of Oddi motility evaluation, EUS and ERCP may assist in the diagnosis.

The therapeutic options for ARP need to be tailored as per the etiology and include cholecystectomy, endoscopic clearance of common bile duct, and eventually endoscopic biliary and/or pancreatic sphincterotomy will be curative in majority of the cases.

CONCLUSION

Acute pancreatitis, because of its complications, is a dreadful disease; if not diagnosed and managed timely, it may result in high mortality. Necrosis and infection further increase the morbidity and mortality. The revised Atlanta classification has lucidly described the severity of the disease and its various complications and guides appropriate management. Treatment of infected pancreatic necrosis has undergone a sea change from aggressive open necrosectomy to more minimally invasive techniques with improved results.

REFERENCES

1. Banks PA, Freeman ML. Practice guidelines in acute pancreatitis. Am J Gastroenterol. 2006;101:2379-400.
2. Singh VK, Wu BU, Bollen TL, et al. A prospective evaluation of the bedside index for severity in acute pancreatitis score in assessing mortality and intermediate markers of severity in acute pancreatitis. Am J Gastroenterol. 2009;104:966-71.
3. Sarr MG. 2012 revision of the Atlanta classification of acute pancreatitis. Pol Arch Med Wewn. 2013;123(3):118-24.
4. Wu BU, Johannes RS, Sun X, et al. The early prediction of mortality in acute pancreatitis: a large population-based study. Gut. 2008;57:1698-703.
5. Banks PA, Bollen TL, Dervenis C, et al. Classification of acute pancreatitis: 2012—revision of the Atlanta classification and definitions by international consensus. Gut. 2013;62(1):102-11.
6. Busireddy KK, AlObaidy M, Ramalho M, et al. Pancreatitis-imaging approach. World J Gastrointest Pathophysiol. 2014;5(3):252-70.
7. Campos T, Parreira JG, Utiyama E, et al. Pesquisa nacional sobre condutas na pancreatite aguda. Revista do Colégio Brasileiro de Cirurgiões. 2008;35(5):304-10.
8. Bakker OJ, van Santvoort H, Besselink MGH, et al. Extrapancreatic necrosis without pancreatic parenchymal necrosis: a separate entity in necrotising pancreatitis? Gut. 2013;62:1475-80.
9. Mofidi R, Duff MD, Wigmore SJ, et al. Association between early systemic inflammatory response, severity of multiorgan dysfunction and death in acute pancreatitis. Br J Surg. 2006;93:738-44.
10. Zhao K, Adam SZ, Keswani RN, et al. Acute Pancreatitis: Revised Atlanta Classification and the Role of Cross-Sectional Imaging. Am J Roentgenol. 2015; 205:W32-41.
11. McKay CJ, Imrie CW. The continuing challenge of early mortality in acute pancreatitis. Br J Surg. 2004;91:1243-4.
12. Blum T, Maisonneuve P, Lowenfels AB, et al. Fatal outcome in acute pancreatitis: its occurrence and early prediction. Pancreatology. 2001;1:237-41.
13. Buter A, Imrie CW, Carter CR, et al. Dynamic nature of early organ dysfunction determines outcome in acute pancreatitis. Br J Surg. 2002;89:298-302.
14. Johnson CD, Abu-Hilal M. Persistent organ failure during the first week as a marker of fatal outcome in acute pancreatitis. Gut. 2004;53:1340-4.
15. Hack CE, Zeerleder S. The endothelium in sepsis: source of and a target for inflammation. Crit Care Med. 2001;29:S21-7.
16. Vege SS, Gardner TB, Chari ST, et al. Low mortality and high morbidity in severe acute pancreatitis without organ failure: a case for revising the Atlanta classification to include "moderately severe acute pancreatitis". Am J Gastroenterol. 2009;104:710-5.

17. Cobb JP, O'Keefe GE. Injury research in the genomic era. Lancet. 2004;363:2076-83.
18. Petrov MS, Shanbhag S, Chakraborty M, et al. Organ failure and infection of pancreatic necrosis as determinants of mortality in patients with acute pancreatitis. Gastroenterology. 2010;139:813-20.
19. Tee YS, Fang HY, Kuo IM, et al. Serial evaluation of the SOFA score is reliable for predicting mortality in acute severe pancreatitis. Medicine (Baltimore). 2018;97(7):e9654.
20. Gravante G, Garcea G, Ong SL, et al. Prediction of mortality in acute pancreatitis: a systematic review of the published evidence. Pancreatology. 2009;9(5):601-14.
21. Greenberg JA, Hsu J, Bawazeer M, et al. Clinical practice guideline: management of acute pancreatitis. Can J Surg. 2016;59(2):128-40.
22. Windsor JA, Hammodat H. Metabolic management of severe acute pancreatitis. World J Surg. 2000;24:664-72.
23. Lenhart DK, Balthazar EJ. MDCT of acute mild (non-necrotizing pancreatitis): abdominal complications and fate of fluid collections. Am J Roentgenol. 2008;190:643-9.
24. Grace P, Williamson R. Modern management of pancreatic pseudocysts. Br J Surg. 1993;80:573-81.
25. Ocampo C, Oria A, Zandalazini H, et al. Treatment of acute pancreatic pseudocysts after severe acute pancreatitis. J Gastrointest Surg. 2007;11:357-63.
26. Chen J, Fukami N, Li Z. Endoscopic approach to pancreatic pseudocyst, abscess and necrosis: review on recent progress. Dig Endosc. 2012;24:299-308.
27. Rau B, Pralle U, Uhl W, et al. Management of sterile necrosis in instances of severe acute pancreatitis. J Am Coll Surg. 1995;181:279-88.
28. Rau B, Pralle U, Mayer JM, et al. Role of ultrasonographically guided fine-needle aspiration cytology in the diagnosis of infected pancreatic necrosis. Br J Surg. 1998;85:179-84.
29. Horvath K, Brody F, Davis B, et al. Minimally invasive management of pancreatic disease. Surg Endosc. 2007;21:367-72.
30. Beger HG, Bittner R, Block S, et al. Bacterial contamination of pancreatic necrosis. A prospective clinical study. Gastroenterology. 1986;91:433-8.
31. Rau B, Bothe A, Beger HG. Surgical treatment of necrotizing pancreatitis by necrosectomy and closed lavage: changing patient characteristics and outcome in a 19-year, single-center series. Surgery. 2005;138:28-39.
32. Isenmann R, Schwarz M, Rau B, et al. Characteristics of infection with *Candida* species in patients with necrotizing pancreatitis. World J Surg. 2002;26:372-6.
33. Appelros S, Lindgren S, Borgström A. Short and long term outcome of severe acute pancreatitis. Eur J Surg. 2001;167:281-6.
34. Da Costa DW, Boerma D, van Santvoort HC, et al. Staged multidisciplinary step-up management for necrotizing pancreatitis. Br J Surg. 2014;101:e65-79.
35. Connor S, Raraty MG, Neoptolemos JP, et al. Does infected pancreatic necrosis require immediate or emergency debridement? Pancreas. 2006;33:128-34.
36. Wittau M, Mayer B, Scheele J, et al. Systematic review and meta-analysis of antibiotic prophylaxis in severe acute pancreatitis. Scand J Gastroenterol. 2011;46:261-70.

37. Van Santvoort HC, Besselink MG, Bakker OJ, et al. A step-up approach or open necrosectomy for necrotizing pancreatitis. N Engl J Med. 2010;362(16): 1491-502.
38. Horvath K, Freeny P, Escallon J, et al. Safety and efficacy of video-assisted retroperitoneal debridement for infected pancreatic collections: a multicenter, prospective, single-arm phase 2 study. Arch Surg. 2010;145:817-25.
39. John BJ, Swaminathan S, VenkataKrishnan L, et al. Management of infected pancreatic necrosis-the "step up" approach and minimal access retroperitoneal pancreatic necrosectomy. Indian J Surg. 2014;77(Suppl 1):125-7.
40. Adams DB, Zellner JL, Anderson MC. Arterial haemorrhage complicating pancreatic pseudocyst: Role of angiography. J Surg Res. 1993;54:150-6.
41. Suzuki T, Ishida H, Komatsuda T, et al. Pseudoaneurysm of the gastroduodenal artery ruptured into the superior mesenteric vein in a patient with chronic pancreatitis. J Clin Ultrasound. 2003;31:278-82.
42. Bergert H, Dobrowolski F, Caffier S, et al. Prevalence and treatment in bleeding complications in chronic pancreatitis. Langenbecks Arch Surg. 2004;389: 504-10.
43. Andersson E, Ansari D, Andersson R. Major haemorrhagic complications of acute pancreatitis. Br J Surg. 2010;97:1379-84.
44. Butler JR, Eckert GJ, Zyromski NJ, et al. Natural history of pancreatitis-induced splenic vein thrombosis: a systematic review and meta-analysis of its incidence and rate of gastrointestinal bleeding. HPB (Oxford). 2011;13:839-45.
45. Aranha GV, Prinz RA, Greenlee HB, et al. Gastric outlet and duodenal obstruction from inflammatory pancreatic disease. Arch Surg. 1984;119:833-5.
46. Winton TL, Birchard R, Nguyen KT, et al. Esophageal obstruction secondary to mediastinal pancreatic pseudocyst. Can J Surg. 1986;29:376-7.
47. Browman MW, Litin SC, Binkovitz LA, et al. Pancreatic pseudocyst that compressed the inferior venacava and resulted in edema of the lower extremities. Mayo Clin Proc. 1992;67:1085-8.
48. Stone MM, Stone NN, Meller S, et al. Bilateral ureteral obstruction: An unusual complication of pancreatitis. Am J Gastroenterol. 1989;84:49-51.
49. Baranyai Z, Jakab F. Pancreatic pseudocyst propagating into retroperitoneum and mediastinum. Acta Chir Hung. 1997;36:16-7.
50. Lee FY, Wang YT, Poh SC. Congestive heart failure due to a pancreatic pseudocyst. Cleve Clin J Med. 1994;61:141-3.
51. Cameron JL, Anderson RD, Zuidema G. Pancreatic ascites. Surg Gynecol Obstet. 1967;125:328.
52. Cameron JL. Chronic pancreatic ascites and pancreatic pleural effusions. Gastroenterology. 1978;74:134-40.
53. Lipsett PA, Cameron JL. Internal pancreatic fistula. Am J Surg. 1992;163:216-20.
54. Varadarajulu S, Noone TC, Tutuian R, et al. Predictors of outcome in pancreatic duct disruption managed by endoscopic transpapillary stent placement. Gastrointest Endosc. 2005;61:568-75.
55. De Waele JJ, Leppäniemi AK. Intra-abdominal hypertension in acute pancreatitis. World J Surg. 2009;33:1128-33.

56. Kirkpatrick AW, Roberts DJ, De Waele J, et al. Intra-abdominal hypertension and the abdominal compartment syndrome: updated consensus definitions and clinical practice guidelines from the World Society of the Abdominal Compartment Syndrome. Intensive Care Med. 2013;39:1190-206.
57. Inkeles DM, Walsh JB. Retinal fat emboli as sequela to acute pancreatitis. Am J Ophthalmol. 1975;80(5):935-8.
58. Testoni PA. Acute recurrent pancreatitis: Etiopathogenesis, diagnosis and treatment. World J Gastroenterol. 2014;20(45):16891-901.

Chapter 4

Management of Colon Cancer: Changing Trends, Recent Advances and Current Practices

Vikram Kate, R Kalayarasan, S Suresh Kumar, Sajal Rai, N Ananthakrishnan

INTRODUCTION

Recent trends in published literature on colon cancer worldwide have shown several important and significant changes from what was existing information on this topic earlier. These advances have included changes in perception of epidemiology focusing not only an awareness of increasing incidence worldwide but a better perception of the differences between right and lefts sided colonic cancers which have therapeutic implications, changes in suggestions for preoperative workup impacting management decisions, a movement from open to minimally invasive and robotic surgery with reviews of oncological outcomes, greater clarity on approach to obstructed colonic cancers presenting as emergencies, a better understanding of approach to patients with stage IV disease at presentation including timing and role of surgery for metastatic disease with better neoadjuvant and adjuvant care, a greater awareness of the role and limitations of monoclonal antibodies in targeted therapy and some research which may impact the diagnosis and management of these cancers in future.

All these have been summarized in this chapter with particular emphasis on what is new, what is still in a phase of evaluation and how the diagnosis and care of these cancers is likely to be impacted by these advances.

EPIDEMIOLOGY: CHANGING TRENDS

A recent trend observed in the United States is a decrease in the incidence of cancer in people more than 50 years of age compared to those less than 50 years.[1] Hence in 2018, the American Cancer Society has recommended reducing the age for colorectal cancer screening down to 45 years.[2] Recent epidemiological studies have shown an increase in the incidence of right colon cancer.[3] Right and left colon cancer have distinct histopathology,

Management of Colon Cancer

Table 1: Differences between right-and left-sided colon cancer.

S. No	Characteristics	Right colon cancer	Left colon cancer
1.	Age	Older > younger age group	Younger > older age group
2.	Sex	Females > males	Males > females
3.	Histology	Sessile serrated adenomas, poorly differentiated mucinous adenocarcinoma	Tubular, villous adenocarcinoma
4.	Morphology	Flat type that makes detection during screening difficult	Polypoid type that facilitates detection during screening colonoscopy
5.	Mutation	Microsatellite Instability (MSI)-high and mismatch repair deficient tumors	Chromosomal instability (CIN)-high tumors
6.	Immunogenicity	High with T cell infiltration	Low
7.	Response to adjuvant therapy	Due to high antigen load respond well to immunotherapy	Respond well to conventional chemotherapy and targeted therapy
8.	Site of metastases	Peritoneal	Liver and lung
9.	Prognosis	Relatively poor. However, early stage (stage I and II) tumors have better prognosis compared to similar stage tumors of left due to high MSI observed in these stage tumors	Relatively better especially in late stage (stage III and IV) tumors

molecular pathway and prognosis.[3-5] These differences are summarized in Table 1.

PREOPERATIVE INVESTIGATIONS

Colonoscopy versus Computed Tomography Colonography

Colonoscopy is the preferred investigation for diagnosis of colon cancer since it permits direct visualization of the tumor, detects synchronous lesions, facilitates removal of polyps and allows a biopsy from the tumor. A randomized study from the UK Special Interest Group in Gastrointestinal and Abdominal Radiology (SIGGAR) in which 1610 patients with symptoms suggestive of colorectal cancer were randomly assigned to colonoscopy (n = 1072) or computed tomography (CT) colonography (n = 538).[6] The need for an additional colonic investigation to detect colorectal cancer or large (>1 cm) polyps was used as the primary endpoint. Both investigations had a similar yield to detect colorectal cancer or large polyps (10.7% vs. 11.4%). However, patients undergoing CT colonography more often required additional colonic investigations (30% vs. 8%).[6] Procedural acceptance is more with CT colonography as it is noninvasive. However, this advantage is offset by the need for additional colonoscopy in the CT colonography group. Currently, CT colonography is primarily indicated in patients with incomplete colonoscopy due to a non-obstructive cause. CT colonography cannot replace incomplete colonoscopy in patients with obstructed left colon cancer as both procedures require bowel preparation.[7,8] Use of fecal tagging to facilitate CT colonography in patients with a loaded colon is associated with poor sensitivity and specificity.

Computed Tomography of Chest in Colon Cancer

Contrast enhanced CT abdomen and pelvis is the primary investigation for staging in patients with colon cancer. CT is more sensitive to detect distant spread than regional lymph node metastasis or depth of tumor infiltration. Since 2007, the National Comprehensive Cancer Network (NCCN) guidelines for colon cancer recommend chest CT in addition to abdomen and pelvis CT although, the role of routine chest CT in colon cancer patients remains controversial.[9] Kim et al. retrospectively reviewed CT chest findings in 319 consecutive colon cancer patients without liver metastasis and with a normal chest X-ray.[10] Lung metastasis was detected in only 6.3% of patients without liver metastasis and a negative chest X-ray. CT-detected lymph node metastasis was identified as the risk factor for lung metastasis.[10] Also, routine chest CT may result in increased detection of incidental and indeterminate lung nodules requiring further evaluation thereby delaying definitive therapy.[11] Based on current evidence routine CT chest is not recommended in colon cancer patients with no liver metastasis and is selectively indicated only in patients with advanced T and N stage tumor.[12]

Role of Positron Emission Tomography-Computed Tomography in Colon Cancer

Positron emission tomography-computed tomography (PET-CT) is more sensitive than conventional CT in detecting metastatic disease. However, its additional value in staging of colon cancer is not well defined. In the current NCCN guidelines, PET-CT is not recommended for the primary staging of colon cancer in patients without any evidence of distant metastasis on conventional CT abdomen and pelvis.[9] As PET-CT scan is usually done without contrast and multiple slicing, it does not obviate the need for additional contrast-enhanced CT and it is primarily indicated in patients with doubtful metastatic lesions on contrast-enhanced CT.[9,12]

The role of PET-CT in patients with liver metastasis is not clearly defined. Ruers et al. randomized 150 patients with colorectal liver metastases selected for hepatic resection to triple-phase contrast-enhanced CT only or CT plus a separate PET scan.[13] The authors reported that the addition of PET significantly reduced the number of non-therapeutic laparotomies (28% vs. 45%). However, in another trial by Moulton et al., 404 patients with potentially resectable liver metastases were randomized to triple-phase contrast-enhanced CT only or PET-CT.[14] Of the 263 patients randomized to the PET-CT arm the extent of surgery was modified in only 8% of patients. More importantly, the addition of PET-CT avoided non-therapeutic laparotomy in only 2.7% of patients leading to the conclusion that the addition of PET-CT to conventional CT alone did not result in a frequent change in surgical management.[14] However, in this study, a significant proportion of patients received neoadjuvant chemotherapy that is known to reduce the yield of fluorodeoxyglucose positron emission tomography (FDG-PET) by reducing the metabolic activity of the metastatic tumor. NCCN guidelines recommend that PET-CT should be performed before planned curative resection for liver metastasis.[9] PET-CT is also used in the postoperative surveillance of patients with rising serum carcinoembryonic antigen (CEA) level and non-diagnostic conventional imaging evaluation following primary treatment and in detecting synchronous tumors in patients with obstructed left colon cancer.[15,16]

PREOPERATIVE MANAGEMENT

Mechanical Bowel Preparation

Proposed advantages of bowel preparation include easy bowel handling, aesthetic surgical field and the ability to palpate a small tumor or polyps. It also facilitates intraoperative colonoscopy if needed. The potential disadvantages are that presence of liquid stools secondary to incomplete bowel preparation might increase the risk of contamination and secondly patient discomfort associated with mechanical preparation. Multiple randomized controlled trials (RCTs) and meta-analysis have concluded that mechanical bowel preparation has no significant effect in reducing the incidence of surgical site infection or anastomotic complications and in many enhanced recovery after surgery (ERAS) protocols for colon cancer, mechanical bowel preparation has been omitted.[17,18] A limitation in the majority of these RCTs is that oral antibiotic prophylaxis was not administered along with mechanical bowel preparation. Administration of mechanical bowel preparation alone without oral antibiotics has no significant effect on colonic bacterial count. Mechanical bowel preparation by reducing the volume of feces facilitates delivery of oral antibiotics to the colonic mucosa.[19-21] An updated meta-analysis published in 2018 concluded that oral antibiotic prophylaxis, in combination with mechanical bowel preparation and parenteral antibiotics, is superior to mechanical bowel preparation and parenteral antibiotic prophylaxis alone in reducing surgical site infection in elective colorectal surgery.[22] The role of mechanical gut preparation, therefore, remains controversial.

Preoperative Fasting

The standard practice in elective colonic surgery is preoperative fasting from midnight of the day prior to surgery. However, multiple studies have shown that intake of fluids up to 2 hours before surgery does not increase the risk of aspiration and may accelerate postoperative recovery.[23] It reduces preoperative thirst, hunger, anxiety and allows the patients to undergo surgery in a metabolically fed state.[24] Preoperative carbohydrate loading minimizes postoperative insulin resistance, negative nitrogen balance, protein loss, maintains lean body mass and muscle strength.[25] However, milk-based fluids should be avoided as they tend to reduce gastric emptying.[26] Similarly, the safety of oral fluids in diabetics, who are at high risk of gastroparesis, is not conclusively proven.[25]

Current ERAS society guidelines are clear fluids should be allowed up to 2 hours and solids up to 6 hours before induction of anesthesia.[18] Specific safety measures should be taken at the time of induction of anesthesia in those patients in whom gastric emptying may be delayed. A routine use of preoperative oral carbohydrate treatment is recommended. In diabetic patients, preoperative oral carbohydrate treatment can be given along with the diabetic medication, although evidence for this recommendation is low.[18]

Prophylaxis against Deep Vein Thromboembolism

Patients with colon cancer are at high risk of deep vein thrombosis with a fatal pulmonary embolism. Mechanical prophylaxis with compression stockings and intermittent pneumatic compression device is strongly recommended.[27] Pharmacological prophylaxis with low molecular weight heparin should be given to these patients.[18,28] In patients receiving low molecular weight heparin, the timing should be adjusted so that epidural catheter is not placed or removed within twelve hours of the last dose of heparin.[18,27,28]

SURGERY FOR COLON CANCER

Principle of Optimal Colonic Cancer Surgery

Total mesorectal excision (TME) for rectal cancer which has improved the oncological outcome was based on the concept that sharp dissection between the visceral or mesorectal fascia and parietal or endopelvic fascia ensures complete removal of a tumor with the draining lymphatics and lymph nodes.[29] The rectal TME plane extends to the sigmoid and descending colon and further from the descending colon, it extends to the pancreas and around the spleen on the left side. On the right side, it extends to include the head of the pancreas, duodenum, ascending colon, cecum and the root of the mesentery.[30] The concept that mesorectum and mesocolon are continuous structures was proved in a recent histological and electron microscopy study.[31] In colon cancer like rectal cancer, lymphatics follow the arteries supplying that portion of the colon and run along the mesocolon, which is in turn covered by visceral fascia on both sides like an envelope. Identification of this plane is easy in sigmoid and transverse colon cancers as they have a distinct mesocolon. In ascending and descending colon, the mesocolic fascia is closely opposed to the retroperitoneal fascia.

The main component of complete mesocolic excision (CME) is to identify the distinct plane between the mesocolic fascia and retroperitoneal fascia by sharp dissection. This plane is marked by a single layer of fascia (Toldt's fascia) (Figs. 1A to C). A good CME prevents the breach in mesocolic fascia and the potential tumor spread. The second important component is to identify and ligate the feeding arteries at the origin to ensure maximal harvest of the regional lymph nodes. The third component of CME is a dissection of the pericolic lymph nodes at least 10 cm on either side of tumor (10 cm rule) as longitudinal lymphatic spread is rarely seen beyond 10 cm.[32] This technique ensures the integrity of mesocolon and improves lymph node yield and thereby survival in colon cancer. In open surgery, lateral to medial approach is used for CME whereas in the laparoscopic and robotic surgery a medial to lateral approach is preferred.[30]

Hohenberger et al. reported that CME with central vascular ligation (CVL) reduced recurrence rate from 6.5% to 3.2% in 1329 patients of colon cancer operated from 1978 to 2002.[30] Bertelsen et al. in a retrospective study compared the oncological outcomes of 364 patients who underwent CME with 1031 patients who underwent non-CME colonic resection.[33] The 4-year disease-free survival rate was significantly higher in the CME Group (85.8% vs. 75.9%, P = 0.001) with multivariate analysis identifying CME surgery as an independent prognostic factor. Other studies have also shown that CME with CVL is associated with higher lymph node yield, R0 resection rate and overall survival.[34,35]

CME with CVL versus D3 Dissection

The Japanese Society for Cancer of the Colon and Rectum recommends D2 lymph node dissection for tumors restricted to submucosa and D3 lymph node dissection for tumor reaching muscularis propria or in patients with clinical evidence of lymph node metastasis irrespective of the depth of invasion.[36] For the right colon cancer in D2 dissection, the ileocolic vessels are tied to the right of superior mesenteric vessels without removing the lympho-adipose tissue over the superior mesenteric vessels whereas in D3

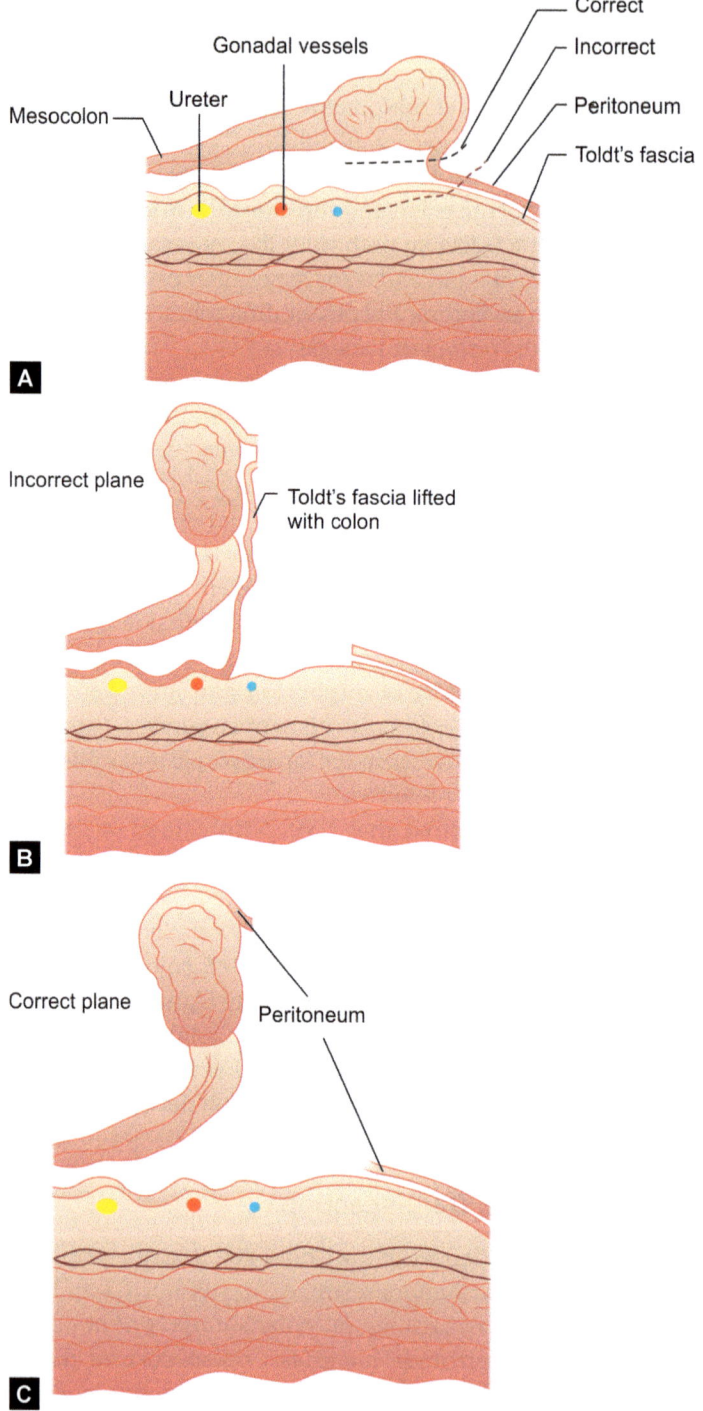

Figs. 1A to C: Plane for complete mesocolic excision (A). Lifting of Toldt's fascia increases the risk of injury to retroperitoneal structures (B). The correct plane is superficial to Toldt's fascia (C).

dissection for right colon cancer, the ileocolic vessels are divided at the origin after clearing the lympho-adipose tissue over the superior mesenteric vessels and exposing them.[37] With respect to the level of vascular ligation, both CME with CVL and D3 dissection are similar.[37] However, the longitudinal length of the specimen is shorter in patients undergoing D3 dissection compared to CME with CVL as Japanese studies have shown that the longitudinal lymphatic spread is rarely seen beyond 10 cm from the tumor.[32,37] Hence, the number of mesenteric nodes removed is more in CME with CVL compared to D3 dissection.[37] Both CME with CVL and D3 dissection result in comparable oncological specimens and outcomes that are superior to conventional colon surgery.[37] Hence, the current recommended treatment for locally advanced colon cancer is either CME with CVL or D3 dissection.

Open versus Laparoscopic Surgery for Colon Cancer

In one of the earliest RCTs, Milsom et al. reported that patients who underwent laparoscopic colectomy (n = 55) had less postoperative pain, pulmonary complications and earlier return of bowel function compared to open colectomy (n = 54).[38] However, in malignancy, more than the short-term benefits it is important to document oncological equivalence. Since the follow up was relatively short (1.5 years) in their study evidence was insufficient to document oncological safety.

The oncological safety of laparoscopic colectomy was documented in an RCT reported by Lacy et al.[39] At a median (range) follow-up of 43 (27–85) months, there was no difference in the overall survival of patients who underwent laparoscopic and open colectomy. However, disease-specific survival was better in the laparoscopy group possibly due to reduced surgical stress and less tumor manipulation during laparoscopic colectomy.[39] Other RCTs also documented the oncological safety of laparoscopic colectomy.[40,41] Port site recurrence is not increased after laparoscopic colectomy with the incidence of port site recurrence being similar to the reported rates of incision site recurrence after open colectomy (0.8–1%).[39-41]

Since the introduction of the concept of CME with CVL for colon cancer, there is a renewed debate whether these could be safely accomplished using a laparoscopic approach. Also, the safety of laparoscopic surgery in locally advanced colon cancer (stage II and III) remains controversial. Recently Kitano et al. reported the results of an open-label, multi-institutional, randomized, two-arm phase 3 trial involving 1057 patients from 30 hospitals in Japan.[41] Similar five-year overall survival in both groups (90.4% vs. 91.8%) confirmed the feasibility and oncological safety of laparoscopic D3 dissection (like CME with CVL) for colon cancer. The excellent survival in both groups also documented the superiority of D3 dissection compared to conventional surgery.

While the oncological safety of laparoscopic surgery has been documented, its role in patients with T4 cancer remains controversial. In the JCOG0404 trial, patients with T4 tumors who underwent laparoscopic surgery had inferior survival compared to the patients who underwent open colectomy possibly due to increased tumor manipulation and violation of the no-touch principle.[41] The feasibility and oncological safety of resecting T4 tumors without adjacent organ involvement have been shown in a few retrospective or prospective non-randomized trials.[42,43]

Laparoscopy versus Robotic Surgery

Robotic surgery has overcome some of the mechanical and visual constraints associated with laparoscopic surgery such as limited degree of freedom of movement, exaggerated tremors and 2D vision. Park et al. in an RCT comparing robot-assisted versus conventional laparoscopic right colectomy reported that hospital stay, surgical complications, postoperative pain score, resection margin and the number of lymph nodes harvested were similar in both groups.[44] Robot-assisted colectomy was associated with prolonged duration of surgery (195 versus 130 min; $P < 0.001$) and higher overall hospital costs (US $12,235 versus $10,320; $P = 0.013$) despite similar duration of hospital stay primarily due to more expensive consumables.[44] A meta-analysis of trials comparing robotic and laparoscopic colectomy confirmed that robotic colectomy did not offer a significant advantage in perioperative and postoperative outcomes compared to laparoscopic colectomy while at the same time contributing to prolonged operative duration and high cost.[45] The primary reason for the lack of benefit with robotics in colonic surgery is that robotic systems are primarily designed to enhance maneuverability, facilitate precise dissection and suturing in narrow confined spaces whereas, colonic surgery is usually a multi-quadrant operation involving a relatively large dissection area. The stable vision and ambidextrous capability of robotics facilitates vascular control and lymph node dissection. However, these potential benefits do not translate to clinical advantage in the trial setting when compared to laparoscopic surgery performed by the experienced surgeon. Hence, robotic surgery is not recommended as a superior option to minimally invasive colon surgery. However, the double console in current robotic systems facilitates learning by resident by allowing them to actively participate in the surgical procedure right from the commencement of their surgical experience and hence may shorten the learning curve.

Management of Obstructed Colonic Cancer

Resection and primary anastomosis is the preferred option for obstructing right colon cancer. Studies have shown that even in the emergency setting, primary anastomosis is associated with a less than 5% anastomotic leak rate.[46,47] The mobility and better blood supply of small bowel contributes to a low anastomotic leak rate in right colon cancer.[46,47] In patients with a poor general condition or prolonged obstruction, ileocolic resection with proximal ileostomy and distal colonic mucus fistula is recommended.[48] Stoma creation (ileostomy) or ileotransverse bypass is reserved for patients with unresectable tumors.[49] Percutaneous cecostomy is an option in poor risk patients although it is often associated with inadequate decompression.[50] Self-expanding metal stent (SEMS) as a bridge to elective surgery is not recommended for obstructed right colonic cancers.[51,52] However, it is an option in the palliative setting.[52]

For patients with obstructed left colon cancer, the choice lies between a single stage vs. a staged procedure and loop colostomy vs. SEMS as a bridge for elective colonic resection. As RCTs comparing various options are lacking, decision making should be based on available evidence from various retrospective and prospective non-randomized studies.

Primary Resection and Anastomosis versus Hartmann's Procedure

The German study group of colorectal carcinoma database reported that postoperative mortality was less in patients undergoing Hartmann's procedure compared to patients undergoing resection with primary anastomosis (7.2% vs. 9%) despite higher preoperative risk factors in patients undergoing the Hartmann's procedure.[53] The primary disadvantage with Hartmann's procedure is the need for a second stage procedure which requires a formal laparotomy. In contrast to rectal tumors where Hartmann's reversal is a challenging procedure due to the short rectal stump, it is a relatively straightforward option following left colectomy.

No RCT has evaluated the role of a diverting stoma in patients undergoing resection anastomosis in the emergency setting. In a series of 743 patients who underwent emergency surgery for obstructed left colon cancer, 58% of patients underwent primary resection anastomosis and 12% of patients underwent resection anastomosis with diverting stoma.[54] There was no significant difference in the rate of the anastomotic leak or the need for reoperation in both the groups.[54] In the absence of bowel preparation, leakage of the anastomosis into the peritoneal cavity will result in peritonitis. This might explain the lack of a protective effect of a diverting stoma in the emergency setting.

Based on the available evidence, use of primary resection anastomosis should be restricted to patients with uncomplicated obstructed left colonic cancer without any risk factors. Use of protective stoma is unlikely to reduce anastomotic leak rate or its severity in patients with a loaded colon. In most of the patients who undergo resection, end colostomy with Hartmann's procedure seems to be a reasonable option.

Subtotal Colectomy versus Segmental Colectomy

In the past, subtotal colectomy has been advocated in patients who undergo resection for obstructed left colonic cancer as it obviates the need to use an unprepared colon for the anastomosis.[55-57] Limitations with subtotal colectomy include prolonged operative time and poor functional result due to increased stool frequency. In the SCOTIA (Subtotal Colectomy versus On-Table Irrigation and Anastomosis) trial 91 patients from 12 different centers were randomized to undergo either subtotal colectomy or segmental colectomy with on-table lavage (47 vs. 44 patients).[58] There was no significant difference in the morbidity and mortality; however, functional outcomes were worse in patients who underwent subtotal colectomy.[58] In patients with loaded colon planned for segmental colectomy and anastomosis, the proximal bowel can be cleared using intraoperative colonic irrigation or manual decompression.[56-59] Both RCTs and systematic reviews of papers comparing intraoperative colonic irrigation with manual decompression have reported similar anastomotic leak rates and mortality.[59,60] However, manual decompression was simpler and took less time compared to intraoperative colonic irrigation.[60] Based on current evidence, segmental colectomy is preferred over subtotal colectomy in patients undergoing emergency resection for obstructed left colonic cancer with subtotal colectomy being reserved for patients with synchronous colonic cancer and in patients with evidence of colonic ischemia or cecal tear/perforation secondary to obstruction.[61]

Loop Colostomy versus SEMS as a Bridge for Elective Colonic Resection

Both diversion colostomy and SEMS allow colonic decompression thereby facilitating bowel preparation and resection anastomosis at a second stage, besides facilitating accurate staging including evaluation for synchronous tumors. However, both the procedures have their advantages and limitations. The advantage of SEMS is that it does not require surgical decompression. Placement of SEMS is associated with complications like stent-induced perforation.[62] Patients who underwent SEMS had poor oncological outcomes.[63] Possible reasons are that the peritumoral inflammation induced by the stent may promote lympho-vascular invasion and lymph node metastasis. Also, microperforations and tumor manipulation caused by radial dilatation of SEMS, facilitates tumor dissemination.[64] RCTs and meta-analysis on stent as a bridge to surgery, report lower short-term overall morbidity.[64,65] However, it is important to remember that two RCTs on stents as a bridge to surgery had to be prematurely stopped due to a high incidence of complications.[66,67] Also, oncologic outcomes of the Dutch Stent-In 2 trial showed that 5 of 6 patients with a stent-related perforation experienced tumor recurrence.[68] In two meta-analysis, the long-term recurrence was more in the stent group compared to emergency surgery, although the difference did not reach statistical significance.[64,65] Hence, based on current evidence, stent as a bridge to surgery should be used only in selected poor risk candidates. Diversion colostomy is preferable over SEMS till more evidence on long-term oncological outcomes from Enteral Stents for Colonic Obstruction (ESCO) and Colo Rectal Endoscopic Stenting Trial (CREST) trials are available.

APPROACH TO PATIENTS WITH METASTATIC DISEASE

Patients suspected of having synchronous metastasis should undergo a metastatic workup including chest, abdominal and pelvic CT.[69] In selected cases potentially curable by surgical resection, a PET-CT may be considered to rule out distant metastasis.[69,70] It is currently recommended that all the patients with metastatic colon cancer should undergo genetic testing including K-ras (KRAS), neuroblastoma RAS (NRAS) and B-Raf (BRAF) mutations (which makes the patients unresponsive to cetuximab and panitumumab).[71-73] The management of metastatic colon cancer primarily depends on three factors, viz. the resectability of the primary colonic tumor, resectability of the extra-colonic organ metastasis and the presence of potentially "convertible to resectable" secondaries.[9] To consider for potentially curative surgery, the following criteria needs to be fulfilled, viz. (a) primary should be resectable with R0 resection, (b) no unstable extrahepatic or extrapulmonary metastasis and (c) likelihood of adequate function of the liver or lung after the resection of metastatic tumor.

Any surgery lesser than R0 resection such as a debulking procedure is not recommended.[9] Patients with unresectable tumors should be re-evaluated at the end of two months of neoadjuvant therapy and every two months thereafter for potential conversion to resectability.[9,74] Liver/lung metastasis can be considered for either synchronous resection of both primary and metastatic tumor or staged colectomy depending on the complexity involved in the liver/lung resection, comorbidity of the patient, expertise of the surgeon and the exposure required during the surgery. Trials have evaluated three types of management protocols with respect to timing of the resection of lung/liver metastasis.[9,74] These include the following:

1. Concurrent or staged colectomy and resection of liver/lung secondary.
2. Neoadjuvant chemotherapy with FOLFOX/CapOX for 2–3 months followed by concurrent or staged colectomy and resection of liver/lung metastasis.
3. Colectomy followed by chemotherapy with FOLFOX/CapOX for 2–3 months and resection of liver/lung secondary.

Presently all the above protocols have shown to be equally effective in terms of disease-free survival and overall survival.[75] It is recommended to give six months of perioperative (neoadjuvant/adjuvant) chemotherapy to patients with metastatic colon cancer.[9] Local ablative therapy such as image guided radiation therapy (IGRT) and stereotactic body radiation therapy (SBRT) may be considered in highly select patients with oligometastatic liver or lung disease.[76,77] Patients with synchronous abdominal/peritoneal metastasis presenting with nonobstructive disease may be considered for intensive systemic chemotherapy depending on the general condition.[73,74] Obstructing lesions are managed either by colonic resection/ diversion stoma or stenting followed by systemic therapy.

ADJUVANT AND NEOADJUVANT THERAPY

For stage I colon cancer which includes node negative T1 and T2 lesions, no adjuvant chemotherapy is recommended following curative R0 resection. There is no consensus on the effect of adjuvant therapy in offering overall survival and disease-free survival benefit in stage II patients. Considering the lack of evidence from RCTs, higher cost and potential toxicity, routine chemotherapy following R0 curative resection should not be administered in these groups.

Recommendations for stage II colon cancer patients is based on identifying risk factors which include inadequate lymph node sampling (<12 nodes), poorly differentiated histology, lymphatic invasion, vascular invasion, perineural invasion, patients presenting with obstruction or perforation, close/indeterminate or positive margins and pT4 tumors. Presence of one or more of these risk factors puts the patient in the high-risk group for recurrence. Though absolute risk reduction with respect to recurrence is not very clear, select group of patients in low risk stage II can be considered for single regime adjuvant therapy with capecitabine or 5-FU/leucovorin.[78] High-risk stage II warrants adjuvant chemotherapy with single agent 5FU/leucovorin or capecitabine. 5-FU or oxaliplatin based duration of six months.[78,79] In patients with stage II colon cancer particularly T3 lesions, microsatellite instability (MIS) and mismatch repair (MMR) testing is recommended especially in cancers proximal to the splenic flexure where deficient mismatch repair occurs in up to 25% of cancers. Right-sided serrated polyps are precursors to sporadic microsatellite unstable colon cancers and have a high rate of synchronous and metachronous lesions.[80] Thus, testing for MIS will help in guiding chemotherapy, as recurrence in the tumors with deficient mismatch repair is 50% lesser with good prognosis and they do not benefit from 5-FU adjuvant therapy.[81,82] However, presence of other high-risk factors should be considered before the decision to discontinue adjuvant therapy in these patients.

All stage III node positive colon cancer patients should receive 5-FU and oxaliplatin based combination therapy. FOLFOX or CapOX (capecitabine and oxaliplatin) or FLOX (5-FU, leucovorin and oxaliplatin) combination regimes have been proven to result in improved disease-free survival and overall survival in stage III colon cancer compared to 5-FU/leucovorin or capecitabine single agent therapy although there are concerns regarding the absolute benefit of oxaliplatin in the subset of elderly population older than 70 years.[73,83,84] When a combination regime is not tolerated, 5-FU as single agent can be used as an alternative. Haller et al. in their recent analysis of pooled data from four randomized controlled trials (AVANT, X-ACT, XELOXA and NSABP C-08) found survival advantage with combined 5-FU and oxaliplatin based combination therapy irrespective of the age and co-morbidity.[85]

Stage IV metastatic resectable synchronous liver and/or lung metastasis is treated with synchronous or staged colectomy along with liver and/or lung resection followed by six months of adjuvant therapy with FOLFOX or CapOX. Alternatively, neoadjuvant FOLFIRI or FOLFOX or CapOX with bevacizumab for 2-3 months followed by synchronous or staged colectomy along with resection of metastasis is recommended. Colectomy followed by 2-3 months of FOLFIRI or FOLFOX or CapOX with bevacizumab followed by resection of metastatic disease has also been reported.

ROLE FOR RADIATION THERAPY IN COLON CANCER

Neoadjuvant radiotherapy along with concurrent 5-FU based chemotherapy regime may be considered in select patients with T4 tumors with penetration to fixed structures (locally unresectable) to aid resection.[9,85] Patients who are medically unfit for surgery and patients with recurrent disease are also candidates for radiotherapy. The recommended dose of radiotherapy is 45-50 Gy in 25-28 fractions.[9] Intraoperative radiotherapy (IORT) has been shown to be beneficial in providing an additional booster dose of radiotherapy to the target anatomical part.[86,87] If facility for IORT is not available, an additional dose of 10-15 Gy can be given as external beam radiotherapy or as brachytherapy. Intensity modulated radiation therapy (IMRT) should be considered only for patients who have been already treated and present with recurrent disease.[88] The option of intra-arterial catheter therapy with yttrium-90 microspheres can be considered in highly select patients with chemotherapy resistant tumors and those with predominantly liver metastasis.[9] Radiotherapy can be considered for metastatic sites in patients with limited number of liver and lung metastasis. However, such modality should be considered only in the setting of a clinical trial and should not be considered as an alternate for surgical resection of metastatic lesion.[73,86]

USE OF MONOCLONAL ANTIBODIES

Epidermal growth factor receptor (EGFR) and vascular endothelial growth factor (VGEF) antibodies have been studied for targeted therapy either as monotherapy or in combination with systemic chemotherapy.[89-92] Addition of anti-VEGF monoclonal antibody bevacizumab and anti-EGFR monoclonal antibody cetuximab/panitumumab with FOLFOX/CapOX for stage II/III disease in the NSABP C-08 and AVANT trials was found to yield no additional benefit. Hence, these targeted drugs are not recommended for adjuvant therapy in stage II/III colon cancer.[93-95]

It is recommended that all patients with metastatic colorectal tumor should have genetic testing to assess for mutation in the signaling pathway.[71,72] Mutation of exon 2 (codons 12 and 13), exon 3 (codons 59 and 61) and exon 4 (codons 117 and 146) of *KRAS or NRAS* gene and V600E mutation of BRAF gene all have been shown to be associated with no response or at times adverse response with EGFR targeted therapy. Patients with KRAS, NRAS, BRAF mutations should not be treated with cetuximab or panitumumab.[96-100] Recent trials have shown resistance to anti-EGFR targeted therapy in patients with BRAF mutation can be overcome by adding BRAF inhibitors.[101,102] Targeted therapy against EGFR and VEGF are shown to have similar overall survival proving lack of superiority of one over the other.[103] Hence, the choice of the agent should be based on tolerability and side effect of the agent. Due to significant improvement in the median survival shown in many trials, monoclonal antibodies are now recommended as first line chemotherapy for metastatic colorectal cancer.[73,103] Newer monoclonal antibodies against various target genes and kinases involved in the signaling pathway have been studied in limited trials and are currently not recommended outside the trial setting.[104-106]

SURVEILLANCE

Guidelines for surveillance are available with National Comprehensive Cancer Network (NCCN), American Society of Clinical Oncology (ASCO), American Society of Colon and Rectal Surgeons (ASCRS), Cancer Care Ontario (CCO) and others. The goal of surveillance in patients after curative radical resection is to detect asymptomatic recurrence when it is still amenable for further curative treatment, to identify appearance of new polyps, which can be removed by endoscopic means, and to detect metachronous cancer, which may occur in up to 2% of colon cancer patients. Surveillance also helps in focusing on quality of life, urinary or sexual problems after surgery and stoma related complications. Study of genetic and familial association helps in formulating guidelines on genetic testing and screening protocols.

Up to 40% of colon cancer patients develop recurrence after curative resection with 80% of the recurrence occurring in the first two years and almost 95% within 5 years.[107] Since surveillance aims at finding recurrence curable either by surgical or adjuvant modality, patients who are not candidates for such interventions due to advanced age or uncontrolled comorbidities need not be subjected to follow up investigations which may involve unnecessary radiation hazards. Risk stratification should be considered to select those who could potentially benefit by an intense surveillance strategy.[108]

Six meta-analyses including a Cochrane Database review are available on the surveillance of colorectal cancer patients after R0 resection. Data from these shows improved survival and increase in curative resection for recurrence with intense surveillance.[109-115] To date no tumor marker other than carcinoembryonic antigen (CEA) has been shown to be effective for follow-up in colonic cancer patients.[73,116] There is no evidence to include fecal occult blood testing and liver function tests in the surveillance protocol or for the inclusion of routine positron emission tomography (PET) imaging in the follow-up.[73,116] However, it is a useful investigation when there is a serial rise of CEA and conventional investigations do not show any evidence of recurrence.

Majority of randomized controlled trials on surveillance of colorectal cancer patients included stage I-III without stage stratification. Some recent RCTs have excluded stage I patients. ASCO and CCO have not recommended any surveillance for stage I patients.[116] However, the Clinical Outcomes of Surgical Therapy (COST) trial comparing laparoscopic versus open colon cancer surgery showed a similar recurrence pattern between early and late stage colon cancer patients.[117] The trial demonstrated similar benefit for early stage patients after post-recurrence treatment and recommended surveillance for stage I and II A patients as well. Identifying patients with high risk of developing recurrence may be a reasonable follow-up strategy. Risk factors include lympho-vascular invasion, positive margins, poor differentiation, and T2 tumors.[116] These patients should receive a surveillance protocol similar to the stage II patients. NCCN recommends a colonoscopy at one year, 3 years and every 5 years thereafter following the curative surgery for stage I colonic cancer.[9]

In Stage II patients' guidelines differ on follow-up interval. ASCRS and NCCN recommends 3-6 monthly clinical examination and CEA testing for 2 years followed by 6 monthly clinical examination and CEA testing for up to 5 years.[73,116] ASCO recommends physical examination and CEA testing 3-6 monthly for up to 5 years, whereas CCO recommends physical examination and CEA testing every 6 months for up to 5 years.[117-119] Gilardoni et al. tried optimizing the surveillance for early stage tumor and found that left side or double colon cancer, vascular invasion, less than 12 lymph nodes sampled and stage IIB are risk factors which significantly lower the disease free and overall survival.[120] They observed that all patients who had recurrence were asymptomatic and were detected only on CT. Hence it was recommended that an intense follow-up strategy with CT imaging should be carried out in this subset of patients. NCCN recommends 6–12 monthly CT for patients with high risk for recurrence (poorly differentiated histology, lymphatic invasion and vascular invasion). Stage III patients are followed up similar to high-risk stage II patients.[9]

Only limited data is available on the follow-up protocol for Stage IV patients, which are inadequate to frame guidelines. Both ASCO and CCO do not recommend surveillance for stage IV colon cancer [117,119] although, improved long-term survival has been shown by some studies in patients with isolated metastatic disease. In view of this fact, ASCRS and NCCN recommend similar surveillance strategy for stage III and IV.[73,116]

ONGOING RESEARCH WHICH MAY IMPACT FUTURE PRACTICE

Prediction of the response and toxicity for systemic chemotherapy recently gained interest following discovery of KRAS and BRAF mutations which has influenced a change of view from giving systemic therapy for all stages to individualized therapy.[121] UGT1A1-28/UGT1A1-6 (uridine diphosphate glucuronosyltransferase) polymorphism has been shown to produce severe toxicity with irinotecan and hence patients who are candidates for irinotecan therapy are recommended for this screening.[121,122] Similarly, thymidine phosphorylase (TP) and dihydropyrimidine dehydrogenase (TPD) have been shown to have better predictive ability for response to systemic therapy and have the potential for targeted therapy.[123,124]

Nanotechnology has been shown to have potential in the early detection and treatment of colorectal cancer. Nanoparticle based identification of specific tumor location, biologically targeted contrast agents (Ironoxide nanocrystal contrast agent in MRI) and drug delivery system (PLGA Nanoparticle as a 5-FU carrier at the point of DNA damage) have been studied.[125,126] This has a potential for future diagnostic and therapeutic role in colon cancer patients. Significant advantage of near infrared (NIR) fluorescence imaging using NIR fluorescent nanoparticles has been shown in experimental models. This has the potential to replace invasive colonoscopy.[127]

CONCLUSION

In summary, review of recent advances in the field of colon carcinoma leads to several conclusions. Currently, CT colonography is primarily indicated in patients with incomplete colonoscopy due to a non-obstructive cause and cannot replace incomplete colonoscopy in patients with obstructed left colon cancer as both procedures require bowel preparation. Use of fecal tagging to facilitate CT colonography in patients with a loaded colon is associated with poor sensitivity and specificity. Current evidence does not support use of routine CT chest in colon cancer patients with no liver metastasis and is selectively indicated only in patients with advanced T and N stage tumors. PET-CT does not obviate the need for additional contrast-enhanced CT and is primarily indicated in patients with doubtful metastatic lesions on contrast-enhanced CT. PET-CT is also indicated in the postoperative surveillance of patients with rising serum CEA level and non-diagnostic conventional imaging following primary treatment and in detecting synchronous tumors in patients with obstructed left colon cancer. The role of mechanical gut preparation remains controversial.

Studies have shown that CME with CVL is associated with a higher lymph node yield, R0 resection rate and overall survival. Hence, the current recommended treatment for locally advanced colon cancer is either CME with CVL or D3 dissection as per Japanese practice. While the oncological safety of laparoscopic surgery has been documented, its role in patients with T4 cancer remains controversial. In the JCOG0404 trial, patients with T4 tumors who underwent laparoscopic surgery had inferior survival compared to patients who underwent open colectomy possibly due to increased tumor manipulation and violation of the no-touch principle. The potential benefits of robotic surgery do not translate into clinical advantage when compared to laparoscopic surgery performed by the experienced surgeon. Hence, robotic surgery is not recommended as a superior option to minimally invasive colon surgery. All three protocols for metastatic disease, viz. concurrent or staged colectomy and resection of liver/lung secondary, neoadjuvant chemotherapy with FOLFOX/CapOX for 2–3 months followed by concurrent or staged colectomy and resection of liver/lung metastasis or colectomy followed by chemotherapy with FOLFOX/CapOX for 2–3 months and resection of liver/lung secondary, all have shown to be equally effective in terms of disease-free survival and overall survival. Obstructing right colon cancers are best treated by primary resection and anastomosis. Use of SEMS as a bridge to surgery in obstructed left colon cancer may be associated with additional morbidity and a poor oncological outcome.

There is no role of adjuvant and neoadjuvant chemotherapy in Stage I patients. High-risk patients with Stage II disease with risk factors such as microsatellite instability and mismatch repair can be selected for chemotherapy. Stage III node positive and Stage IV patients are definite candidates for adjuvant therapy including RT in selected T4 cases. Monoclonal antibodies are recommended as first line therapy for metastatic colon cancer patients after appropriate genetic testing to rule out non-responders. Surveillance strategies for follow-up after treatment have changed in recent years with recommendation for intense surveillance for stage I–III patients which may result in survival benefits. Significant research is on-going in predicting response or toxicity in patients to chemotherapy and use of nanotechnology in diagnosis and therapy.

REFERENCES

1. Peterse EFP, Meester RGS, Siegel RL, et al. The impact of the rising colorectal cancer incidence in young adults on the optimal age to start screening: Microsimulation analysis I to inform the American Cancer Society colorectal cancer screening guideline. Cancer. 2018;124:2964-73.
2. Smith RA, Andrews KS, Brooks D, et al. Cancer screening in the United States, 2018: A review of current American Cancer Society guidelines and current issues in cancer screening. CA Cancer J Clin. 2018;68:297-316.
3. Baran B, Mert Ozupek N, Yerli Tetik N, et al. Difference between left-sided and right-sided colorectal cancer: A focused review of literature. Gastroenterology Res. 2018;11:264-73.
4. Lim DR, Kuk JK, Kim T, et al. Comparison of oncological outcomes of right-sided colon cancer versus left-sided colon cancer after curative resection: Which side is better outcome? Medicine (Baltimore). 2017;96:e8241.
5. Yahagi M, Okabayashi K, Hasegawa H, et al. The worse prognosis of right-sided compared with left-sided colon cancers: A systematic review and meta-analysis. J Gastrointest Surg. 2016;20:648-55.
6. Atkin W, Dadswell E, Wooldrage K, et al. Computed tomographic colonography versus colonoscopy for investigation of patients with symptoms suggestive of colorectal cancer (SIGGAR): A multicentre randomised trial. Lancet. 2013;381: 1194-202.
7. Ojidu H, Palmer H, Lewandowski J, et al. Patient tolerance and acceptance of different colonic imaging modalities: An observational cohort study. Eur J Gastroenterol Hepatol. 2018;30:520-5.
8. Heuschmid M, Luz O, Schaefer JF, et al. Computed tomographic colonography (CTC): Possibilities and limitations of clinical application in colorectal polyps and cancer. Technol Cancer Res Treat. 2004;3:201-7.
9. Benson AB 3rd, Venook AP, Al-Hawary MM, et al. NCCN Guidelines Insights: Colon Cancer, Version 2.2018. J Natl Compr Canc Netw. 2018;6:359-69.
10. Kim HY, Lee SJ, Lee G, et al. Should preoperative chest CT be recommended to all colon cancer patients? Ann Surg. 2014;259:323-8.
11. Pavoor RS, Shukla PJ, Milsom JW. The importance of preoperative staging with chest CT scan in patients with colorectal cancer. Ann Surg Oncol. 2011;18: S224-5.
12. Pellino G, Warren O, Mills S, et al. Comparison of western and Asian guidelines concerning the management of colon cancer. Dis Colon Rectum. 2018;61: 250-9.

13. Ruers TJ, Wiering B, van der Sijp JR, et al. Improved selection of patients for hepatic surgery of colorectal liver metastases with 18F-FDG PET: A randomized study. J Nucl Med. 2009;50:1036-41.
14. Moulton CA, Gu CS, Law CH, et al. Effect of PET before liver resection on surgical management for colorectal adenocarcinoma metastases: A randomized clinical trial. JAMA. 2014;311:1863-9.
15. Zhang Y, Feng B, Zhang GL, et al. Value of ^{18}F-FDG PET-CT in surveillance of postoperative colorectal cancer patients with various carcinoembryonic antigen concentrations. World J Gastroenterol. 2014;20:6608-14.
16. Hojo D, Tanaka T, Takahashi M, et al. Efficacy of 18-fluoro deoxy glucose-positron emission tomography computed tomography for the detection of colonic neoplasia proximal to obstructing colorectal cancer. Medicine (Baltimore). 2018; 97:e11655.
17. Guenaga KF, Matos D, Wille-Jorgensen P. Mechanical bowel preparation for elective colorectal surgery. Cochrane Database Syst Rev. 2011;(9):CD001544.
18. Gustafsson UO, Scott MJ, Schwenk W, et al. Enhanced Recovery After Surgery (ERAS) Society, for Perioperative Care; European Society for Clinical Nutrition and Metabolism (ESPEN); International Association for Surgical Metabolism and Nutrition (IASMEN). Guidelines for perioperative care in elective colonic surgery: Enhanced Recovery After Surgery (ERAS (®)) Society recommendations. World J Surg. 2013;37:259-84.
19. Klinger AL, Green H, Monlezun DJ, et al. The role of bowel preparation in colorectal surgery: Results of the 2012-2015 ACS-NSQIP Data. Ann Surg. 2017.
20. Koller SE, Bauer KW, Egleston BL, et al. Comparative effectiveness and risks of bowel preparation before elective colorectal surgery. Ann Surg. 2018;267: 734-42.
21. Sadahiro S, Suzuki T, Tanaka A, et al. Comparison between oral antibiotics and probiotics as bowel preparation for elective colon cancer surgery to prevent infection: prospective randomized trial. Surgery. 2014;155:493-503.
22. McSorley ST, Steele CW, McMahon AJ. Meta-analysis of oral antibiotics, in combination with preoperative intravenous antibiotics and mechanical bowel preparation the day before surgery, compared with intravenous antibiotics and mechanical bowel preparation alone to reduce surgical-site infections in elective colorectal surgery. BJS Open. 2018;2:185-94.
23. Brady M, Kinn S, Stuart P. Preoperative fasting for adults to prevent perioperative complications. Cochrane Database Syst Rev. 2003;(4):CD004423.
24. Svanfeldt M, Thorell A, Hausel J, et al. Randomized clinical trial of the effect of preoperative oral carbohydrate treatment on postoperative whole-body protein and glucose kinetics. Br J Surg. 2007;94:1342-50.
25. Nygren J, Thorell A, Ljungqvist O. Preoperative oral carbohydrate nutrition: An update. Curr Opin Clin Nutr Metab Care. 2001;4:255-9.
26. Ljungqvist O, Nygren J, Thorell A. Modulation of post-operative insulin resistance by pre-operative carbohydrate loading. Proc Nutr Soc. 2002;61:329-36.
27. Kwon S, Meissner M, Symons R, et al. Surgical care and outcomes assessment Program Collaborative. Perioperative pharmacologic prophylaxis for venous thromboembolism in colorectal surgery. J Am Coll Surg. 2011;213:596-603.

28. Erem HH, Kiran RP, Remzi FH, et al. Venous thromboembolism in colorectal surgery: skip SCIP or comply? Tech Coloproctol. 2014;18:719-24.
29. Heald RJ, Ryall RD. Recurrence and survival after total mesorectal excision for rectal cancer. Lancet. 1986;1:1479-82.
30. Hohenberger W, Weber K, Matzel K, et al. Standardized surgery for colonic cancer: complete mesocolic excision and central ligation–technical notes and outcome. Colorectal Dis. 2009;11:354-64.
31. Culligan K, Walsh S, Dunne C, et al. The mesocolon: A histological and electron microscopic characterization of the mesenteric attachment of the colon prior to and after surgical mobilization. Ann Surg. 2014;260:1048-56.
32. Japanese Society for Cancer of the Colon and Rectum. Japanese classification of colorectal carcinoma; 2nd Edition. Tokyo: Kanehara-shuppan Co.; 2009.
33. Bertelsen CA, Bols B, Ingeholm P, et al. Can the quality of colonic surgery be improved by standardization of surgical technique with complete mesocolic excision? Colorectal Dis. 2011;13:1123-9.
34. Mori S, Baba K, Yanagi M, et al. Laparoscopic complete mesocolic excision with radical lymph node dissection along the surgical trunk for right colon cancer. Surg Endosc. 2015;29:34-40.
35. Siani LM, Pulica C. Laparoscopic complete mesocolic excision with central vascular ligation in right colon cancer: Long-term oncologic outcome between mesocolic and non-mesocolic planes of surgery. Scand J Surg. 2015;104:219-26.
36. Watanabe T, Muro K, Ajioka Y, et al. Japanese Society for Cancer of the Colon and Rectum. Japanese Society for Cancer of the Colon and Rectum (JSCCR) guidelines 2016 for the treatment of colorectal cancer. Int J Clin Oncol. 2018; 23:1-34.
37. West NP, Kobayashi H, Takahashi K, et al. Understanding optimal colonic cancer surgery: comparison of Japanese D3 resection and European complete mesocolic excision with centralvascular ligation. J Clin Oncol. 2012;30:1763-9.
38. Milsom JW, Böhm B, Hammerhofer KA, et al. A prospective, randomized trial comparing laparoscopic versus conventional techniques in colorectal cancer surgery: a preliminary report. J Am Coll Surg. 1998;187:46-54.
39. Lacy AM, García-Valdecasas JC, Delgado S, et al. Laparoscopy-assisted colectomy versus open colectomy for treatment of non-metastatic colon cancer: A randomised trial. Lancet. 2002;359:2224-9.
40. Deijen CL, Vasmel JE, de Lange-de Klerk ESM, et al. COLOR (Colon cancer Laparoscopic or Open Resection) study group. Ten-year outcomes of a randomised trial of laparoscopic versus open surgery for colon cancer. Surg Endosc. 2017;31:2607-15.
41. Kitano S, Inomata M, Mizusawa J, et al. Survival outcomes following laparoscopic versus open D3 dissection for stage II or III colon cancer (JCOG0404): a phase 3, randomised controlled trial. Lancet Gastroenterol Hepatol. 2017;2:261-8.
42. Kim IY, Kim BR, Kim YW. The short-term and oncologic outcomes of laparoscopic versus open surgery for T4 colon cancer. Surg Endosc. 2016;30:1508-18.
43. Yang ZF, Wu DQ, Wang JJ, et al. Short- and long-term outcomes following laparoscopic vs open surgery for pathological T4 colorectal cancer: 10 years of experience in a single center. World J Gastroenterol. 2018; 24:76-86.

44. Park JS, Choi GS, Park SY, et al. Randomized clinical trial of robot-assisted versus standard laparoscopic right colectomy. Br J Surg. 2012;99:1219-26.
45. Petrucciani N, Sirimarco D, Nigri GR, et al. Robotic right colectomy: A worthwhile procedure? Results of a meta-analysis of trials comparing robotic versus laparoscopic right colectomy. J Minim Access Surg. 2015;11:22-8.
46. Faucheron JL, Paquette B, Trilling B, et al. Emergency surgery for obstructing colonic cancer: A comparison between right-sided and left-sided lesions. Eur J Trauma Emerg Surg. 2018;44:71-7.
47. Hsu TC. Comparison of one-stage resection and anastomosis of acutecomplete obstruction of left and right colon. Am J Surg. 2005;189:384-7.
48. Lee YM, Law WL, Chu KW, et al. Emergency surgery for obstructing colorectal cancers: a comparison between right-sided and left-sided lesions. J Am Coll Surg. 2001;192:719-25.
49. Yeo HL, Lee SW. Colorectal emergencies: Review and controversies in the management of large bowel obstruction. J Gastrointest Surg. 2013;17:2007-12.
50. Tewari SO, Getrajdman GI, Petre EN, et al. Safety and efficacy of percutaneous cecostomy/colostomy for treatment of large bowel obstruction in adults with cancer. J Vasc Interv Radiol. 2015;26:182-8.
51. Kye BH, Lee YS, Cho HM, et al. Comparison of long-term outcomes between emergency surgery and bridge to surgery for malignant obstruction in right-sided colon cancer: A multicenter retrospective study. Ann Surg Oncol. 2016; 23:1867-74.
52. Amelung FJ, de Beaufort HW, Siersema PD, et al. Emergency resection versus bridge to surgery with stenting in patients with acute right-sided colonic obstruction: A systematic review focusing onmortality and morbidity rates. Int J Colorectal Dis. 2015;30:1147-55.
53. Meyer F, Marusch F, Koch A, et al. German Study Group "Colorectal Carcinoma (Primary Tumor)". Emergency operation in carcinomas of the left colon: Value of Hartmann's procedure. Tech Coloproctol. 2004;8 Suppl 1:s226-9.
54. Kube R, Granowski D, Stubs P, et al. Surgical practices for malignant left colonic obstruction in Germany. Eur J Surg Oncol. 2010;36:65-71.
55. Arnaud JP, Bergamaschi R. Emergency subtotal/total colectomy with anastomosis for acutely obstructed carcinoma of the left colon. Dis Colon Rectum. 1994; 37:685-8.
56. Torralba JA, Robles R, Parrilla P, et al. Subtotal colectomy vs. intraoperative colonic irrigation in the management of obstructed left colon carcinoma. Dis Colon Rectum. 1998;41:18-22.
57. Hennekinne-Mucci S, Tuech JJ, Brehant O, et al. Emergency subtotal/total colectomy in the management of obstructed left colon carcinoma. Int J Colorectal Dis. 2006;21:538-41.
58. Group, T.S.S. Single-stage treatment for malignant left-sided colonicobstruction: A prospective randomized clinical trial comparing subtotalcolectomy with segmental resection following intraoperative irrigation. The SCOTIA Study Group. Subtotal Colectomy versus On-table Irrigation and Anastomosis. Br J Surg. 1995;82:1622-7.

59. Lim JF, Tang CL, Seow-Choen F, et al. Prospective, randomized trial comparing intraoperative colonic irrigation with manual decompression only for obstructed left-sided colorectal cancer. Dis Colon Rectum. 2005;48:205-9.
60. Kam MH, Tang CL, Chan E, et al. Systematic review of intraoperative colonic irrigation vs. manual decompression in obstructed left-sided colorectal emergencies. Int J Colorectal Dis. 2009;24:1031-7.
61. Pisano M, Zorcolo L, Merli C, et al. 2017 WSES guidelines on colon and rectal cancer emergencies: Obstruction and perforation. World J Emerg Surg. 2018; 13:36.
62. Kim SJ, Kim HW, Park SB, et al. Colonic perforation either during or after stent insertion as a bridge to surgery for malignant colorectal obstruction increases the risk of peritoneal seeding. Surg Endosc. 2015;29:3499-506.
63. Huang X, Lv B, Zhang S, et al. Preoperative colonic stents versus emergency surgery for acute left-sided malignant colonic obstruction: A meta-analysis. J Gastrointest Surg. 2014;18:584-91.
64. Ribeiro IB, Bernardo WM, Martins BDC, et al. Colonic stent versus emergency surgery as treatment of malignant colonic obstruction in the palliative setting: A systematic review and meta-analysis. Endosc Int Open. 2018;6:E558-67.
65. Arezzo A, Passera R, Lo Secco G, et al. Stent as bridge to surgery for left-sided malignant colonic obstruction reduces adverse events and stoma rate compared with emergency surgery: Results of a systematic review and meta-analysis of randomized controlled trials. Gastrointest Endosc. 2017;86:416-26.
66. van Hooft JE, Fockens P, Marinelli AW, et al. Dutch Colorectal Stent. Early closure of a multicentre randomized clinical trial of endoscopic stenting versus surgery for stage IV left-sided colorectal cancer. Endoscopy. 2008;40:184-91.
67. Pirlet IA, Slim K, Kwiatkowski F, et al. Emergency preoperative stenting versus surgery for acute left-sided malignant colonic obstruction: A multicenter randomized controlled trial. Surg Endosc. 2011;25:1814-21.
68. Sloothaak DA, van den Berg MW, Dijkgraaf MG, et al. collaborative Dutch Stent-In study group. Oncological outcome of malignant colonic obstruction in the Dutch Stent-In 2 trial. Br J Surg. 2014;101:1751-7.
69. Niekel MC, Bipat S, Stoker J. Diagnostic imaging of colorectal liver metastases with CT, MR imaging, FDG PET, and/or FDG PET/CT: A meta-analysis of prospective studies including patients who have not previously undergone treatment. Radiology. 2010;257:674-84.
70. Van Kessel CS, Buckens CF, van den Bosch MA, et al. Preoperative imaging of colorectal liver metastases after neoadjuvant chemotherapy: A meta-analysis. Ann Surg Oncol. 2012;19:2805-13.
71. Van Cutsem E, Köhne CH, Láng I, et al. Cetuximab plus irinotecan, fluorouracil, and leucovorin as first-line treatment for metastatic colorectal cancer: Updated analysis of overall survival according to tumor KRAS and BRAF mutation status. J Clin Oncol. 2011;29:2011-9.
72. Ye LC, Liu TS, Ren L, et al. Randomized controlled trial of cetuximab plus chemotherapy for patients with KRAS wild-type unresectable colorectal liver-limited metastases. J Clin Oncol. 2013;31:1931-8.

73. Zheng P, Liang C, Ren L, et al. Additional biomarkers beyond RAS that impact the efficacy of cetuximab plus chemotherapy in mCRC: A retrospective biomarker analysis. J Oncol. 2018;2018:5072987.
74. Ludwig EB, Arya R, Wu Y, et al. Role of adjuvant radiotherapy in locally advanced colonic carcinoma in the modern chemotherapy era. Ann Surg Oncol. 2016; 23:856-62.
75. Lee KC, Ou YC, Hu WH, et al. Meta-analysis of outcomes of patients with stage IV colorectal cancer managed with chemotherapy/radio-chemotherapy with and without primary tumor resection. Onco Targets Ther. 2016;9:7059-69.
76. Takeda A, Sanuki N, Kunieda E. Role of stereotactic body radiotherapy for oligometastasis from colorectal cancer. World J Gastroenterol. 2014;20:4220-9.
77. Chapelle N, Matysiak-Budnik T, Douane F, et al. Hepatic arterial infusion in the management of colorectal cancer liver metastasis: Current and future perspectives. Dig Liver Dis. 2018;50:220-5.
78. Quasar Collaborative Group, Gray R, Barnwell J, et al. Adjuvant chemotherapy versus observation in patients with colorectal cancer: A randomised study. Lancet. 2007;370:2020-9.
79. Labianca R, Nordlinger B, Beretta GD, et al Early colon cancer: ESMO clinical practice guidelines for diagnosis, treatment and follow-up. Ann Oncol. 2013; 24:vi64-72.
80. Ananthakrishnan N, Maroju NK, Kate V. Polyps of the gastrointestinal tract. In: Chattopadhyay TK (ed.) G.I. Surgery, Annual Vol 17. New Delhi: Byword, 2010: 10-35.
81. Sinicrope FA, Foster NR, Thibodeau SN, et al. DNA mismatch repair status and colon cancer recurrence and survival in clinical trials of 5-fluorouracil-based adjuvant therapy. J Natl Cancer Inst. 2011;103:863-75.
82. Sargent DJ, Marsoni S, Monges G, et al. Defective mismatch repair as a predictive marker for lack of efficacy of fluorouracil-based adjuvant therapy in colon cancer. J Clin Oncol. 2010;28:3219-26.
83. Schmoll HJ, Twelves C, Sun W, et al. Effect of adjuvant capecitabine or fluorouracil, with or without oxaliplatin, on survival outcomes in stage III colon cancer and the effect of oxaliplatin on post-relapse survival: A pooled analysis of individual patient data from four randomised controlled trials. Lancet Oncol. 2014;15: 1481-92.
84. McLeay NJ, Meyerhold JA, Green E, et al. Impact of age on the efficacy of newer adjuvant therapies in patients with stage II/III colon cancer: Findings from the ACCENT database. J Clin Oncol. 2013;31:2600-6.
85. Haller DG, O'Connell MJ, Cartwright TH, et al. Impact of age and medical comorbidity on adjuvant treatment outcomes for stage III colon cancer: A pooled analysis of individual patient data from four randomized, controlled trials. Ann Oncol. 2015;26:715-24.
86. Mirnezami R, Chang GJ, Das P, et al. Intraoperative radiotherapy in colorectal cancer: systematic review and meta-analysis of techniques, long-term outcomes, and complications. Surg Oncol. 2012; 22:22-35.
87. Cantero-Muñoz P, Urién MA, Ruano- Ravina A. Efficacy and safety of intraoperative radiotherapy in colorectal cancer: A systematic review. Cancer Lett. 2011; 306:121-33.

88. Hong TS, Ritter MA, Tomé WA, et al. Intensity-modulated radiation therapy: emerging cancer treatment technology. Br J Cancer. 2005;92:1819-24.
89. Downward J. Targeting RAS signalling pathways in cancer therapy. Nat Rev Cancer. 2003;3:11-22.
90. Recondo G Jr, Díaz-Cantón E, de la Vega M, et al. Advances and new perspectives in the treatment of metastatic colon cancer. World J Gastrointest Oncol. 2014; 6:211-24.
91. Karkkainen MJ, Petrova TV. Vascular endothelial growth factor receptors in the regulation of angiogenesis and lymphangiogenesis. Oncogene. 2000;19:5598-605.
92. Goel HL, Mercurio AM. VEGF targets the tumour cell. Nat Rev Cancer. 2013; 13:871-82.
93. Allegra CJ, Others G, O'Connell MJ, et al. Phase III trial assessing bevacizumab in stages II and III carcinoma of the colon: results of NSABP protocol C-08. J Clin Oncol. 2011;29:11-16.
94. De Gramont A, Van Cutsem E, Schmoll HJ, et al. Bevacizumab plus oxaliplatin-based chemotherapy as adjuvant treatment for colon cancer (AVANT): A phase 3 randomised controlled trial. Lancet Oncol. 2012;13:1225-33.
95. Alberts SR, Sargent DJ, Nair S, et al. Effect of oxaliplatin, fluorouracil, and leucovorin with or without cetuximab on survival among patients with resected stage III colon cancer: A randomized trial. JAMA. 2012;307:1383-93.
96. Van Cutsem E, Köhne CH, Hitre E, et al. Cetuximab and chemotherapy as initial treatment for metastatic colorectal cancer. N Engl J Med. 2009;360:1408-17.
97. Douillard JY, Oliner KS, Siena S, et al. Panitumumab-FOLFOX4 treatment and RAS mutations in colorectal cancer. N Engl J Med. 2013;369:1023-34.
98. Tol J, Nagtegaal ID, Punt CJ. BRAF mutation in metastatic colorectal cancer. N Engl J Med. 2009;361:98-9.
99. De Roock W, Claes B, Bernasconi D, et al. Effects of KRAS, BRAF, NRAS, and PIK3CA mutations on the efficacy of cetuximab plus chemotherapy in chemotherapy-refractory metastatic colorectal cancer: A retrospective consortium analysis. Lancet Oncol. 2010;11:753-62.
100. Yang H, Higgins B, Kolinsky K, et al. Antitumor activity of BRAF inhibitor vemurafenib in preclinical models of BRAF-mutant colorectal cancer. Cancer Res. 2012;72:779-89.
101. Hong DS, Morris VK, El Osta B, et al. Phase IB study of vemurafenib in combination with irinotecan and cetuximab in patients with metastatic colorectal cancer with BRAFV600E mutation. Cancer Discov. 2016;6:1352-65.
102. Lee SY, Cheul-Oh S. Advances of targeted therapy in treatment of unresectable metastatic colorectal cancer. Biomed Res Int. 2016;2016:7590245.
103. Wilhelm SM, Dumas J, Adnane L, et al. Regorafenib (BAY 73-4506): A new oral multikinase inhibitor of angiogenic, stromal and oncogenic receptor tyrosine kinases with potent preclinical antitumor activity. Int J Cancer. 2011;129: 245-55.
104. Santoro A, Comandone A, Rimassa L, et al. A phase II randomized multicenter trial of gefitinib plus FOLFIRI and FOLFIRI alone in patients with metastatic colorectal cancer. Ann Oncol. 2008;19:1888-93.

105. Tournigand C, Chibaudel B, Samson B. Bevacizumab with or without erlotinib as maintenance therapy in patients with metastatic colorectal cancer (GERCOR DREAM; OPTIMOX3): A randomised, open-label, phase 3 trial. Lancet Oncol. 2015;16:1493-505.
106. American Cancer Society. Colorectal Cancer Facts & Figures: 2011-2013. Atlanta: American Cancer Society; 2011. [online] Available from https://www.cancer.org/content/dam/cancer-org/research/cancer-facts-and-statistics/colorectal-cancer-facts-and-figures/colorectal-cancer-facts-and-figures-2011-2013.pdf [Accessed December 2018].
107. Tong LL, Gao P, Wang ZN, et al. Is pT2 subclassification feasible to predict patient outcome in colorectal cancer? Ann Surg Oncol. 2011;18:1389-96.
108. Tjandra JJ, Chan MK. Follow-up after curative resection of colorectal cancer: A meta-analysis. Dis Colon Rectum. 2007;50:1783-99.
109. Bruinvels DJ, Stiggelbout AM, Kievit J, et al. Follow-up of patients with colorectal cancer: A meta-analysis. Ann Surg. 1994;219:174-82.
110. Rosen M, Chan L, Beart RW Jr, et al. Follow-up of colorectal cancer: A meta-analysis. Dis Colon Rectum. 1998;41:1116-26.
111. Jeffery GM, Hickey BE, Hider P. Follow-up strategies for patients treated for non-metastatic colorectal cancer. Cochrane Database of Syst Rev. 2002(1): CD002200.
112. Renehan AG, Egger M, Saunders MP, et al. Impact on survival of intensive follow up after curative resection for colorectal cancer: Systematic review and meta-analysis of randomised trials. BMJ. 2002;324:813.
113. Figueredo A, Rumble RB, Maroun J, et al. Follow-up of patients with curatively resected colorectal cancer: a practice guideline. BMC Cancer. 2003;3:26.
114. Jeffery M, Hickey BE, Hider PN. Follow-up strategies for patients treated for non-metastatic colorectal cancer. Cochrane Database Syst Rev. 2007(1): CD002200.
115. Steele SR, Chang GJ, Hendren S, et al. Practice guideline for the surveillance of patients after curative treatment of colon and rectal cancer. Dis Colon Rectum. 2015;58:713-25.
116. Meyerhardt JA, Mangu PB, Flynn PJ, et al. Follow-up care, surveillance protocol, and secondary prevention measures for survivors of colorectal cancer: American Society of Clinical Oncology clinical practice guideline endorsement. J Clin Oncol. 2013;31:4465-70.
117. Tsikitis VL, Malireddy K, Green EA, et al. Postoperative surveillance recommendations for early stage colon cancer based on results from the clinical outcomes of surgical therapy trial. J Clin Oncol. 2009;27:3671-6.
118. Earle C, Annis R, Sussman J, et al. Follow-up Care, Surveillance Protocol, and Secondary Prevention Measures for Survivors of Colorectal Cancer. Toronto (ON): Cancer Care Ontario; 2012 Feb 3. Program in Evidence-based Care Evidence-Based Series No.: 26-2. [online] Available from http://www.southlakeregional.org/doc.aspx?id=900 [Accessed December 2018].
119. Gilardoni E, Bernasconi DP, Poli S, et al. Surveillance for early stages of colon cancer: potentials for optimizing follow-up protocols. World J Surg Oncol. 2015; 13:260.

120. Rodrigues D, Longatto-Filho A, Martins SF. Predictive biomarkers in colorectal cancer: From the single therapeutic target to a plethora of options. Biomed Res Int. 2016;2016:6896024.
121. Liu X, Cheng D, Kuang Q, et al. Association between UGT1A1*28 polymorphisms and clinical outcomes of irinotecan-based chemotherapies in colorectal cancer: A meta-analysis in Caucasians. PLoS One. 2013;8:e58489.
122. Cheng L, Li M, Hu J, et al. UGT1A1*6 polymorphisms are correlated with irinotecan-induced toxicity: A system review and meta-analysis in Asians. Cancer Chemother Pharmacol. 2014;73:551-60.
123. Ye DJ, Zhang JM. Research development of the relationship between thymidine phosphorylase expression and colorectal carcinoma. Cancer Biol Med. 2013;10:10-5.
124. Omura K. Clinical implications of dihydropyrimidine dehydrogenase (DPD) activity in 5-FU-based chemotherapy: Mutations in the DPD gene, and DPD inhibitory fluoropyrimidines. Int J Clin Oncol. 2003;8:132-8.
125. Espinosa A, Di Corato R, Kolosnjaj-Tabi J, et al. Duality of iron oxide nanoparticles in cancer therapy: Amplification of heating efficiency by magnetic hyperthermia and photothermal bimodal treatment. ACS Nano. 2016;10:2436-46.
126. Kuo CY, Liu TY, Chan TY, et al. Magnetically triggered nanovehicles for controlled drug release as a colorectal cancer therapy. Colloids Surf B Biointerfaces. 2016;140:567-73.
127. Kolitz-Domb M, Cohen S, Salkmon EC, et al. Design of Near Infra-Red Fluorescent Functional Nanoparticles Diagnosis of Colon Cancer. [online]. Available from http://www.avidscience.com/book/recent-advances-in-colon-cancer/ [Accessed December 2018].

Chapter 5

Management of Intestinal Obstruction

Sunil Kumar, Arunima Verma

INTRODUCTION

Intestinal obstruction (IO) is a common surgical emergency and challenging problem for surgeons. Global data suggests 1% of all hospital admissions are accounted by intestinal obstruction. In the West, the incidence is decreasing while in tropical countries, IO continues to impose a substantial burden on the healthcare system. Prevalence of IO is nearly 20% among all surgical emergencies that present to a hospital.[1] Intestinal obstruction is defined as "interference in the passage of food, liquids and content of the intestine either due to mechanical or neurological cause". Peritoneal adhesion and hernia remain the most common causes. All patients with IO are potential candidates for surgical intervention. Various factors affect the decision of operative versus conservative management. Surgery in emergency setting entails high morbidity and mortality; while on the other hand, prolongation of conservative trial at times may prove deleterious to the patient. Hence, it becomes imperative to diagnose the probable cause early. With improved diagnostic facilities, it is possible to choose appropriate patients for timely intervention.[2]

CLASSIFICATION OF INTESTINAL OBSTRUCTION[3]

In majority (80%) of patients with IO, the cause remains in the small bowel. Despite the liberal use of laparoscopy, postoperative abdominal adhesion continues to be the commonest (2/3rd) etiology for small bowel obstruction (SBO). Adhesion related complications are responsible for 20% re-admissions in the first postoperative year and 30% within 10 years of primary abdominal surgery. These are fibrous bands and are part of wound healing. The formation of adhesion is significantly affected by type of surgery, duration of procedure, contamination and contact with the intestinal contents, use of prosthesis and technique of surgery. Laparoscopic surgery has decreased the incidence of intra-abdominal adhesions following gastrointestinal procedures by 25%, reduced the average adhesive grade (Table 1) by 1.7 points and also need for re-intervention for adhesive SBO as compared to open surgery. Other important mechanical causes (Table 2) of SBO include hernia (10-15%), Tuberculosis and Crohn's disease (~10%) and malignancy (5-7%).

The common causes of mechanical large bowel obstruction include left sided malignancy (most common), diverticulitis, sigmoid and cecal volvulus (Table 2). Diverticulitis is more common in Western countries, while sigmoid volvulus is an important cause in developing countries. It is important to classify the obstruction according to cause (intraluminal or extraluminal), grade of obstruction (partial or complete), site of obstruction, duration of symptoms (acute/subacute/chronic) and viability of bowel (simple/strangulated or closed loop) as these factors decide the course of action. It is indispensable to recognize the development of peritonitis (strangulated hernia/perforation proximal to the obstruction/ischemia) in case of intestinal obstruction as it mandates surgery.

Table 1: Grades of intra-abdominal adhesions.

Adhesion grade	Definition
Grade 0	No adhesion
Grade 1	Filmy adhesions that are avascular and separate spontaneously
Grade 2	Firm and limited vascular adhesions that separate by traction
Grade 3	Dense adhesion that require sharp dissection to separate

Table 2: Causes of intestinal obstruction.

Small bowel obstruction (80%)	Colonic obstruction (20%)
Common Causes	
Adhesive obstruction (60–70%) Hernia (10–15%) Crohn's disease in West/ Tuberculosis in Asia and Africa (10%) Malignancy (5–7%)	Colorectal malignancy (60–80%) *Volvulus (10–15%)*: Common in Asia and Africa • Sigmoid (90%) • Cecum (5%) • Transverse colon (<5%) *Diverticulitis (5–10%)*: Common in West
Other Causes (5%)	
Volvulus Intussusception Gallstone ileus Superior mesenteric artery syndrome Ascariasis Enteroliths/Bezoars	Inflammatory bowel disease Tuberculosis Fecal impaction Hernia Radiation proctitis Anastomotic stricture Pseudo-obstruction (old age)

PATHOPHYSIOLOGY

Small bowel is responsible for digestion of ingested food and absorption of fluid, nutrients and electrolytes through the mucosa. In IO, bowel proximal to the point of obstruction dilates from accumulated swallowed air, intestinal fluid and ingested food materials.[4] Distal to obstruction the bowel shows normal peristalsis and absorption until it become empty and collapse.[5] Stasis in the proximal loop promotes bacterial growth and fermentation of food. The final result is fluid sequestration in the lumen, mucosal edema, decrease in absorptive capacity and transudative loss of fluid into the peritoneal cavity. Emesis from the proximal segment of bowel in addition to decreased absorption results in loss of fluid and electrolytes. If the deficit is not replaced in time, dehydration leads to decreased renal perfusion, renal failure and metabolic acidosis. Progressive bowel dilatation increases the intramural pressure adversely affecting the perfusion of the intestinal wall. If the contents are not decompressed, bowel ischemia ensues resulting in perforation in the dilated segment.[6] Loss of mucosal integrity due to ischemia and bowel edema promotes translocation of bacteria across the bowel wall into the bloodstream leading to sepsis.[7] In closed loop obstruction, the bowel is obstructed both proximally and distally and causes torsion of arterial inflow and venous drainage. It rapidly leads to bowel ischemia and perforation.

CLINICAL MANIFESTATIONS

The clinical symptoms of intestinal obstruction include colicky abdominal pain, vomiting, abdominal distension and constipation, which form the classic tetrad.[8]

Abdominal pain: It is the most prominent initial symptom in intestinal obstruction, which is usually sudden in onset, intermittent and colicky in nature. The intensity of pain may decrease with the bowel fatigue or bowel decompression through nasogastric tube. The pain becomes intense and unremitting once ischemia sets in or perforation occurs. Closed-loop obstruction often presents with pain out of proportion to the abdominal signs because of concurrent mesenteric ischemia.[9]

Vomiting: Vomiting is more common with small bowel obstruction and is late phenomenon in colonic obstruction. The nature of vomitus is often bilious and turns feculent as time elapses.[10,11]

Abdominal distension: Abdominal distension is a prominent feature of distal small bowel and colonic obstruction. This is more marked in complete obstruction. Periodic measurement of abdominal girth may help to gauge the severity and help in decision making.[12]

Table 3: Clinical features of small and large bowel obstruction.

Small intestinal obstruction	Large intestinal obstruction
• Abdominal pain associated with visible peristaltic waves in upper and mid abdomen	• Intermittent lower abdominal pain
• Upper and central abdominal distension	• Generalized abdominal distension including the flanks
• Nausea and early profuse vomiting	• Minimal or no vomiting even in late phase
• Obstipation	• Obstipation or ribbon-like stools
• Sever fluid and electrolyte imbalance	• Fluid and electrolyte imbalance is less likely
• Metabolic alkalosis initially due to gastric acid loss followed by metabolic acidosis due to dehydration and renal derangement	• Metabolic acidosis

Constipation: Constipation is a late symptom because residual gas and stool in bowel distal to the obstruction may continue to evacuate. Complete non-passage of flatus or stool is termed as obstipation.

Other symptoms: The clinical presentation of patients with IO varies with the degree of obstruction. In severe case with presence of ischemia and mucosal translocation of bacteria, the patients develop bacteremia, pyrexia and later on sepsis with shock.[13] Subtle differences between small and large bowel obstruction are enlisted in Table 3. Past history of similar symptoms, past surgical history and duration of symptoms should always be an integral part of patient's history.

Signs of Intestinal Obstruction

The patient with intestinal obstruction presents with tachycardia followed by hypotension which indicates development of shock. Early in the course of obstruction, the abdomen is distended. Visible bowel peristalsis is not uncommon. Tympanic note on percussion can be appreciated. On auscultation, high pitched hyperactive bowel sounds may be heard as a result of propulsive efforts of bowel to overcome the obstruction. With advanced IO, the bowel gets fatigued and the abdomen becomes silent. The patients should be periodically evaluated to detect development of tenderness and thus early detection of strangulation or perforation. Abdominal malignancies may present with lump. Examination remains incomplete without per rectal examination. It may reveal presence of fecal impaction or rectal mass. Presence of stool in the rectum may suggest partial or non-mechanical obstruction, while presence of blood in the rectum may suggest malignancy or development of intestinal ischemia.

DIAGNOSIS

Laboratory Tests

Laboratory changes are nonspecific in IO. Patients present with hemoconcentration and electrolyte imbalance (hyponatremia, hypokalemia, hypochloremia). Total leukocyte count may show a rise with neutrophilia. With progressive dehydration and renal impairment, blood urea nitrogen and creatinine show a rise. With the development of ischemia, serum lactate, creatine kinase (CK) and lactate dehydrogenase (LDH) may rise. They are nonspecific indicators of bowel hypoperfusion. However, lactate is highly sensitive (90–100%) for bowel ischemia, though the specificity is low (40–85%). Hence, an increase in lactate is good guide to proceed with urgent surgery.[14]

Plain X-ray Abdomen

The accuracy of diagnosis of the intestinal obstruction on plain abdominal radiographs is estimated to be approximately 60%.[15] Positive predictive value of high grade intestinal obstruction is 80%.[16] Characteristic findings on supine radiographs are dilated loops of small intestine, i.e. more than 3 cm in diameter. Upright radiographs demonstrate multiple air fluid levels, with more than 2.5 cm in length and differential air fluid level (>5 mm difference in height of the air fluid levels.).[17] Differences in appearance of small bowel and large bowel on X-ray have been described in Table 4. Plain abdominal films are not reliable to detect the site of obstruction. They can appear normal in early obstruction, in high jejunal or duodenal obstruction.

It is important to note the presence or absence of gas in the pelvis to differentiate between partial (paralytic ileus or passable stricture) and complete obstruction. Free gas under the diaphragm in the upright films suggests pneumoperitoneum (perforation). A large pneumoperitoneum may present with dark dome appearance in the upper abdomen even on supine film – Football Sign. The double wall sign or Rigler's sign, i.e. both sides of bowel wall is visible when gas is on the inside as well as outside the bowel loop. Visualization of the falciform on radiographs is termed as Silver sign. In severe sepsis, gas in portal vein is an ominous sign.

Contrast Radiographs

Contrast studies are useful in recurrent IO or low-grade obstruction to define the obstructed segment and degree of obstruction precisely. The use of water-soluble contrast material is not only diagnostic, but may also be therapeutic in patients with partial small bowel obstruction.[18] Barium studies including

Table 4: Differences in appearance of small and large bowel on radiographs.

Small bowel	Large bowel
The gas filled loops are centrally located in the abdomen	Gas shadows are located peripherally in the abdomen
Arranged in a step-ladder pattern	Haustrations (incomplete mucosal folds) present in the walls placed at different levels
Valvulae conniventes (complete mucosal folds) in the walls	

barium meal follow through and enteroclysis is the investigation of choice in subacute and intermittent small bowel obstruction. It is a dynamic study to define the site of strictures especially in Crohn's disease and tuberculosis. Typical features include multiple partial strictures (Hourglass sign), single long stricture (String sign) and retracted fibrosed cecum with dilated ileum (Goose neck deformity). These signs are nonspecific and can be present in both tuberculosis and Crohn's disease.

Ultrasonography of Abdomen

Ultrasonography remains a valuable investigation for unstable patients with an ambiguous diagnosis and in patients for whom radiation exposure is contraindicated, such as pregnant women.[19] Transabdominal ultrasonography is less accurate in evaluation of small bowel obstruction due to poor sonologic window in presence of excessive intestinal gas.[20] The sonographic findings include dilated fluid-filled bowel loops with hyperechoic spots of gas moving within the fluid. Thickness of bowel wall should be more than 4 mm and hypoperistalsis in presence of mechanical obstruction suggest development of ischemia and are indications for urgent surgery.

Computed Tomography

Computed tomography (CT) is the most versatile investigation in acute as well as chronic IO. It should be performed in all patients with IO if not contraindicated (pregnancy, renal failure, and contrast allergy). It can reliably determine the etiology, site of obstruction, any organic lesion, signs of ischemia or perforation. It is the best investigation to distinguish between partial or complete obstruction. In a meta-analysis, conventional CT had a sensitivity of 92% (range 81–100%) and specificity of 93% (range 68–100%) in detecting complete obstruction.[21] Multidetector CT (MDCT) has high sensitivity in diagnosing high-grade obstruction but has relatively low sensitivity in diagnosing low-grade obstruction. It also identifies other causes of intestinal obstruction, such as volvulus or intestinal strangulation. Classical finding in SBO is dilated small bowel measuring more than 3 cm and colonic loops less than 6 cm, while in colonic pathology, the cecum is dilated (>6 cm) as well.

Use of oral contrast (Diatrizoate meglumine and diatrizoate sodium) is beneficial in partial obstruction. The osmolarity of contrast agent is six times that of extracellular fluid. Its administration promotes fluid shift into the bowel lumen, resulting in decrease in bowel edema and facilitates movement of intestinal contents forward. The presence of contrast into the colon within 24 hours predicts success of conservative management with more than 90% accuracy. It can be helpful to avoid urgent surgery but does not influence the rate of SBO recurrence. If bowel ischemia is suspected then positive oral contrast can obscure findings of wall ischemia on CT. In such cases, negative or neutral oral contrast should be used. Decreased or absent mural enhancement predicts bowel ischemia with a sensitivity of 60% and specificity of 95%. Other signs on CT, which suggest hypoperfusion of the bowel wall, include: thumb printing (due to submucosal edema), mesenteric edema and pneumatosis intestinalis (intramural gas produced by the bacteria). Free intraperitoneal gas seen under the anterior abdominal wall suggests perforation.

Some important CT findings include:

Transition point: It is the abrupt change in the caliber of the bowel lumen, representing the site of obstruction. Marked change in gut diameter suggests complete obstruction and predicts the need for early surgery.

Whirl sign: It is due to the twisting of mesentery and the gut around an axis, evident in volvulus. Luminal narrowing produces an appearance of a "beak". Presence of whirl sign mandates early intervention – colonoscopic or surgical procedure for sigmoid volvulus and urgent laparotomy for SBO.

Small bowel feces sign: It is due to accumulation of food material over a long period of time resembling the colonic content. This suggests near complete obstruction in a chronic disease.

Most of the time, plain X-ray abdomen usually gives diagnosis of bowel obstruction, however further evaluation is required in 20% to 30% of patients. CT examination is particularly useful in patients with history of abdominal malignancy, postsurgical patients, and patients who have no history of abdominal surgery and present with symptoms of bowel obstruction.

Magnetic Resonance Imaging

Magnetic resonance imaging (MRI) is time consuming and more variable in image quality as compared to CT. CT scan is superior in detection of free air. MRI is useful for Crohn's disease, evaluation of pelvis in rectal malignancy and in case where CT is contraindicated.[22,23]

MANAGEMENT OF INTESTINAL OBSTRUCTION

Management of Intestinal obstruction consists of conservative treatment, supportive treatment and surgical treatment depending upon the cause of intestinal obstruction.

Fluid Resuscitation

Patients of acute IO require aggressive fluid resuscitation and correction of electrolyte imbalance. As the hydration improves, pulse and blood pressure improves. Serial electrolytes, urine output and vitals should be monitored.

Intravenous Antibiotics

Broad-spectrum antibiotics are used prophylactically to counter the bacteremia due to intestinal overgrowth of bacteria and translocation across the bowel wall.[24] But the role of antimicrobials in nontoxic patients is minimal. Antibiotics are administered preoperatively if the patient requires surgery.

Role of Bowel Decompression

Nasogastric (NG) suction with a tube in IO is a standard of care. Suction with a nasogastric tube empties the stomach and reduces the complications (aspiration of vomitus). It relieves the symptoms of pain partially and decreases the bowel distension. Hence, it helps to break the vicious cycle of bowel edema by lowering the intramural pressure. Use of long nasoenteral tubes for direct and effective decompression of small bowel especially in adhesive obstruction has not been found to be superior to NG tube.

In inflammatory bowel disease, use of steroids and immunomodulators may alleviate the symptoms. Hyperbaric oxygen has been suggested to relieve obstruction in adhesive bowel disease. The conservative trial should not be extended for more than 3–5 days. Regular patient surveillance should continue to detect the signs of bowel perforation or strangulation early. Surgery delayed by more than 72 hours increases the mortality threefold.

Surgical Management

Clinical picture, laboratory and radiographic findings all should be considered when taking decision for surgical intervention in bowel obstruction.[25] Small bowel obstruction in young age, obstrution in virgin abdomen and large bowel obstruction needs early intervention (within 48 hours). Abdominal wall hernia is responsible for bowel obstruction in 26.8% in absence of previous intervention.[26] In adhesive intestinal obstruction, the conservative management is usually continued up to 48 to 72 hours in the hope of spontaneous resolution.

Indications for early surgical intervention:
- Obstructed hernia
- Suspected intestinal strangulation
- Obstructive features in a virgin abdomen.

The principles of surgical intervention for obstruction are: to identify the site of obstruction, status of proximal bowel and the cause of obstruction. The abdomen should be accessed through midline laparotomy for adequate exposure and better visualization of the bowel segments. Once identification of cause and site is over, proximal bowel is decompressed to allow easy diaphragmatic movement. At the time of decompression care must be taken to avoid spillage of the intestinal contents into the peritoneal cavity.

Viability of the bowel is assessed (Table 5). The definitive step depends on the cause and may vary from simple band division to resection and anastomosis.

Management of Internal Hernia

Internal hernia is a rare cause of small bowel obstruction but once diagnosed necessitates timely intervention. Internal hernia is difficult to diagnose pre-operatively both clinically and radiologically, though CT scan comes handy in this situation.[27] The diagnosis of internal hernia most commonly is done by laparoscopy as an incidental finding.[28] Internal hernia can either be congenital or acquired. Paraduodenal hernias are the most common type of congenital hernia. Acquired hernias are most common after bariatric surgeries.[29] Treatment of obstructed internal hernia is to release the constricting agent and check the bowel viability. If the bowel is ischemic, resection and anastomosis should be performed.

Adhesive Small Bowel Obstruction

This is the most frequently encountered cause of SBO. Evaluation involves detailed history, examination and diagnostic work-up including CECT. Postoperative adhesions are more common following pelvic surgery and surgery for malignancy. Conservative trial including oral contrast, NG decompression, correction of electrolytes and hyperbaric oxygen therapy is often useful. The success rate of conservative treatment for ileus caused by postoperative adhesions is between 73% and 90%. Adhesive intestinal obstruction requiring surgical intervention can be associated with serious complications when surgery is unusually delayed more than 48 hours.[30] The mortality rate in uncomplicated intestinal obstruction is only around 5% but it rises to 30% in patients with strangulation of the small intestine.[31]

Common causes of intra-abdominal adhesions:
- Acute inflammation
- Abdominal tuberculosis
- Peritonitis
- Crohn's disease
- Foreign material.

Good surgical technique, removal of clots with saline wash after completion of procedure, reduced contact time of gauze with bowel are

Table 5: Differentiation between viable and non-viable intestine.

Viable intestine	Non-viable intestine
• Looks shiny	• Dull appearance
• Possible visible pulsations in mesenteric arteries	• No pulsations
• Firm intestinal musculature	• Flabby, thin intestinal musculature
• Peristalsis can be seen	• No peristalsis

some of the factors which help in reducing the postoperative adhesion formation.[32] Patients who do not settle with conservative management may require surgery—either laparotomy or laparoscopic adhesolysis. Laparoscopy is being increasingly used. Only contraindication is presence of pneumoperitoneum/peritonitis and severe cardiopulmonary disorder.

Success of the procedure is predicted by the following factors:
- Less than 3 previous laparotomies
- Non-median laparotomy
- Experienced surgeon
- Intervention within 24 hours of symptoms
- No sign of peritonitis.[33]

It is more important to prevent abdominal adhesions following a procedure. Various techniques have been described includes gentle handling of the tissue, prevention of gross contamination by avoiding spillage of contents, reduced laparoscopy ports and specimen extraction via natural orifices, avoid closure of the peritoneum and use of anti-adhesive barriers. Anti-adhesive barriers aim to separate the injured peritoneum from the serosa of the bowel till the healing occurs. Hyaluronate carboxymethylcellulose (Seprafilm) has been shown to reduce the incidence of adhesive obstruction following colorectal surgery without any adverse effect. Another barrier, oxidized regenerated cellulose (Interceed) is used in open gynecological surgery. The disadvantage of these two products is that they cannot be employed through a trocar in laparoscopy. Icodextrin 4% (2000 mL) at the end of the procedure has been evaluated after minimal invasive procedures and has shown to decrease recurrence of adhesive SBO significantly in the study group. No adverse event including blood loss, anastomotic dehiscence or infection episodes were documented with the use of Icodextrin.[34]

Obstruction due to Ascariasis

Ascaris lumbricoides is the largest and most prevalent of the human helminths. Heavy infestation is common in low socioeconomic group in South-East Asian countries.[35] Most common site of obstruction is terminal ileum. Delay in the management of the intestinal obstruction can lead to bowel perforation with spillage of the worms and eggs into the peritoneal cavity. Patients who complain of low grade or no fever, mild abdominal distension, and diffuse pain can be managed conservatively. In presence of significant obstruction with perforation, the patients present with high grade fever and severe dehydration. Abdominal examination may reveal signs of peritonitis in late phase. Diagnosis can be easily established on USG or CT scan. The typical findings on sonography is bull's eye appearance in transverse section and tram-track appearance in longitudinal section. Plain X-ray abdomen erect shows multiple air-fluid levels.

Laparotomy is usually required if patient do not respond to conservative management or there are features suggestive of peritonitis. The surgical procedure is dependent on the viability of bowel and findings at the time of operation. If worms are loaded in terminal ileum milking of the worms into cecum is attempted. If worms are loaded in jejunum, enterotomy should be performed to release the obstruction. The incision should be closed transversally with great care to avoid contamination of the peritoneal cavity by the worms or eggs. If the bowel is nonviable or perforation is identified then resection and primary anastomosis should be considered.

SUPERIOR MESENTERIC ARTERY SYNDROME

It is also known as Wilkie's syndrome, cast syndrome, and aortomesenteric syndrome.[36] It is a rare cause of intestinal obstruction. Superior mesenteric artery syndrome is caused by external compression of the third portion of the duodenum between the superior mesenteric artery and the abdominal aorta. The mean angle between the SMA and the abdominal aorta is approximately 45°. Many precipitating factors that narrow the aorto-mesenteric angle by approximately 6–25° can cause this syndrome. The classical presentation is recurrent postprandial pain, nausea, vomiting, bloating, abdominal discomfort, or pain and tenderness. Typical features include pain aggravated by a supine position and relieved by prone or left lateral decubitus, or even by a knee-chest position.

Precipitating factors for SMA syndrome

- Malnourished patients
- Prolonged bed bound patients
- Thin built persons
- Advanced lumbar lordosis
- Spinal deformity and spinal trauma
- Anatomical abnormalities like insufficient rotation of duodenum and short ligament of Trietz.

Computed tomography scan or CT angiography, magnetic resonance angiography, conventional angiography, ultrasonography, and endoscopy are helpful in the diagnosis.

Radiological criteria for diagnosing SMA syndrome

- Dilatation of the first and second part of the duodenum, with or without gastric dilatation
- Vertical and oblique compression of mucosal folds
- Anti-peristaltic flow of barium proximal to the obstruction.

Surgical procedures

These procedures are used either to resolve or bypass the duodenal compression.
- Gastrojejunostomy
- Duodenojejunostomy—operation of choice to relieve the obstruction
- Strong's operation—duodenal mobilization with duodenal derotation to alter the aortomesenteric angle and place the third and fourth portions of the duodenum to the right of the superior mesenteric artery.

Management of Cecal and Sigmoid Volvulus

Cecal volvulus is a rare cause of acute intestinal obstruction with the incidence of 1 to 1.5%.[37] It is most common in middle-aged females and is a surgical emergency. In cecal volvulus, there is an axial twist of the cecum and terminal ileum around their mesentery leading to vascular compromise and strangulation, which may necessitate resection. If bowel is viable, the volvulus should be reduced followed by cecal fixation to right iliac fossa or a cecostomy. Limited right hemicolectomy is also one of the choices for cecal volvulus.

Ideal management of sigmoid volvulus still remains unclear.[38] It is responsible for 15% of all causes of complete bowel obstruction. In suspected volvulus, flexible endoscopy is diagnostic as well as therapeutic.[39] The diagnosis can be made from history, clinical examination and plain X-ray abdomen. In sigmoid volvulus patient presents with severe colicky abdominal pain, constipation and rapid abdominal distension. Plain X-ray abdomen shows bent inner tube or omega sign. It also shows two fluid levels in dilated colon and narrow base of the involved segment. In the absence of peritonitis, flatus tube, hydrostatic enema or colonoscopic reduction and simple derotation are procedures of choice but if the bowel is gangrenous the endoluminal procedures are contraindicated. High recurrence rate following colonoscopic reduction is also the disadvantage of this procedure.

Sigmoidopexy: Simple fixation of the colon to the intra-abdominal structures is an effective procedure in a viable bowel. The morbidity and mortality is almost nil with sigmoidopexy.[40] However, this procedure is also associated with high recurrence rate.

Resection and primary anastomosis: Resection and primary anastomosis is possible especially in younger patients and viable colon.[41] The main complication with this procedure is anastomotic leak. Hartmann's operation is a lifesaving procedure in emergency situation when the bowel is nonviable and gangrenous where distal stump is closed and proximal stump is brought out as colostomy. The stoma is usually closed after two to three months.

Management of Cancer-related Intestinal Obstruction

Gastrointestinal and ovarian tumors are most common intra-abdominal primary malignancies responsible for intestinal obstruction.[42] The incidence of IO in ovarian tumors ranges from 5% to 50%. Primary gastrointestinal tumors are associated with IO in 10–28%. Left sided colonic primaries are most common cause for obstruction. Splenic flexure is most common site to be involved. Mechanical obstruction most commonly affects the small bowel in isolation (61%), but may also affect only the large bowel (33%) or both simultaneously (20%).[43] True mechanical obstruction occurs secondary to diffuse peritoneal malignancy causing either direct obstruction, or secondary to malignant adhesions.

CHOICE OF SURGICAL PROCEDURES

Resection and primary anastomosis for obstructed right colonic cancers is recommended. Obstructing left colonic primaries have been traditionally treated with a two-stage procedure of resection and defunctional colostomy (Hartmann's procedure) followed by re-anastomosis at later date.[44] One-stage procedures necessitates a subtotal colectomy with ileorectal anastomosis (IRA). Various studies have shown poor functional outcomes with IRA. In such cases, metallic stents can be used as a bridge to planned surgery.

Self-expanding Metallic Stents

When a short segment obstruction is identified in the left colon or rectum on cross-sectional imaging, endoscopic stenting can tide over the acute crisis. The patients are symptomatically relieved, improved on general condition, planned for neoadjuvant therapy and taken up for surgery after adequate bowel preparation as a single stage curative procedure. Perforation and stent migration has been reported in 5% and 10% respectively. Use of metallic stent as evaluated in random clinical trials (RCTs) and meta-analysis has shown to increase the chances of recurrence and lymphatic metastasis due to peri-stent inflammation. Current recommendation on the use of stents is limited to candidates with poor general status. Diversion colostomy is preferred over stenting to tide over the obstruction crisis.

In 2007, Tinley in his review documented that colonic stenting could offer effective palliation for malignant unrescetable bowel obstruction, with short hospital stay and low rate of stoma formation, although there was no advantage in long-term survival.[45] Other nonsurgical treatments used for palliation with limited effectiveness include balloon dilatation, endoscopic laser ablation, and decompression tubes.

Role of Laparoscopy in Management of Intestinal Obstruction

With technical advancements and improving skills, laparoscopy is being increasingly used in the management of acute intestinal obstruction.[46] Bastug et al. reported the first laparoscopic lysis of a single adhesive band causing intestinal obstruction.[47] Laparoscopy has been proposed as an effective management although the conversion rate is high. Common reasons for conversion include inadequate visualization due to distended small bowel, iatrogenic perforations, gangrenous small bowel, and the inability to adequately relieve obstruction laparoscopically.

Patient criteria for laparoscopic selection:
- Early presentation with intestinal obstruction
- Proximal obstruction
- Suspected cases of single band
- Localized dilated bowel loops in plain X-ray abdomen
- Suspected partial intestinal obstruction
- Good general condition of the patient.

Contraindications for laparoscopy:
- Complete obstruction
- Suspected patient with malignancy
- Hemodynamically unstable patients
- Suspected closed loop obstruction or perforation
- Patients with severe comorbidities such as cardiovascular, respiratory and hemostatic disease
- Inexperienced laparoscopic skills.

Advantages of the laparoscopic procedure:[48]
- Short recovery time
- Decreased postoperative complications like incision site pain, infection
- Short hospital stay
- Faster return to normal diet
- Faster return to work or normal activity.

Complications

Iatrogenic injury is the dangerous complication with laparoscopic management of bowel obstruction. However, recent reports have shown similar risk of bowel injury with open or laparoscopic adhesiolysis.[49] Duration of surgery is definitely longer in laparoscopic management than open surgery.

Inflammatory Bowel Disease and Tuberculosis

Small bowel and ileocecal strictures are common in inflammatory bowel disease (IBD) and Tuberculosis (TB). Though Crohn's disease (CD) is uncommon in India, abdominal TB is frequently encountered. It is responsible for nearly 20% of all causes of acute abdomen presenting to the emergency in India. The presentation is usually subacute with a protracted history of intermittent pain and vomiting. Diagnosis can be established with CECT, Barium studies and endoscopic biopsy. Nonoperative management is usually successful. Surgical options include resection anastomosis of affected segment (significant narrowing of the lumen involving a short segment or multiple strictures over a short length of bowel or obstruction associated with perforation), stricturoplasty (in short to long stricture with luminal narrowing less than 50% and possibility of short bowel syndrome), bypass in presence of poor functional status or adhesiolysis in presence of bands. Surgery entails high morbidity and mortality with chances of anastomotic leak up to 20% especially in CD. The chance of re-stricture remains high. Yamamoto et al. first described the use of double balloon enteroscopic dilatation of strictures (DBE) to avoid surgery in majority. In a systemic review by Baars et al., DBE dilatation could avoid surgery in >80% of patients of CD with small bowel stricture.[50,51] The complication rate of the procedure was less than 5%. About 50% of the population did not require a second procedure on an average of over 2.5 years follow-up. This procedure is possible under fluoroscopy or direct endoscopic vision under sedation. The balloon is inflated for 30–60 seconds up to a maximum diameter of 20 mm. It is suitable for short (<5 cm) strictures with no acute angulation of bowel. It is contraindicated in presence of ulcer or fistula.

Pseudo-obstruction

Pseudo-obstruction or Ogilvie's syndrome is a phenomenon, which is caused by attenuated or un-coordinated colonic muscular contractions. The delayed intestinal transit occurs in the absence of a mechanical cause of obstruction or acute intra-abdominal inflammatory disease. Various causes of pseudo-obstruction are enlisted in Table 6. It produces severe colonic dilatation. Small

Table 6: Causes of pseudo-obstruction.

- Metabolic causes:
  - Diabetes
  - Hypokalemia
  - Uremia
  - Intermittent porphyria
- Drugs:
  - Laxatives overuse
  - Tricyclic antidepressants
  - Phenothiazines
- Idiopathic causes
- Retroperitoneal hematoma and tumor
- Prolonged bed bounded patient
- Severe traumatic injury

bowel is usually normal in caliber. No transit point is visible on imaging. It is important to determine the cause.

Detailed medical treatment history is of prime importance. Diagnosis is confirmed by colonic transit studies. Two methods are widely reported. One method uses radiopaque markers and other uses radiolabeled (Indium) liquid phase meals. The movement of the markers through the length of bowel is detected by serial imaging or gamma-cameras at 24, 48 and 72 hours. Excretion time in normal subjects is 72 hours. Retention of more than 20% markers after 5 days is diagnostic of delayed transit time.[52] Conservative treatment and holding the drug responsible is effective in 53-96% of cases with a perforation risk of less than 2.5% and a mortality of 0-14%. Neostigmine is effective in 3/4th of patients after a first dose. Second dose is effective in another 40% to 100% of cases. It should be administered with continuous monitoring of pulse and cardiac status in old age. Colonoscopic decompression is safe and effective with a success rate of 60-100% with perforation in less than 5% and mortality in less than 5%. Polyethylene glycol is useful to prevent recurrence after successful treatment with neostigmine or endoscopic decompression. In refractory cases, cecostomy is highly effective in colonic decompression but entails a high mortality.[53]

CONCLUSION

Intestinal obstruction is one of the most common surgical emergencies. CECT abdomen with oral contrast is the most useful investigation. It may play a therapeutic role in partial obstruction. Conservative management should not be extended beyond 3-5 days. Delay in recognition of ischemic changes can be deleterious. Morbidity and mortality can be significantly decreased with early detection and prompt management.

REFERENCES

1. Balouch NA, Baber KM, Mengal MA, et al. Spectrum of mechanical obstruction. JSP (Int). 2007;7:7-9.
2. Zinner MJ, Ashley SW. Maingot's Abdominal Operations, 11th edition. New York: McGraw Hill; 2007. pp. 128-33.
3. Kulaylat MN, Doerr RJ. Small bowel obstruction. Gastrointest Endosc Clin N Am. 2007;2:323-9.
4. Wright HK, O'Brien JJ, Tilson MD. Water absorption in experimental closed segment obstruction of the ileum in man. Am J Surg. 1971;121:96-9.
5. Shelton BK. Intestinal obstruction. AACN Clin Issues. 1999;10:478-91.
6. Rana SV, Bhardwaj SB. Small intestinal bacterial overgrowth. Scand J Gastroenterol. 2008;43:1030-7.
7. Wangensteen OH. Understanding the bowel obstruction problem. Am J Surg. 1978;135:131-49.

8. Frager DH, Baer JW, Rothpearl A, et al. Distinction between postoperative ileus and mechanical small-bowel obstruction: value of CT compared with clinical and other radiographic findings. Am J Roentgenol.1995;164:891-4.
9. Cappell MS, Batke M. Mechanical obstruction of the small bowel and colon. Med Clin North Am. 2008;92:575-97.
10. Williams NS, Bulstrode CJK, O'Connel PR. Clinical features of intestinal obstruction. In: Bailey & Love's Short Practice of Surgery, 25th edition. Hodder Arnold, England; 2008. pp:1188-1203.
11. Cuschieria. Clinical features of intestinal obstruction, acute abdomen. In: Clinical Surgery, 2nd edition. USA: Blackwell, 2003. pp.166-180.
12. Ellis H. The cause and prevention of postoperative intraperitoneal adhesions; Collective review. Surg Gynecol Obset. 1971;133:497-511.
13. Stringer, Pablot SM, Brereton RJ. Paediatric intussusception. Br J Surg. 1992;79: 867-76.
14. Lange H, Jackel R. Usefulness of plasma lactate concentration in diagnosis of acute abdominal disease. Eur J Surg. 1994;160:381-4.
15. Maglinte DD, Heitkamp DE, Howard TJ, et al. Current concepts in imaging of small bowel obstruction. Radiol Clin North Am. 2003;41:263-83.
16. Lappas JC, Reyes BL, Maglinte DD. Abdominal radiography findings in small-bowel obstruction: Relevance to triage for additional diagnostic imaging. Am J Roentgenol. 2001;176:167-74.
17. Brunicardi FC. Small intestine. In: Tavakkoli A, Ashley SW, Zinner MJ (Eds). Schwartz's Principles of Surgery, 9th edition. USA: McGraw Hill; 2010. pp. 980-1012.
18. Choi HK, Chu KW, Law WL. Therapeutic value of gastrografin in adhesive small bowel obstruction after unsuccessful conservative treatment: A prospective randomized trial. Ann Surg. 2002;236:1-6.
19. Lim JH, Ko YT, Lee DH, et al. Determining the site and causes of colonic obstruction with sonography. Am J Roentgenol. 1994;163:1113-7.
20 Kohn A, Cerro P, Miltie G, et al. Prospective evaluation of transabdominal bowel sonography in the diagnosis of intestinal obstruction in Crohn's disease: comparison with plain abdominal film and small bowel enteroclysis. Inflamm Bowel Dis. 1999;5:153-7.
21. Mallo RD, Salem R, Lalani T et al. Computed tomography diagnosis of ischemia and complete obstruction in small bowel obstruction: A systematic review. J Gastrointest Surg. 2005;9:690-4.
22. Taylor I, Johnson CD. Intra-abdominal Adhesions Formation and Management. Recent Advances in Surgery, 24th edition. 2001; USA. pp. 1-19.
23. Wiarda BM, Horsthuis K, Dobben AC, et al. Magnetic resonance imaging of the small bowel with the true FISP sequence: intra- and inter-observer agreement of enteroclysis and imaging without contrast material. Clin Imaging. 2009;33:267-73.
24. Sagar PM, MacFie J, Sedman P, et al. Intestinal obstruction promotes gut translocation of bacteria. Dis Colon Rectum. 1995;38:640-4.
25. Zielinski MD, Eiken PW, Bannon MP, et al. Small bowel obstruction-who needs an operation? A multivariate prediction model. World J Surg. 2010;34:910-9.

26. Lo OS, Law WL, Choi HK, et al. Early outcomes of surgery for small bowel obstruction: Analysis of risk factors. Langenbecks Arch Surg. 2007;392:173-8.
27. Blachar A, Federle MP, Brancatelli G, et al. Radiologist performance in the diagnosis of internal hernia by using specific CT findings with emphasis on transmesenteric hernia. Radiology. 2001:221:422-8.
28. Blachar A, Federle MP, Dodson SF. Internal hernia: Clinical and imaging findings in 17 patients with emphasis on CT criteria. Radiology. 2001;218:68-74.
29. Al-Mansour MR, Mundy R, Canoy JM, et al. Internal hernia after laparoscopic antecolic Roux-en-Y gastric bypass. Obes Surg. 2015;25:2106-11.
30. Sosa J, Gardner B. Management of patients diagnosed as acute intestinal obstruction secondary to adhesions. Am Surg. 1993;59:125-8.
31. Ellis H. The clinical significance of adhesions: focus on intestinal obstruction. Eur J Surg Suppl.1997;577:5-9.
32. Seror D, Feigin E, Szold A, et al. How conservatively can postoperative small bowel obstruction be treated? Am J Surg. 1993;165:125-6.
33. Farinella E, Cirocchi R, La Mura F, et al. Feasibility of laparoscopy for small bowel obstruction. World J Emerg Surg. 2009;4:3.
34. Catena F, Ansaloni L, Di Saverio S, et al. P.O.P.A. study: Prevention of postoperative abdominal adhesions by icodextrin 4% solution after laparotomy for adhesive small bowel obstruction. A prospective randomized controlled trial. J Gastrointest Surg. 2012;16:382-8.
35. Mokoena T, Luvuno FM. Conservative management of intestinal obstruction due to Ascaris worms in adult patients: A preliminary report. JR Coll Surg Edinb. 1988;33:318-21.
36. Welsch T, Büchler MW, Kienle P. Recalling superior mesenteric artery syndrome. Dig Surg. 2007;24:149-56.
37. Katoh T, Shigemori T, Fukaya R, et al. Cecal volvulus: Report of cecal and review of Japanese literature. World J Gastroenterol. 2009;15:2547-9.
38. Lou Z, Yu ED, Zhang W, et al. Appropriate treatment of acute sigmoid volvulus in the emergency setting. World J Gastroenterol. 2013;19:4979-83.
39. Atamanalp SS. Sigmoid volvulus: Diagnosis in 938 patients over 45.5 years. Tech Coloproctol. 2013;17:419-24.
40. Connolly S, Brannigan AE, Heffeman E. Sigmoid volvulus: A 10-year-audit. Ir J Med Sci. 2002;171:216-7.
41. Dulger N. Management of sigmoid colon volvulus. Hepatogastroenterology. 2000;47:1280-3.
42. Feuer DJ, Broadley KE, Shepard JH, et al. Systematic review of surgery in malignant bowel obstruction in advanced gynecological and gastrointestinal cancer. The Systematic Review Steering Committee. Gynecol Oncol. 1999;75:313-22.
43. Ripamonti C, Twycross R, Baines M, et al. Clinical-practice recommendations for the management of bowel obstruction in patients with end-stage cancer. 2001;9:223-33.
44. Kruschewski M, Runkel N, Buhr HJ. Radical resection in obstructing colorectal carcinomas. Int J Colorectal Dis. 1998;13:247-50.
45. Tan CJ, Dasari BV, Gardiner K. Systematic review and meta-analysis of randomized clinical trials of self-expanding metallic stents as a bridge to surgery

versus emergency surgery for malignant left-sided large bowel obstruction. Br J Surg. 2012;99:469-76.
46. Liauw JJ, Cheah WK. Laparoscopic management of acute small bowel obstruction. Asian J Surg. 2005;28:185-8.
47. Bastug DF, Trammell SW, Boland JP, et al. Laparoscopic adhesiolysis for small bowel obstruction. Surg Laparosc Endosc. 1991;1:259-62.
48. Chopra R, McVay C, Phillips E, et al. Laparoscopic lysis of adhesions. Am Surg. 2003;69:966-68.
49. Wullstein C, Gross E. Laparoscopic compared with conventional treatment of acute adhesive small bowel obstruction. Br J Surg. 2003;90:1147-51.
50. Baars JE, Theyventhiran R, Aepli P, et al. Double-balloon enteroscopy -assisted dilatation avoids surgery for small bowel strictures: A systemic review. World J Gastroenterol. 2017;23(45):8073-81.
51. Yamamoto H, Sekine Y, Sato Y, et al. Total enteroscopy with a nonsurgical steerable double-balloon method. Gastrointest Endosc. 2001;53:216-20.
52. Kim ER, Rhee PL. How to interpret a functional or motility test—Colon Transit Study. J Neurogastroenterol Motil. 2012;18(1):94-9.
53. Ben Ameur H, Boujelbene S, Beyrouti MI. Treatment of acute colonic pseudo-obstruction (Ogilvie's Syndrome): Systematic review. Tunis Med. 2013;91(10): 565-72.

Chapter 6

Barrett's Esophagus

Rajinder Parshad, Aditya Kumar, Gaurav Joshi

INTRODUCTION

Barrett's esophagus (BE) is a disease in which the normal squamous lining of the esophagus is replaced by metaplastic columnar epithelium. It appears as salmon colored mucosa into the esophagus for a distance more than or equal to 1 cm above gastroesophageal junction (GEJ). It develops as a consequence of long-standing gastroesophageal reflux disease (GERD) and predisposes to esophageal adenocarcinoma (EAC).[1] The condition is named after an Australian-born British surgeon Norman Barrett who described abnormalities in the lower esophagus but misdiagnosed this condition as a congenitally foreshortened esophagus. This was later clarified by Allison and Johnstone as a columnar-lined esophagus. After 7 years, Barrett's accepted this theory in his paper "The lower esophagus lined by columnar epithelium."[2]

The main limitation in BE is the optimal management, inability to accurately identify, and correctly stratify the individuals who are at risk of developing EAC. In nondysplastic BE (NDBE), the risk of EAC is 0.3% annually, which increases to 0.5% in BE with low-grade dysplasia (LGD) and 7% with high-grade dysplasia (HGD). Traditionally, HGD and intramucosal cancer (IMC) were treated by esophagectomy. However in last two decades, endoscopic methods are widely being used and have lower morbidity and long-term survival rate similar to esophagectomy.

EPIDEMIOLOGY

The actual prevalence of disease in the general population is not known. However, increase in GERD is accompanied by increased prevalence of BE. The exact prevalence of BE in different population is difficult to assess as this condition itself remains asymptomatic and diagnosed only when an endoscopy is performed. It is estimated that 5–15% patients with GERD in the US suffer from BE with a population prevalence of 0-2%.[3] A recent meta-analysis including 453,147 patients of Asian origin showed a pooled prevalence of 7.8% for endoscopic Barrett's in patients suffering from GERD. Of these, 1.3% had histologically proven Barrett's suggesting that the prevalence may be similar to the western population.[4]

RISK FACTORS

The predominant risk factor for BE is GERD. The risk appears to be correlated with the severity and duration of GERD. Other predisposing factors include male gender, white race, cigarette smoking, and central adiposity. Patients with Barrett's are usually aged 50-65 years with male preponderance. Patients with obesity, body mass index (BMI) more than 30 kg/m² or a hip waist ratio of more than or equal to 0.9 in males and more than or equal to 0.85 in females are at increased risk.[5,6] Erosive esophagitis is an independent risk factor for BE, with a fivefold increased risk of Barrett's at 5-year follow-up.[7] Patients with a peptic stricture have a higher prevalence of BE than those without strictures. Familial association is seen in up to 28% of first-degree relatives of patients with adenocarcinoma. Germline mutations in *MSR1*, *ASCC1*, and *CTHRC1* genes have been associated with the presence of BE and EAC,[8] and one large genome-wide association study identified genetic variants associated with Barrett's at chromosomes 6p21 and 16q24.[9]

NATURAL HISTORY OF THE DISEASE

The natural history of BE, that is the course of disease, when left untreated is difficult to quantify. Early surveillance and use of proton pump inhibitors (PPIs) have largely rendered this impossible. Though BE is a precursor to formation of EAC, the natural course from no dysplasia to LGD to HGD to EAC is not consistent. A recent multicenter cohort study in the US evaluated 1,791 patients with NDBE of less than 1 cm (irregular Z-line/"ultra-short segment") at index endoscopy and followed them for development of HGD/EAC. At a median follow-up of 4.8 years, none of the patients developed HGD/EAC.[10] This forms an interesting finding for the further need for surveillance/follow-up in these patients.

The natural history of LGD is even poorly understood. The incidence of EAC is approximately 0.54% annually.[11] It is a slowly progressing lesion with even possibility of regression to nondysplastic mucosa. This could be explained by overdiagnosis of LGD by variable sampling, difficulty in differentiating reactive from dysplastic or possibly actual neoplastic regression. The highest prevalence of cancer in BE is noted in patients with high-grade dysplasia. When patients with HGD undergo esophagectomy, malignancy was reported in up to 40%.[12] However, other studies have not shown progression to carcinoma on long-term follow-up leading to ongoing debate.[13] The high risk supports the need for intervention in these patients. The extent of involvement of HGD may also influence risk of EAC with decreased risk reported with focal lesions as compared to diffuse lesions by some studies.[14,15] The risk of progression to HGD or EAC is very low in short-segment BE (<3 cm). However, increase risk is reported with increase in BE length. The risk of combined HGD and EAC was 0.31 per year for length of BE segment less than 3 cm and increased to 1.28-fold for every cm to 2.41% for those with BE segment more than 13 cm. the use of PPI is associated with 7% reduced risk of HGD or EAC. It is also reported that statins and nonsteroidal anti-inflammatory drugs (NSAIDs) alone or in combination reduces the risk of progression.

CLINICAL FEATURES

The metaplastic mucosa causes no specific symptoms. The patients are evaluated initially for symptoms associated with GERD such as heartburn, regurgitation, and dysphagia. Epigastric pain, hematemesis, and odynophagia are rarer symptoms associated with the disease.

DIAGNOSIS

The diagnosis of BE is made by visible change in the lining of the distal esophagus and histological confirmation of columnar epithelium. Thus, the component of diagnosis includes endoscopy, targeted biopsy, and histological confirmation.

Endoscopic Diagnosis

Transoral endoscopy is the diagnostic test for evaluation of BE and salmon-colored columnar mucosa seen more than or equal to 1 cm above the GEJ is diagnostic. It is recommended that Prague C&M classification should be used for standardized reporting of endoscopic findings (Fig. 1). It includes the maximum extent and circumferential extent above the GEJ in centimeters.[16]

Endoscopy must include identification of three important landmarks:
1. *The GEJ*: Proximal margin of gastric folds
2. *Diaphragmatic pinch*: Point where diaphragmatic crura constrict/pinch esophagus (important landmark to identify hiatal defects)
3. *Squamocolumnar junction*: Junction between esophageal-stratified squamous epithelium and gastric columnar epithelium. Barrett's is considered when it is more than or equal to 1 cm above GEJ.

More recently, the role of transnasal endoscopy is being evaluated for its potential use as a screening tool. The benefits include better patient tolerance/

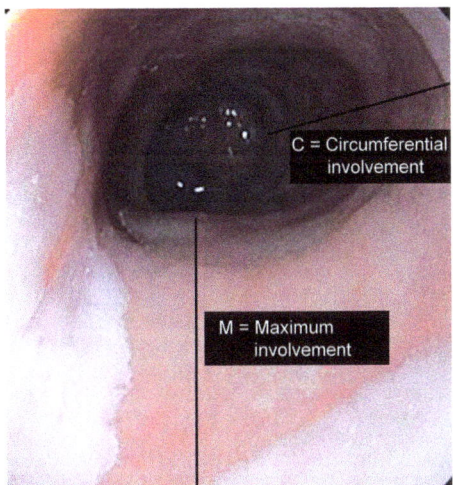

Fig. 1: Endoscopic image of Barrett's esophagus (BE) where salmon-colored mucosal changes can be appreciated. The maximum and circumferential involvements are marked according to the Prague C&M classification.

acceptability, no need for sedatives, cost-effectiveness, and possible use in periphery. However, it is not yet recommended for surveillance due to limited field of view, image quality, and inadequate size of biopsy.[17,18]

Histological Diagnosis

The final and important component in the diagnosis of BE is histological confirmation. It shows a mosaic of columnar cells including intestinal metaplasia (IM), gastric fundic, and gastric cardia type mucosa. Pathologist plays an important role in surveillance of BE by evaluating biopsies for features of dysplasia. Dysplasia is defined as neoplastic epithelium with cytologic and architectural atypia confined to the epithelium. The features evaluated include surface maturation, glandular architecture, cytologic atypia, and presence of inflammation/erosions as seen in Figures 2A to D.

Chances of neoplastic change increases with IM; however, few studies are available that support the fact. It is also emphasized that the finding of IM increases with the length of BE segment and number of biopsy sample taken. There is controversy with the definition of BE with different societies. The American society defines it as columnar change in the distal esophageal mucosa with IM (presence of goblet cells) on biopsy.[4,5] The British Society of Gastroenterology (BSG) does not consider IM in defining BE.[19]

The current consensus guidelines, therefore, recommend that two GI pathologists should evaluate the report of samples suspected to have BE. Standardized reporting of the findings should be in concordance to the Vienna Classification (Table 1).[20]

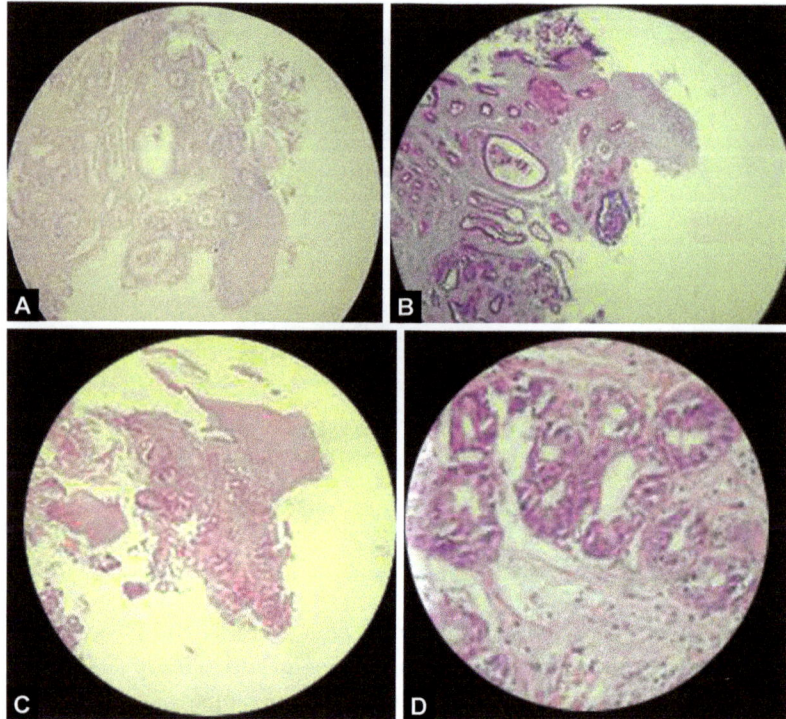

Figs. 2A to D: Pathology slides shown above are of: (A) Barrett's esophagus (BE) without dysplasia; (B) Alcian blue stain of BE without dysplasia; (C) BE with low-grade dysplasia (LGD); (D) BE with LGD (40× magnification).

Source: Dr Kirti Jangra, Pathologist, All India Institute of Medical Sciences, New Delhi, India.

Table 1: Vienna classification for Barrett's esophagus.

Category	Description
Category 1	No dysplasia
Category 2	Indefinite for dysplasia
Category 3	Noninvasive low-grade neoplasia (low-grade adenoma/dysplasia)
Category 4	Noninvasive high-grade neoplasia
Category 4.1	High-grade adenoma/dysplasia
Category 4.2	Noninvasive carcinoma (carcinoma *in situ*)
Category 4.3	Suspicion of invasive carcinoma
Category 5	Invasive epithelial neoplasia
Category 5.1	Intramucosal cancer
Category 5.2	Submucosa cancer

Biopsy for BE should be taken in accordance to the Seattle protocol with four-quadrant biopsy at 1-cm intervals. The 1-cm interval recommendation evolved from a study comparing serial biopsies taken at 1 cm versus 2 cm. It found that 29% of all patients with EAC and 50% of patients with EAC from Barrett's mucosa without endoscopically viable lesions were missed using the 2 cm biopsy protocol.[21]

Adherence to Seattle protocol has been variable. A Dutch study showed a decrease in adherence from 79% in lesions up to 5 cm to 30% in lesions 10–15 cm from GEJ.[22] Further increase in the diagnostic yield has been noted by increasing the number of biopsies. Increasing from 4 to 8 and 16 cores, the yield increases from 34.7% to 67.9% to 100%.[17]

Role of Biomarkers

Various biomarkers are being evaluated in Barrett's esophagus, which might be used in different ways like assessing the risk of cancer development, predicting the treatment response, and estimating the prognosis. Biomarkers, which predict progression of BE to EAC, include MCM2 expression pattern, LOH on distinct gene loci, especially at 17p, hypermethylation of p16 and the expression pattern of P53. Similarly, prognostic biomarkers being studied include, cyclin D1, Ki-67, transforming growth factor-α, adenomatous polyposis coli, cyclooxygenase-2, telomerase, and vascular endothelial growth factor. Kastelein et al. did an analysis of more than 12,000 from 635 patients with BE. They noted an increased cancer risk in patients with aberrant p53 expression and the risk was more so when there was a loss of p53 expression compared to p53 over expression [adjusted relative risk (RR) 14.0, 95% confidence interval (CI)].[23] These biomarkers are promising but need further validation.[24]

Cytosponge: Trefoil Factor-3

The cytosponge is an ingestible gelatin capsule containing a compressed mesh sponge with a string attached. On swallowing, gelatin dissolves in stomach within 5 minutes and release 3 cm diameter spherical mesh sponge. The string attached is pulled through mouth by traction, which scrapes off the esophageal cells. The mesh captures up to 1 million cells lining the esophagus. The cytology specimen is further analyzed for cellular markers. Trefoil factor-3 (TFF-3) is a cellular marker of intestinalization and is measured to detect Barrett's metaplasia. This cytosponge is used in screening for BE. The initial cohort study [Barrett's Esophagus Trial 1 (BEST-1)] evaluating the role of cytosponge included 504 patients of BE. It was found that cytosponge had a sensitivity of 73% and specificity of 94% in patients with more than

1 cm circumferential Barrett's.[25] A follow-up study [Barrett's Esophagus Trial 2 (BEST-2)] with 1,110 patients evaluated patients diagnosed with Barrett's and patients with GERD who were not investigated for Barrett's. Cytosponge was seen to be as accurate as endoscopy, easier to swallow (93% and preferred over endoscopy by 90% patients).[26] The Barrett's Esophagus Trial 3 (BEST-3) is a multicenter RCT currently underway to compare cytosponge with endoscopic biopsy.[27]

Advanced Imaging for Barrett's Esophagus

Advanced imaging techniques are being evaluated to detect early mucosal changes and identification of malignancy in patients with BE.

Narrow-band Imaging

It is a high-resolution endoscopic technique that enhances the structure of the mucosal surface. The principle of use is based on the fact that wavelength of light is proportional to the depth of penetration. Blue light penetrates superficially and provides better visualization of the mucosa and superficial vasculature by absorption. A meta-analysis of eight studies with 446 patients with 2,194 lesions revealed a pooled sensitivity and specificity of 94% and 65% for Barrett's and 96% and 94% for HGD concluding that narrow-band imaging (NBI) with magnification has high diagnostic precision for diagnosis of HGD in Barrett's.[28]

Chromoendoscopy

Chromoendoscopy stains to enhance tissue localization, characterization, and diagnosis. Dyes presently used include—methylene blue, indigo carmine, crystal violet, and acetic acid. A meta-analysis on methylene blue chromoendoscopy revealed no added benefit over random biopsy.[29] However, another meta-analysis including 1,379 patients using acetic acid chromoendoscopy with targeted biopsy showed superior results as compared to random biopsy with a pooled sensitivity and specificity of 92% and 96% for HGD/esophageal carcinoma (EC) and has a high diagnostic accuracy. Even though sensitivity is high (96%), the specificity is low (69%) for specialized intestinal metaplasia (SIM) warranting a biopsy in these cases.[30]

Confocal Laser Endomicroscopy

It uses high magnification and resolution images of the esophageal mucosa. It is based on tissue illumination with a low-power laser with subsequent detection of the fluorescence of light reflected from the tissue through a pinhole.[31] Two systems are used:

1. Probe-based confocal laser endomicroscopy (pCLE) system comprises a fiberoptic bundle with an integrated distal lens that is connected to a laser scanning unit. The probe-based system to date has a fixed focal length and so it can only scan in a single plane unlike current microscope systems that can create cross-sectional images at different depths.
2. Endoscope-based CLE (eCLE) uses a confocal microscope with a diameter of 12.8 mm, and the tip length is increased to accommodate the laser microscope so that there is a 5-cm rigid portion.

Contrast agents used are intravenous fluorescein or topical spray of acriflavine hydrochloride, tetracycline, or cresyl violet. A randomized double-blind controlled cross-over trial conducted in Johns Hopkins evaluated the yield of CLE with targeted mucosal biopsy when compared to standard endoscopy with a four-quadrant, random biopsy protocol. Overall, 39 patients completed the study protocol. It was found that CLE with targeted biopsy almost doubled the diagnostic yield for neoplasia (34% vs 17%) and was equivalent to the standard protocol for the final diagnosis of neoplasia.[32]

Autofluorescence

In this method, tissues are exposed to short wavelength light which cause fluorophores (endogenous biological substances) to get excited leading to fluorescence, this phenomenon is referred to as autofluorescence. This helps in differentiating tissues based on differential emission of fluorescence. This variability is due to presence of collagen, nicotinamide adenine dinucleotide hydrate (NADH), aromatic amino acids, and porphyrins with differential amounts of fluorophores.[33] Two modalities described include autofluorescence spectroscopy and autofluorescence endoscopy. These have shown to detect higher numbers of HGD/EAC but have poor imaging and high false positive rates (51%).[34]

Volumetric laser endomicroscopy (VLE) and iScan are the other upcoming modalities needing validation. VLE is a second-generation optical coherence tomography (OCT) that provides high-resolution cross-sectional imaging of esophageal mucosa using near-infrared light. Its principle is similar to endosonography but image formation in OCT depends on the variations in the reflection of light from different tissue layers rather than ultrasonic waves. The images are obtained from mucosa to the depth of 3 mm and have resolution of 7 μm, which is quite comparable to low-power microscopy. They can be seen on console with cross-sectional and longitudinal views.[35,36]

Endoscopy and biopsy sampling remains the mainstay of diagnosis of BE. However, focus is shifting from white light endoscopy to real time imaging with selective sampling to increase the yield as compared to random biopsy. The major advantage of advanced imaging is in reducing the interobserver variation. The main challenge in their application is the expertise of use which may not be available and thus standardized protocols can not be made. Therefore, till now, they are mostly used for selective patients and in specialized centers only.

MANAGEMENT

Screening

The role of screening and the target group has been a controversial topic over decades. Most guidelines suggest screening in patients at risk includes patients suffering from GERD with risk of adenocarcinoma. The common risk factors are age more than 50 years, male gender, Caucasian race, chronic GERD symptoms, obesity, family history of BE, or EAC in first-degree relatives. The recent BSG guidelines recommend screening in chronic GERD patients with three or more risk factors. However, American College of Gastroenterology (ACG) recommends presence of two or more risk factor with chronic and or frequent GERD symptoms in male. In females, screening should be individualized and presence of multiple risk factors is taken as high risk. The guidelines for screening for Barrett's have been listed in Table 2.

Surveillance

The idea of surveillance is to make an early diagnosis of dysplasia and intramucosal carcinoma. The endoscopic surveillance is performed optimally with high-definition white light endoscopy. The development of various advanced imaging for evaluation of BE to detect dysphagia or early cancer is being done. ACG recommend the use of electronic chromoendoscopy

Table 2: Screening guidelines for Barrett's esophagus.

	American Gastroenterology Association[37]	American College of Gastroenterology[38]	British Society of Gastroenterology[19]
Recommendation	Suggest	Consider	Consider
Threshold	Multiple risk factors	Men with chronic GERD + >two risk factors	>Three risk factors
	>50 years Males White race Chronic GERD Hiatus hernia Increased BMI with central obesity	>50 years White race Central obesity Barrett's/adenocarcinoma in first-degree relative Smoking	>50 years White race Male Chronic GERD Obesity Barrett's/adenocarcinoma in first-degree relative

(BMI: body mass index; GERD: gastroesophageal reflux disease)

for the surveillance of BE; however, no other guidelines endorse the use of modern advanced imaging techniques like chromoendoscopy, CLE, VLE, or autofluorescence imaging. Evidence on the role of surveillance is poor because of a lack of randomized controlled trials (RCTs). In 2012, Corley et al.[39] did not demonstrate an association between surveillance and a decreased risk of death in a case-control study of more than 8,000 patients of BE patients with EAC. In a retrospective review of 224 patients, Grant et al.[40] found that those who underwent surveillance had significantly lower stage tumors at the time of diagnosis. In a recent study by Verbeek et al., 9,780 patients were evaluated out of which 791 patients had prior BE, the 2- and 5-year mortality rates were lower in patients undergoing surveillance.[41] Though the evidence in favor of surveillance is weak, given the risk and anxiety associated with possibility of progression to EAC, most of the gastroenterologist recommends surveillance. ACG and other guidelines endorse the surveillance strategy of endoscopy with biopsy every 3–5 years, if there is no dysplasia on index endoscopy in patients with BE, endoscopy and biopsy every 6–12 months for LGD and every 3 months for HGD in the absence of eradication therapy.[38] A multicenter RCT, BOSS trial (Barrett's Esophagus Surveillance vs Surveillance at Need) is on its way to answer whether 2 yearly endoscopy is efficacious compared to endoscopy at need.[42]

Therapy of Barrett's Esophagus with/without Dysplasia

Medical Therapy

Therapy for BE has been ever evolving with newer modalities being attempted for surveillance and cure. Esophagectomy has been the intervention of choice for HGD/EAC traditionally. However, with advances in endoscopic technology and morbidity associated with esophagectomy, endoscopic techniques are now increasingly been used for management. GERD has been the most significant risk factor underlying BE where PPIs are used as first-line therapy.[43] There is conflicting data on whether PPI reduces the risk of disease progression. Earlier reports suggested that long-term use of PPI is associated with increased risk of EAC. However, no causal association could be established with EAC in patients of BE with long-term PPI use, and hence, they are prescribed when required.

In a meta-analysis including 2,813 patients with BE, use of PPIs was associated with a decreased risk of EAC.[44] In another recent meta-analysis including 5,712 patients with BE, PPIs were found to have no association with the risk of EAC and HGD in patients with BE and there is no protective effect of PPI in setting of BE.[45] Thus, PPI improves quality of life by controlling symptoms, but its role in preventing disease progression is debatable.

Surgical Therapy

Both acid and bile refluxate are implicated in the pathogenesis of EAC. PPIs reduce the acid production and thus reduce injury to the epithelial cells. However, they do not prevent reflux. Fundoplication partial or complete decreases both acid and bile reflux and hence should prevent EAC in patients of BE. In a multicenter RCT, The LOTUS trial, PPI therapy was compared to antireflux surgery in patients of BE. In this study, pH study at 6 months follow-up demonstrated significantly improved scores for those randomized to laparoscopic antireflux surgery compared with PPIs (13.2% to 0.4% and 7.4% to 4.9%, respectively; P = 0.002).[46] Another study concluded that dysplasia and IM may regress postantireflux surgery.[47]

A cohort of 946 patients who underwent antireflux surgery when compared to a matched control of GERD patients showed no reduced risk of EAC.[48] In another meta-analysis including 34 studies, incidence of EAC in patients who underwent antireflux surgery was found to be 3.8 per 1,000 patient years compared to 5.3 per 1,000 patient years in patients taking PPI. Given the very low incidence of EAC in BE, this did not reach statistical significance.[49] Finally, recent systematic review and meta-analysis found out incidence rate ratio (IRR) in antireflux surgery arm was significantly lower compared to the medical management arm for EAC.[50] Thus, there is evidence now that antireflux surgery may prevent EAC better than medical management arm in patients with BE. However, even after antireflux procedure risk of EAC is more compared to general population hence continued surveillance is recommended.

Low-grade Dysplasia

In the patients of BE with the diagnosis of LGD in surveillance, confirmation is needed by one additional expert pathologist. When there is doubt of LGD, repeat EGD and biopsy is performed after optimizing PPI therapy, within 6 months. In such cases, if LGD is confirmed then patients may undergo some form of endoscopic therapy for eradication of abnormal mucosa followed by continued surveillance. There is enough evidence now that treatment of BE with LGD by ablation of abnormal mucosa decreases further progression compared to surveillance alone. In a multicenter RCT (SURF trial), which included a total of 136 patients of BE with LGD, radiofrequency ablation (RFA) resulted in reduced risk of progression to HGD or EAC than surveillance alone.[51] Surveillance alone is an alternate to the ablation therapy in such patients in view of slow rate of progression of LGD to EAC.[38]

High-grade Dysplasia

Patients of BE with HGD should undergo endoscopic treatment as the risk of malignant change is very high. Management also depends upon pathological findings, general condition of patient, their estimated life expectancy, and availability of resources. If a patient with biopsy proven HGD has a gross lesion (like mucosal nodularity or an ulcer) on endoscopy, it should be subjected to endoscopic resection first and then endoscopic ablation therapy.[19,52] Vagal-sparing esophagectomy is performed in centers where endoscopic techniques are not available.

Indefinite for Dysplasia

If diagnosis of dysplasia is equivocal on microscopic evaluation pathologist reports such findings as indefinite for dysplasia (IND). Repeat endoscopy and biopsy is recommended after treatment with PPI for 3 months. In a large cohort study, patients with a first diagnosis of IND in BE between 2002 and 2011 were selected from a nationwide registry of histopathology diagnosis in Netherlands. Patients were followed up until treatment for HGD or detection of EAC. In total, 1,258 patients met the inclusion criteria, of whom 842 (66.9%) underwent endoscopic follow-up. Patients were followed for a total of 2,585 person-years. The progression rate from IND to the combined endpoint of HGD or EAC was 2.0 and progression to EAC was 1.2.[53] Treatment summary for Barrett's esophagus is given in Table 3.

Endoscopic Ablative Therapies

The common modalities in endoscopic ablative therapy are RFA, cryoablation, argon plasma coagulation (APC), and photodynamic therapy (PDT).

Radiofrequency Ablation

The RFA is most studied and preferable mode of endoscopic ablation. It consists of series of electrodes, which ablate the Barrett's mucosa by radiofrequency energy. It has ability to deliver uniform ablation to a consistent depth of esophageal wall. The circumferential BE longer than 3 cm (long segment) is ablated by circumferential technique and noncircumferential segments or segment shorter than 3 cm (short segment) are ablated by focal technique. Endoscopy is repeated after 8–12 weeks to ablate any residual areas. A randomized sham-controlled trial concluded that RFA is highly effective at removing all IM evident on histopathology examination. Procedure is safe and compared to controls ablation group had reduced risk of EAC.[54] Recurrence of IM or dysplasia can occur after complete eradication of IM, hence ongoing surveillance is mandatory.

In a meta-analysis of 18 studies including 3,802 patients, complete eradication of IM was achieved in 78% of patients and complete eradication of dysplasia was achieved in 91%. After treatment, IM recurred in 13%.[55]

Table 3: Treatment summary of Barrett's esophagus.

Endoscopy findings at surveillance		Management guidelines as per American College of Gastroenterology (ACG)	Remark
No dysplasia		Repeat endoscopy and biopsy in 3–5-years interval	As per BOB CAT Consensus, routine endoscopy is not indicated
			No surveillance, if life expectancy < 5 years
			As per British Society of Gastroenterologist (BSG) For short (<3 cm) BE endoscopy every 3–5 years, interval may be reduced to 2–3 years if long-segment BE (>3 cm)
IDN (indefinite for dysplasia)		Confirmation by two experienced pathologists. Optimize PPI and repeat endoscopy in 6 months	Endoscopy within 6–12 months as per various consensuses
LGD	Flat mucosa	Confirmation by two expert pathologist Offer RFA, then continued yearly surveillance In case, if patients do not receive any therapy continued 6 monthly surveillance	6 monthly as per BSG, ACG 6–12 months as per BOB-CAT consensus
	Nodular	EMR for staging. If LGD confirmed, offer RFA, then continued yearly surveillance In case if patients do not receive any therapy continued 6 monthly surveillance	6 monthly as per BSG, ACG 6–12 months as per BOB CAT consensus
HGD or T1a stage	Flat mucosa	Confirmation by two expert pathologists. RFA is recommended	Following ablation continued surveillance
	Nodular	EMR of nodule. Confirmation by two expert pathologists RFA is recommended to ablate rest of the BE	

(BOB CAT: Benign Barrett's and CAncer Taskforce; HGD: high-grade dysplasia; LGD: low-grade dysplasia; PPI: proton pump inhibitor; RFA: radiofrequency ablation)

Lugiano et al.[56] did a comprehensive review in 2016, which showed that overall effectiveness of RFA in eradicating dysplasia ranges from 61.5% to 100%; whereas, the success of eradication of IM ranges from 61.5% to 91%. Post-treatment stricture formation is a most common complication (5–6%). The other complications include chest pain (3–5%), bleeding (1%), ulceration, and perforation (rare).

Cryotherapy

Cryotherapy involves the principle of rapid freezing and slow thawing of tissue in multiple cycles leading to immediate cellular injury. The cryogens used in BE ablation are liquid nitrogen, nitrous oxide, and liquid carbon dioxide. Cryotherapy system uses spray catheter through working channel of standard endoscope, which delivers low pressure (<5 psi) liquid nitrogen (−196°C) with 25 W of energy. Rapid cooling and thawing leads to intracellular ice crystal formation and cell rupture. It is less expensive compared to RFA. Cryotherapy can be used in BE refractory to RFA.

In a single-center retrospective study, a total of 32 patients with BE-HGD underwent cryotherapy every 8 weeks until complete eradication of HGD (CE-HGD) and intestinal metaplasia (CE-IM). CE-HGD was 31/32 (97%), and CE-IM was 26/32 (81%).[57] In a retrospective study of 78 patients with neoplastic BE who had not undergone previous ablation (treatment-naïve group) or who had persistent or recurrent neoplasia despite previous treatment (rescue treatment group) were enrolled. At 1 year, the overall complete response rates were 77% for cancer (10/13), 89% for dysplasia (57/64), and 94% for HGD.[58]

Cryotherapy is especially helpful in patients with high-grade dysplasia or intramucosal cancer with a nodular surface in an area in which it is difficult to perform endoscopic resection due to scarring from acid reflux or prior therapy. The disadvantages include difficulty in delivering the liquid nitrogen and gaseous distension leading to perforation. Other challenge is visibility during procedure, which is hampered due to frost created by freezing of the tissues.[59]

Argon Plasma Coagulation

Argon plasma coagulation is also a no contact technique in which ionized argon gas is sprayed to cause tissue coagulation. Depth of necrosis is more predictable compared to cryotherapy. In a RCT of 58 patients with more than 5 years of follow-up, APC demonstrated 95% regression of IM with no incidence of HGD compared to surveillance alone.[60] In a long-term (16 years) follow-up Study by Milashks et al. (NDBE 28, LGD 5), 32 patients underwent multiple treatment (1 to 5) sessions. At 16 years, 16 patients (50%) had sustained eradication, and 11 (35%) had partial eradication. 6% were lost to follow-up. Carcinoma occurred in three patients (9%).[58] The major disadvantage of APC is stricture formation and subsquamous Barrett's. To overcome this problem, a hybrid APC technique was introduced recently, the Barrett epithelium is lifted with a saline injection using a high-pressure water jet, creating a safety cushion under the mucosa thus a safe and complete eradication of Barrett's epithelium is obtained. Hybrid APC has a longer procedural time and technically challenging and it is not preferred in Barrett's more than 5 cm.[61] The complication of APC includes self-limiting odynophagia or dysphagia. Stenosis (3-4%) and perforation (2%) is rare.

Photodynamic Therapy

Photodynamic therapy works on the principle that once a photosensitizer is administered and activated by light, free radicals like superoxide and hydroxyl are produced causing apoptosis of cell. The metaplastic and neoplastic cells have more affinity for photosensitizer, thus it can damage BE epithelium-sparing normal squamous mucosa. The commonly used photosensitizers are porfimer sodium (IV), 5-aminolevulinic acid (orally), and m-tetra(hydroxyphenyl) chlorin (IV). After administration of the photosensitizer, endoscopy is performed and red light is transmitted either by optical fibres or balloon-diffusing fibers through endoscope. In these patients, endoscopy is repeated after 2-3 days, and extent of mucosal damage is assessed. The efficacy of PDT is predicted by the length of BE. Patients with BE more than 3 cm are less likely to have complete eradication in comparison to those with BE less than 3 cm.[62,63]

The most common side effect of PDT is photosensitivity (6%). Patients are advised to apply sunscreen, fully cover the exposed body part in sunlight for 4-6 week. Stricture of esophagus is also reported. The other minor side effects are vomiting, dyspepsia, and chest pain.[62,63]

Endoscopic Resection

Endoscopic resection includes endoscopic mucosal resection (EMR), serial radical endoscopic resection (SRER) involving resection in piecemeal of entire IM and endoscopic submucosal dissection (ESD). EMR is performed by two methods—lift suck cut technique or ligate and cut technique. The ligate and cut technique is commonly used due to shorter resection time and cost-effectiveness. In ligate and cut technique, after introduction of scope into esophagus, the lesion is sucked into a cup and the lesion is resected with snare. In lift suck cut technique, submucosa is lifted by normal saline injection, following which a pseudopolyp is created by suctioning the lesion into the cap and base is cut with snare. The EMR is an effective method of complete eradication of BE. However, studies have also shown good result by combining EMR with PDT or RFA. The CE-IM rate for combined therapy is between 82% and 96%. The complication rates are also low in combined technique for treating BE. Bleeding and stricture with EMR are 1.2% and 1%, respectively. Perforation is rare (0.2-1.3%). Limitation of EMR is that it cannot be used for en bloc resection of lesion greater than 2 cm.[63,64]

Endoscopic submucosal dissection technique was initially developed for the resection of early gastric neoplasm and now is being used for resection of early neoplastic lesions in other parts of gastrointestinal tract (GIT). ESD has advantage over EMR in its ability to resect out lesions en bloc (including large lesions). In this technique, the lesion is marked with electrocautery circumferentially. The submucosa is infiltrated with solution; circumferential incision is made with electrosurgical knife. Then, careful dissection at submucosa results in en bloc removal of lesion. The complete and curative resection rates for ESD are 74.5% and 64.9%, respectively; and incidence of recurrence after complete resection is 0.17%.[63,65]

Endoscopic submucosal dissection has limitations as it is time consuming; requires more training and expertise and steep learning curve. The complication rate of ESD is slightly higher than EMR. Bleeding, perforation, and stricture have been reported as 1.5%, 1.7%, and 11.6%, respectively.[65]

Endoscopic resection has an advantage of providing tissue for histopathological examination and can provide staging information (T stage). In a meta-analysis of 22 studies, efficacy of endoscopic resection and RFA was compared. Dysplasia was eradicated in 95% of patients after EMR and 92% after RFA. After a median follow-up of 23 months for complete EMR and 21 months for RFA, eradication of dysplasia was maintained in 95% of patients treated with complete EMR and 94% treated with RFA. Study reported high rate of stricture formation with EMR.[66]

Chemoprevention

Various chemopreventive agents such as statins, aspirin, and PPI have been used for BE. Recent meta-analysis performed shows reduced risk of EAC with aspirin and statins. Corley et al. performed meta-analysis of nine studies involving 1,813 patients. Study concluded reduced risk of EAC with intake of aspirin (OR = 0.82; CI: 0.67-0.99).[67] In the meta-analysis performed by Alexander et al., it was concluded that intake of statins reduces risk of EAC [pooled effect size of 0.86 (95% CI: 0.78-0.94, P = 0.001, I2 = 0%) for risk of EAC].[68] A large prospective RCT was conducted in UK and Canada—the ASPECT trial. A total of 2,557 patients were enrolled with the primary composite endpoint was time to all-cause mortality, EAC, or HGD. Patients were randomized; only PPI in low dose (n = 705), high dose PPI (n = 704), low-dose PPI and aspirin (571), high dose PPI and aspirin (n = 577). Median follow-up was 8.9 years. It was concluded that high-dose PPI with aspirin had strongest protective effect. Chemoprevention in BE is currently not recommended but may find its place in future when more evidence is available.[69]

CONCLUSION

Barrett's esophagus is a common disease with a potential for developing into EAC. Although the condition has been described since a long time, diagnosis and management strategies are ever evolving. Accurate and early diagnosis of dysplasia and adenocarcinoma are key aspects in the management. Endoscopy and biopsy are still the gold standard for diagnosis although less invasive modalities like cytosponge have shown promising result. Biomarker such as p53 is also under evaluation for predicting malignancy. Endoscopic ablative techniques have widely replaced surgical procedures for management of Barrett's and RFA being the most preferred modality. Role of chemopreventive agents is under evaluation with some encouraging results.

REFERENCES

1. Sharma P, McQuaid K, Dent J, et al. A critical review of the diagnosis and management of Barrett's esophagus: the AGA Chicago Workshop. Gastroenterology. 2004;127(1):310-30.
2. Barrett NR. The lower esophagus lined by columnar epithelium. Surgery. 1957;41(6):881-94.
3. Runge TM, Abrams JA, Shaheen NJ. Epidemiology of Barrett's esophagus and esophageal adenocarcinoma. Gastroenterol Clin North Am. 2015;44(2):203-31.
4. Shiota S, Singh S, Anshasi A, et al. The prevalence of Barrett's esophagus in Asian countries: A systematic review and meta-analysis. Clin Gastroenterol Hepatol Off Clin Pract J Am Gastroenterol Assoc. 2015;13(11):1907-18.
5. Corley DA, Kubo A, Levin TR, et al. Abdominal obesity and body mass index as risk factors for Barrett's esophagus. Gastroenterology. 2007;133(1):34-41; quiz 311.
6. Edelstein ZR, Farrow DC, Bronner MP, et al. Central adiposity and risk of Barrett's esophagus. Gastroenterology. 2007;133(2):403-11.
7. Ronkainen J, Talley NJ, Storskrubb T, et al. Erosive esophagitis is a risk factor for Barrett's esophagus: A community-based endoscopic follow-up study. Am J Gastroenterol. 2011;106(11):1946-52.
8. Orloff M, Peterson C, He X, et al. Germline mutations in MSR1, ASCC1, and CTHRC1 in patients with Barrett esophagus and esophageal adenocarcinoma. JAMA. 2011;306(4):410-9.
9. Su Z, Gay LJ, Strange A, et al. Common variants at the MHC locus and at chromosome 16q24.1 predispose to Barrett's esophagus. Nat Genet. 2012;44(10):1131-6.

10. Thota PN, Vennalaganti P, Vennelaganti S, et al. Low risk of high-grade dysplasia or esophageal adenocarcinoma among patients with Barrett's esophagus less than 1 cm (irregular Z line) within 5 years of index endoscopy. Gastroenterology. 2017;152(5):987-92.
11. Singh S, Manickam P, Amin AV, et al. Incidence of esophageal adenocarcinoma in Barrett's esophagus with low-grade dysplasia: A systematic review and meta-analysis. Gastrointest Endosc. 2014;79(6):897-909.e4; quiz 983.e1, 983.e3.
12. Heitmiller RF, Redmond M, Hamilton SR. Barrett's esophagus with high-grade dysplasia: An indication for prophylactic esophagectomy. Ann Surg. 1996;224(1):66-71.
13. Schnell TG, Sontag SJ, Chejfec G, et al. Long-term nonsurgical management of Barrett's esophagus with high-grade dysplasia. Gastroenterology. 2001;120(7): 1607-19.
14. Dar MS, Goldblum JR, Rice TW, et al. Can extent of high grade dysplasia in Barrett's oesophagus predict the presence of adenocarcinoma at oesophagectomy? Gut. 2003;52(4):486-9.
15. Buttar NS, Wang KK, Sebo TJ, et al. Extent of high-grade dysplasia in Barrett's esophagus correlates with risk of adenocarcinoma. Gastroenterology. 2001;120(7):1630-9.
16. Sharma P, Dent J, Armstrong D, et al. The development and validation of an endoscopic grading system for Barrett's esophagus: The Prague C&M Criteria. Gastroenterology. 2006;131(5):1392-9.
17. Harrison R, Perry I, Haddadin W, et al. Detection of intestinal metaplasia in Barrett's esophagus: An observational comparator study suggests the need for a minimum of eight biopsies. Am J Gastroenterol. 2007;102(6):1154-61.
18. Shariff MK, Varghese S, O'Donovan M, et al. Pilot randomized crossover study comparing the efficacy of transnasal disposable endosheath with standard endoscopy to detect Barrett's esophagus. Endoscopy. 2016;48(2):110-6.
19. Fitzgerald RC, di Pietro M, Ragunath K, et al. British Society of Gastroenterology guidelines on the diagnosis and management of Barrett's oesophagus. Gut. 2014;63(1):7-42.
20. Schlemper R, Riddell R, Kato Y, et al. The Vienna classification of gastrointestinal epithelial neoplasia. Gut. 2000;47(2):251-5.
21. Reid B. Optimizing endoscopic biopsy detection of early cancers in Barrett's high-grade dysplasia. Am J Gastroenterol. 2000;95:3089-96.
22. Curvers WL, Peters FP, Elzer B, et al. Quality of Barrett's surveillance in the Netherlands: a standardized review of endoscopy and pathology reports. Eur J Gastroenterol Hepatol. 2008;20(7):601-7.
23. Kastelein F, Biermann K, Steyerberg EW, et al. Aberrant p53 protein expression is associated with an increased risk of neoplastic progression in patients with Barrett's oesophagus. Gut. 2013;62(12):1676-83.
24. Fouad YM, Mostafa I, Yehia R, et al. Biomarkers of Barrett's esophagus. World J Gastrointest Pathophysiol. 2014;5(4):450-6.
25. Kadri SR, Lao-Sirieix P, O'Donovan M, et al. Acceptability and accuracy of a non-endoscopic screening test for Barrett's oesophagus in primary care: Cohort study. BMJ. 2010;341:c4372.

26. Ross-Innes CS, Chettouh H, Achilleos A, et al. Risk stratification of Barrett's oesophagus using a non-endoscopic sampling method coupled with a biomarker panel: a cohort study. Lancet Gastroenterol Hepatol. 2017;2(1):23-31.
27. Offman J, Muldrew B, O'Donovan M, et al. Barrett's oesophagus trial 3 (BEST3): study protocol for a randomised controlled trial comparing the cytosponge-TFF3 test with usual care to facilitate the diagnosis of oesophageal pre-cancer in primary care patients with chronic acid reflux. BMC Cancer. 2018;18(1):784.
28. Mannath J, Subramanian V, Hawkey CJ, et al. Narrow band imaging for characterization of high grade dysplasia and specialized intestinal metaplasia in Barrett's esophagus: A meta-analysis. Endoscopy. 2010;42(5):351-9.
29. Ngamruengphong S, Sharma VK, Das A. Diagnostic yield of methylene blue chromoendoscopy for detecting specialized intestinal metaplasia and dysplasia in Barrett's esophagus: A meta-analysis. Gastrointest Endosc. 2009;69(6):1021-8.
30. Coletta M, Sami SS, Nachiappan A, et al. Acetic acid chromoendoscopy for the diagnosis of early neoplasia and specialized intestinal metaplasia in Barrett's esophagus: A meta-analysis. Gastrointest Endosc. 2016;83(1):57-67.e1.
31. Chauhan SS, Abu Dayyeh BK, Bhat YM, et al. Confocal laser endomicroscopy. Gastrointest Endosc. 2014;80(6):928-38.
32. Dunbar KB, Okolo P, Montgomery E, et al. Confocal laser endomicroscopy in Barrett's esophagus and endoscopically inapparent Barrett's neoplasia: A prospective, randomized, double-blind, controlled, crossover trial. Gastrointest Endosc. 2009;70(4):645-54.
33. Haringsma J, Tytgat GN. Fluorescence and autofluorescence. Baillieres Best Pract Res Clin Gastroenterol. 1999;13(1):1-10.
34. Kara MA, Peters FP, Ten Kate FJW, et al. Endoscopic video autofluorescence imaging may improve the detection of early neoplasia in patients with Barrett's esophagus. Gastrointest Endosc. 2005;61(6):679-85.
35. Aziz M, Fatima R. Future of diagnosing neoplasia in Barrett's esophagus: volumetric laser endomicroscopy. Clin J Gastroenterol. 2018;11(3):179-83.
36. Swager A, van der Sommen F, Klomp S, et al. Computer-aided detection of early Barrett's neoplasia using volumetric laser endomicroscopy. Gastrointest Endosc. 2017;86:839-46.
37. American Gastroenterological Association, Spechler SJ, Sharma P, et al. American Gastroenterological Association medical position statement on the management of Barrett's esophagus. Gastroenterology. 2011;140(3):1084-91.
38. Shaheen NJ, Falk GW, Iyer PG, et al. ACG clinical guideline: Diagnosis and management of Barrett's esophagus. Am J Gastroenterol. 2016;111(1):30-50.
39. Corley DA, Mehtani K, Quesenberry C, et al. Impact of endoscopic surveillance on mortality from Barrett's esophagus-associated esophageal adenocarcinomas. Gastroenterology. 2013;145(2):312-19.e1.
40. Grant KS, DeMeester SR, Kreger V, et al. Effect of Barrett's esophagus surveillance on esophageal preservation, tumor stage, and survival with esophageal adenocarcinoma. J Thorac Cardiovasc Surg. 2013;146(1):31-7.
41. Verbeek RE, Leenders M, Ten Kate FJW, et al. Surveillance of Barrett's esophagus and mortality from esophageal adenocarcinoma: A population-based cohort study. Am J Gastroenterol. 2014;109(8):1215-22.

42. Old O, Moayyedi P, Love S, et al. Barrett's Oesophagus Surveillance versus Endoscopy at Need Study (BOSS): protocol and analysis plan for a multicentre randomized controlled trial. J Med Screen. 2015;22(3):158-64.
43. Brown CS, Lapin B, Wang C, et al. Reflux control is important in the management of Barrett's Esophagus: results from a retrospective 1,830 patient cohort. Surg Endosc. 2015;29(12):3528-34.
44. Singh S, Garg SK, Singh PP, et al. Acid-suppressive medications and risk of oesophageal adenocarcinoma in patients with Barrett's oesophagus: A systematic review and meta-analysis. Gut. 2014;63(8):1229-37.
45. Hu Q, Sun T-T, Hong J, et al. Proton pump inhibitors do not reduce the risk of esophageal adenocarcinoma in patients with Barrett's esophagus: A systematic review and meta-analysis. PLoS One. 2017;12(1):e0169691.
46. Attwood SE, Lundell L, Hatlebakk JG, et al. Medical or surgical management of GERD patients with Barrett's esophagus: The LOTUS trial 3-year experience. J Gastrointest Surg Off J Soc Surg Aliment Tract. 2008;12(10):1646-54; discussion 1654-1655.
47. Hofstetter WL, Peters JH, DeMeester TR, et al. Long-term outcome of antireflux surgery in patients with Barrett's esophagus. Ann Surg. 2001;234(4):532-8; discussion 538-539.
48. Tran T, Spechler SJ, Richardson P, et al. Fundoplication and the risk of esophageal cancer in gastroesophageal reflux disease: A Veterans Affairs cohort study. Am J Gastroenterol. 2005;100(5):1002-8.
49. Corey KE, Schmitz SM, Shaheen NJ. Does a surgical antireflux procedure decrease the incidence of esophageal adenocarcinoma in Barrett's esophagus? A meta-analysis. Am J Gastroenterol. 2003;98(11):2390-4.
50. Maret-Ouda J, Konings P, Lagergren J, et al. Antireflux surgery and risk of esophageal adenocarcinoma: A systematic review and meta-analysis. Ann Surg. 2016;263(2):251-7.
51. Phoa KN, van Vilsteren FGI, Weusten BLAM, et al. Radiofrequency ablation vs endoscopic surveillance for patients with Barrett's esophagus and low-grade dysplasia: A randomized clinical trial. JAMA. 2014;311(12):1209-17.
52. Standards of Practice Committee, Wani S, Qumseya B, et al. Endoscopic eradication therapy for patients with Barrett's esophagus-associated dysplasia and intramucosal cancer. Gastrointest Endosc. 2018;87(4):907-31.e9.
53. Kestens C, Leenders M, Offerhaus GJA, et al. Risk of neoplastic progression in Barrett's esophagus diagnosed as indefinite for dysplasia: A nationwide cohort study. Endoscopy. 2015;47(5):409-14.
54. Shaheen NJ, Sharma P, Overholt BF, et al. Radiofrequency ablation in Barrett's esophagus with dysplasia. N Engl J Med. 2009;360(22):2277-88.
55. Orman ES, Li N, Shaheen NJ. Efficacy and durability of radiofrequency ablation for Barrett's Esophagus: Systematic review and meta-analysis. Clin Gastroenterol Hepatol Off Clin Pract J Am Gastroenterol Assoc. 2013;11(10):1245-55.
56. Luigiano C, Iabichino G, Eusebi LH, et al. Outcomes of radiofrequency ablation for dysplastic Barrett's esophagus: A comprehensive review. Gastroenterol Res Pract. 2016;2016:1-8.

57. Gosain S, Mercer K, Twaddell WS, et al. Liquid nitrogen spray cryotherapy in Barrett's esophagus with high-grade dysplasia: Long-term results. Gastrointest Endosc. 2013;78(2):260-5.
58. Canto MI, Shin EJ, Khashab MA, et al. Safety and efficacy of carbon dioxide cryotherapy for treatment of neoplastic Barrett's esophagus. Endoscopy. 2015;47(7):582-91.
59. Dumot J. The use of cryotherapy for treatment of Barrett's esophagus. Gastroenterol Hepatol. 2013;9(12):811-3.
60. Bright T, Watson DI, Tam W, et al. Randomized trial of argon plasma coagulation versus endoscopic surveillance for Barrett's esophagus after antireflux surgery: Late results. Ann Surg. 2007;246(6):1016-20.
61. Pech O. (2017). Hybrid Argon Plasma Coagulation in Patients with Barrett's Esophagus. [online] Available from *https://www.ncbi.nlm.nih.gov/pmc/articles/PMC5718177/*. [Accessed December, 2018].
62. Dunn JM, Mackenzie GD, Banks MR, et al. A randomised controlled trial of ALA vs. Photofrin photodynamic therapy for high-grade dysplasia arising in Barrett's oesophagus. Lasers Med Sci. 2013;28:707-15.
63. Singh T, Sanaka MR, Thota PN. Endoscopic therapy for Barrett's esophagus and early esophageal cancer: Where do we go from here? World J Gastrointest Endosc. 2018;10(9):165-74.
64. Desai M, Saligram S, Gupta N, et al. Efficacy and safety outcomes of multimodal endoscopic eradication therapy in Barrett's esophagus-related neoplasia: A systematic review and pooled analysis. Gastrointest Endosc. 2017;85:482-95.e4.
65. Yang D, Zou F, Xiong S, et al. Endoscopic submucosal dissection for early Barrett's neoplasia: A meta-analysis. Gastrointest Endosc. 2018;87:1383-93.
66. Chadwick G, Groene O, Markar SR, et al. Systematic review comparing radiofrequency ablation and complete endoscopic resection in treating dysplastic Barrett's esophagus: A critical assessment of histologic outcomes and adverse events. Gastrointest Endosc. 2014;79(5):718-31.e3.
67. Corley DA, Kerlikowske K, Verma R, et al. Protective association of aspirin/NSAIDs and esophageal cancer: a systematic review and meta-analysis. Gastroenterology. 2003;124(1):47-56.
68. Alexandre L, Clark AB, Cheong E, et al. Systematic review: potential preventive effects of statins against oesophageal adenocarcinoma. Aliment Pharmacol Ther. 2012;36(4):301-11.
69. Jankowski JAZ, de Caestecker J, Love SB, et al. Esomeprazole and aspirin in Barrett's oesophagus (AspECT): A randomised factorial trial. Lancet Lond Engl. 2018;392(10145):400-8.

Chapter 7

Borderline Resectable and Locally Advanced Pancreatic Cancer

Manish S Bhandare, Vikram Chaudhari, Shailesh V Shrikhande

INTRODUCTION

Worldwide, pancreatic cancer accounts for more than 200,000 deaths every year, being the 13th most common cancer and the 8th most frequent cause of death from cancer. 5-year survival in patients with pancreatic cancer, for all stages remains as low as 6–7%. The low survival rate is attributed to several factors, of which perhaps the most important one, apart from aggressive tumor biology, is the late stage at which most patients are diagnosed. Most patients with pancreatic cancer are asymptomatic until the disease develops to an advanced stage. Only 10–20% of patients are eligible for resection at presentation, 30–40% are unresectable/locally advanced and 50–60% are metastatic.[1] In absence of metastatic disease, the most important factor for improving survival and possibly offer cure is to achieve a margin negative resection. Even after potential curative resection, most patients develop recurrences eventually, and 5-year survival of completely resected patients is only up to 25%.[1] The aggressive tumor biology contributes to early recurrence and metastasis, and resistance to chemotherapy and radiotherapy.

Pancreatic cancer has been broadly classified into resectable, locally advanced and metastatic disease. One promising development in recent years has been the description of a new subgroup within the locally advanced tumors of *borderline resectable pancreatic cancer* (BRPC) comprising of approximately 5–10% of total patient population. The term BRPC became more formal after its recognition and inclusion as a unique subcategory by National Comprehensive Cancer Network (NCCN) in 2006. Although its exact definition has been refined over past few years depending on the vascular involvement around the tumor, the term was initially proposed for tumors which are at a high-risk of having margin positivity after resection. This concept was brought in with a view of extending benefit of surgery and improving survival of these advanced tumors, and so far the results are encouraging. This chapter will discuss about diagnosis, evaluation and treatment of borderline resectable and locally advanced unresectable pancreatic cancer.

EVALUATION AND WORKUP

In general, the diagnostic evaluation of a patient with suspected pancreatic cancer includes serologic evaluation and abdominal imaging. Additional testing is then directed based upon the findings of the initial testing as well as patient's clinical presentation and risk factors. All patients presenting with jaundice or epigastric pain should have an assay of serum amino transferases, alkaline phosphatase, and bilirubin to determine if cholestasis is present. In addition, patients with epigastric pain and a history suggestive of acute pancreatitis should also be evaluated with a serum lipase.

- *Tumor markers*: Carbohydrate antigen 19-9 (CA 19-9).

Very high levels at presentation in absence of obstructive jaundice (> 500 U/mL) usually indicates advanced metastatic disease.[2,3]

- *Imaging modalities:*
    - Transabdominal ultrasonography
    - *CT scan*: Multidetector row computed tomography (MD-CT) with triphasic technique and 1-2 mm cuts enables most accurate assessment of resectability, vascular invasion,[4] diagnosis of metastatic lesions and at present, is the imaging modality of choice. The following CT findings aid in the diagnosis of pancreatic cancer.[5] For comprehensive imaging of a suspected pancreas cancer, the patient is usually scanned in several dynamic phases of contrast injection (termed as "pancreas protocol"):
        - The arterial phase of enhancement, which corresponds to the first 30 seconds after the start of the contrast injection, provides excellent opacification of the celiac axis, superior mesenteric artery (SMA), and peripancreatic arteries.
        - An attenuation difference between tumor and normal pancreas, which increases lesion conspicuity, is best achieved after peak enhancement of the aorta in the arterial phase but before peak enhancement of the liver, which occurs in the portal venous phase, at 40-50 seconds after contrast injection. This is sometimes termed the "pancreatic phase".
        - The venous phase, which is obtained at 60-70 seconds after the start of the contrast injection, provides better enhancement of the superior mesenteric vein, splenic and portal veins. In addition, peak hepatic enhancement, which optimizes the detection of hepatic metastases, also occurs in the portal venous phase.

Overall accuracy of MD-CT for diagnosis of pancreatic cancer is about 90%. MD-CT has an accuracy of 85–95% in determining resectability.[6,7]
- *MRI:* It has similar to the sensitivity (83%) and specificity (63–75%) as that of MDCT[8] for assessing the pancreatic lesion.
- *Positron emission tomography (PET):* Fludeoxyglucose (FDG)-PET plus CT has no obvious advantage for diagnosing pancreatic cancer compared with contrast-enhanced MDCT.[9] However, PET-CT in locally advanced lesions will help rule out distant metastases.[10]
- *Endoscopic ultrasonography:* Endoscopic ultrasonography (EUS) is recommended for assessing lesions not clearly detected, but suspected, on CT/MRI and in tumors considered 'borderline resectable' on MDCT to assess vascular involvement and obtain a tissue diagnosis that is essential since neoadjuvant treatment, if more often required in these tumors.

Image-guided or endoscopic biopsy is often performed in the beginning to establish tissue diagnosis, as most patients with borderline resectable and almost all with locally advanced disease will require chemotherapy or some form of neoadjuvant therapy.

DEFINITIONS

Based on the radiological criteria on MDCT images or contrast-enhanced MRI scan, the advanced but non-metastatic tumors are classified as borderline resectable or unresectable/locally advanced. The present anatomical definition of BRPC as proposed in NCCN 2016, divides tumors into pancreatic head/uncinate process and pancreatic body/tail and the extent of vascular invasion is detailed for each of the named veins and arteries. This definition avoided the use of ambiguous terms used in previous definitions such as vascular abutment, impingement, narrowing, encasement, invasion, adherence etc. and the degree of interface between tumor and vessels was defined as "less than 180°" or "180° or more" in an attempt at providing uniformity and standardization in reporting and documentation. Improvements in modern radiology have enabled superior assessment of vascular involvement and resectability in the arterial, pancreatic parenchymal and portal venous phase of the CT scan.

Locally Advanced/Unresectable Tumors

Local unresectability is usually (but not always) due to vascular invasion, particularly superior mesenteric artery (SMA) (Fig. 1A). According to the most widely followed NCCN consensus guidelines,[11] the characteristics that indicate unresectability are depicted in Box 1. Most of these patients will be managed non-surgically with initial chemotherapy with or without

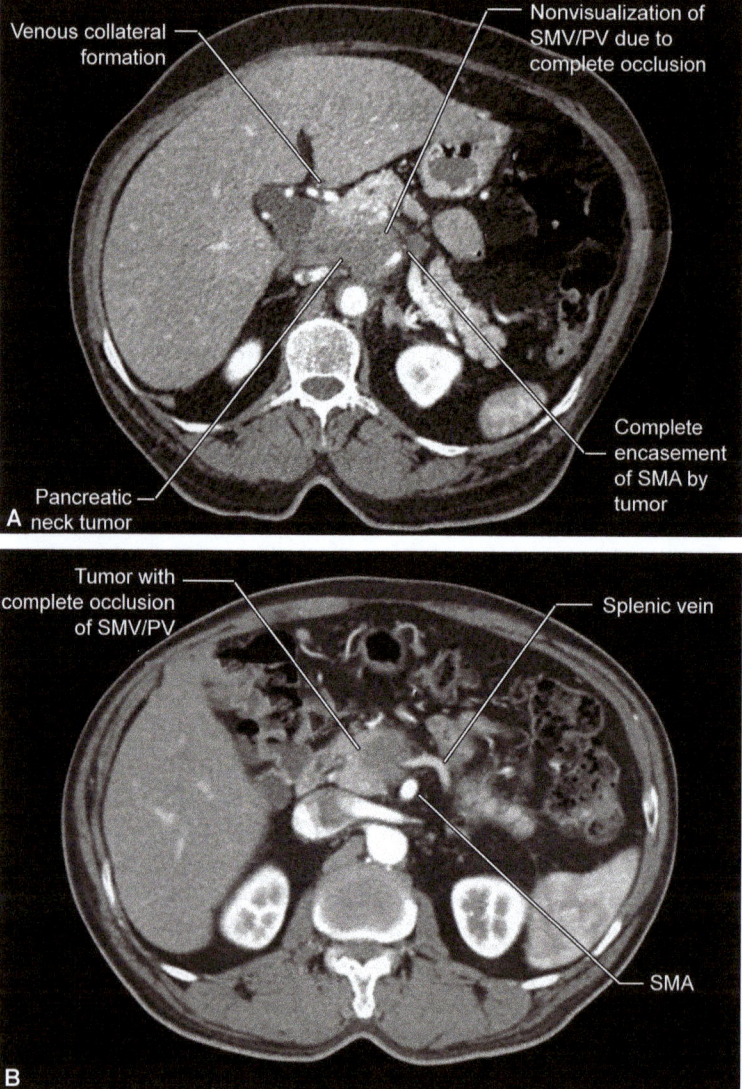

Figs. 1A and B: Radiological appearance: (A) Locally advanced pancreatic cancer; (B) Borderline resectable pancreatic cancer.

chemoradiotherapy, although there are some exceptions. Minority of these patients with excellent downstaging can be considered for surgical therapy.

Borderline Resectable Tumors

The initial definitions for BRPC were based solely on the tumor extension and involvement of the surrounding vasculature, viz. superior mesenteric artery (SMA), superior mesenteric/portal vein (SMV/PV), hepatic artery (HA)

> **Box 1:** Radiological criteria for unresectability.
>
> *For head pancreas lesions:*
> - Solid tumor contact with the superior mesenteric artery (SMA) >180°
> - Solid tumor contact with the celiac axis >180°
> - Solid tumor contact with the first jejunal SMA branch
> - Unreconstructable superior mesenteric (SMV) or portal vein (PV) stump due to tumor involvement
> - Contact with the most proximal draining jejunal branch into the SMV
>
> *Body and tail lesions:*
> - Solid tumor contact of >180° with the SMA or celiac axis
> - Solid tumor contact with the celiac axis and aortic involvement
> - Unreconstructable SMV or PV stump due to tumor involvement

> **Box 2:** Radiological criteria for borderline resectable tumors.
>
> *For tumors of the head or uncinate process*:
> - Solid tumor contact with the superior mesenteric (SMV) or portal vein (PV) of >180° with contour irregularity of the vein or thrombosis of the vein, but with suitable vessel proximal and distal to the site of involvement, allowing for safe and complete resection and vein reconstruction
> - Solid tumor contact with the inferior vena cava
> - Solid tumor contact with the common hepatic artery without extension to the celiac axis or hepatic artery bifurcation, allowing for safe and complete resection and arterial reconstruction
> - Solid tumor contact with the SMA ≤180°
> - Solid tumor contact with variable anatomy (e.g. accessory right hepatic artery, replaced right hepatic artery, replaced common hepatic artery, and the origin of replaced or accessory artery), and the presence and degree of tumor contact should be noted
>
> *For tumors of the body/tail*:
> - Solid tumor contact with the celiac axis of ≤180°
> - Solid tumor contact with the celiac axis >180° without involvement of the aorta and with an intact and uninvolved gastroduodenal artery, thereby permitting a modified Appleby procedure

and celiac artery (CA) seen on MDCT images i.e. anatomical criteria (Box 2), (Fig. 1B). However, the decision about whether a patient is offered a resection should not be based on anatomic criteria alone. The biological behavior of the cancer and the ability of the patient to withstand the physiological stress of complex and demanding surgery should play a very important role in the decision making process. The recent international consensus on definition and criteria of BRPC has defined patients with BRPC according to three distinct dimensions,[12] anatomical (A), biological (B), and conditional (C):

- The anatomical definition of BRPC is a tumor that is at high risk for margin-positive resection (R1 or R2) (Box 2).
- The biological definition of BRPC is when there are findings that raise the possibility (but not certainty) of extrapancreatic metastatic disease (high serum Ca 19-9 levels/radiologically suspected but unproven metastases).

- The conditional definition of BRPC is when the patient has a high risk for morbidity or mortality after surgery because of host-related factors including performance status and comorbidities.

These refinements in the various definitions and their worldwide adoption is expected to ensure standard reporting of outcomes that would ultimately help in establishing the best possible treatment approaches for this unique subset of pancreatic cancer.

PRINCIPLES OF MANAGEMENT

Treatment of borderline resectable and locally advanced pancreatic cancer now requires a multimodal approach ranging from surgery, chemotherapy, and radiation therapy to symptom relief and palliative care. In addition to the stage, baseline performance status, comorbidities, and goals of care should be taken into consideration before planning the treatment. In patients with BRPC, the likelihood of an incomplete (R1) resection is high. Hence, preferred approach is attempted downstaging with neoadjuvant chemotherapy or chemoradiotherapy and then reassessment for possible curative resection. Patients with unresectable/locally advanced disease are managed initially with chemotherapy (uncertain intent or even palliative intent) with or without radiotherapy.

All patients should have a full assessment of symptom burden, psychological status, and social support as early as possible. In most cases, this will indicate a need for formal palliative care consultation.[13] Early initiation of palliative care service improves quality of life and may prolong survival.

Management of Patients with a Borderline Performance Status with Obstructive Jaundice

Patients with elevated serum bilirubin with poor nutritional and overall performance status are particularly challenging. These patients are generally not considered fit to receive any cancer directed therapy at least at presentation. An individualized decision must be made with regard to suitability for neoadjuvant therapy and the specific approach to be used.

- The first step is to relieve jaundice via endoscopic retrograde pancreatography (ERCP) and placement of a short self-expanding metal stent (SEMS). If ERCP is not feasible due to technical considerations, a transhepatic drainage should be performed. When adequate biliary drainage is achieved (serum bilirubin less than 3 mg%), consideration could be given to dose-adjusted FOLFIRINOX or gemcitabine/nab-paclitaxel with close monitoring of toxicities.
- For patients with poor performance status (>2), the first priority is given to perform measures to improve general condition. For instance, to

treat any recent infection (e.g. cholangitis) with adequate antibiotics, to relieve gastric outlet obstruction and improve nutrition by placement of nasojejunal tube, self-expanding metal stents or by performing a gastrojejunostomy. These patients' best subjected to single agent gemcitabine chemotherapy.

Borderline Resectable Pancreatic Cancer

The management of borderline resectable pancreatic cancer (BRPC) is evolving. While precisely defining BRPC is important, the fundamental question "what is best suited treatment approach?" is still unanswered. The current management strategies include:
- Surgery first followed by adjuvant chemotherapy +/– radiotherapy
- Neoadjuvant chemotherapy (NACT) followed by surgery
- Neoadjuvant chemoradiotherapy (NACT–RT) followed by surgery

The International Study Group of Pancreatic Surgery (ISGPS) consensus statement does recommend upfront resection for tumors with isolated venous involvement. On the other hand, neoadjuvant therapy is increasingly utilized and there are numerous published studies which use one or more neoadjuvant regimens, either in the form of chemoradiation or chemotherapy with reported benefits.

When to Consider Neoadjuvant Therapy?

Although the concept of using neoadjuvant therapy is to downsize the tumor and enable margin negative resection, a number of patients with BRPC can also receive an R0 resection without downsizing, e.g. small volume disease with short segment of SMV/PV involvement of less than 180°. These patients if subjected to neoadjuvant therapy are at a risk of disease progression which is reported to be in the range of 10–40%.[14,15] Clearly, there is still a role of upfront surgery in these patients. Our own high-volume experience at the Tata Memorial Hospital seems to suggest that all patients need not receive neoadjuvant treatment and well-selected patients can receive margin negative upfront surgical resections.[16]

However, the rationale for neoadjuvant therapy is not only to minimize the risk of a positive resection margin, but also to treat occult systemic disease. Unfortunately, there have been no randomized clinical trials (RCT) addressing the impact of neoadjuvant therapy on overall survival as against upfront surgery. Lower levels of evidence do suggest improvement in R0 resections but that has not translated into improved overall or disease-free survival. Future clinical trials should be planned to see the actual long-term benefits with neoadjuvant approaches.

Neoadjuvant Chemotherapy or Neoadjuvant Chemoradiotherapy

The type of neoadjuvant regimen is another issue to be addressed in absence of any high level of evidence. A recent systematic review failed to arrive at any conclusion on this and hence the best regimen for neoadjuvant therapy is still unknown.[17] Amongst the chemotherapy options, FOLFIRINOX regimen has been shown to be the most effective protocol resulting in a significantly better resection rate and overall survival than other regimens.[16] Its main drawback is severe adverse events due to toxicity especially in elderly patients with comorbidities approaching about 30–40%. These key findings need to be factored carefully in the light of the new anatomical, biological and conditional definition of BRPC.

The combination of chemotherapy with radiation in neoadjuvant setting is used with a desire of achieving superior response rates and better sterility of margins in BRPC. There have been increasing reports showing improvement in margin negative R0 resections with this approach.[17] Again the problem is toxicity and the treatment completion rates. A recent and the only RCT, using neoadjuvant chemoradiation for BRPC from Korea showed a survival advantage with chemoradiation over upfront surgery.[18] In absence of more such higher level of evidences and the lack of consensus on dose and mode of delivery of radiation [conventional versus stereotactic body radiotherapy (SBRT)], it still cannot be considered as standard of care despite the promising results of the Korean study.

In experienced centers, SBRT could be considered an alternative to conventional fractionation chemoradiotherapy although there is lack of any comparative trials and the general consensus is to use SBRT only in the setting of clinical trial. SBRT is capable of precisely delivering high doses of radiation to small tumor volumes and uses real-time tracking of implanted fiducials to potentially integrate organ motion into real-time therapy. However, substantial local toxicity seen in early reports with SBRT. The phase III Alliance trial A021501 has been deigned to compare neoadjuvant extended chemotherapy to chemotherapy and SBRT. The results of this trial will hopefully solve the issue of the type of neoadjuvant approach for BRPC.[19]

Surgical Management

Surgical resection is regarded as the only treatment for cure and can result in significantly longer survival compared with any other treatment options. Involvement of SMV/PV was previously considered as inoperable. However, curative resection along with SMV/PV with vascular reconstruction has become standard now in specialized high volume centers (Figs. 2A and B).

Consensus-based guidelines from the NCCN define radiological characteristics to define these categories[20] (Box 1 and 2). However, the definitions of these three categories are not uniform because resectability

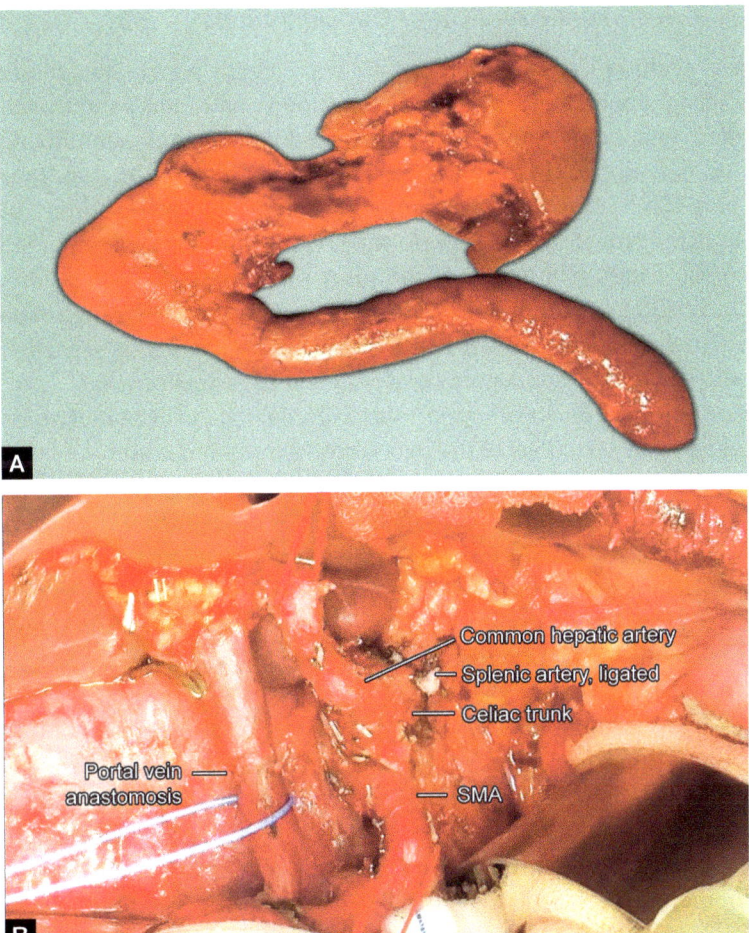

Figs. 2A and B: Radical total pancreaticosplenectomy for borderline resectable pancreatic cancer, post-neoadjuvant chemotherapy: (A) Total pancreaticosplenectomy specimen; (B) Postoperative tumor bed.

depends on surgical experience and techniques. For example, one of the most commonly used definitions of borderline resectable pancreatic cancer (BRPC) includes no distant metastases, venous involvement of the superior mesenteric vein or portal vein, gastroduodenal artery encasement up to the hepatic artery, and tumor abutment of the superior mesenteric artery of less than or equal to 180°. In specialized centers, en bloc resection of the portal vein or superior mesenteric vein, or both, is commonly and safely practiced in the setting of borderline resectable tumors involving these veins.[21] However, when there is tumor abutment of a major artery such as the superior mesenteric artery, surgical resection often results in positive surgical margin and is presently not recommended.[22,23]

Surgical Techniques and Other Considerations

Surgical techniques for pancreatic cancer include pancreaticoduodenectomy, distal pancreatectomy with splenectomy, and total pancreatectomy. Standard lymphadenectomy for pancreatoduodenectomy should include removal of lymph node stations 5, 6, 8a, 12b1, 12b2, 12c, 13a, 13b, 14a, 14b, 17a, and 17b.[24] After pancreaticoduodenectomy, pancreatic stump, biliary and gastric reconstruction is performed. Clinically, relevant postoperative pancreatic fistula (CR-POPF) is the most troublesome complication after pancreatoduodenectomy. Currently, no specific technique can completely eliminate development of CR-POPF. The most commonly used techniques include pancreaticojejunostomy and pancreaticogastrostomy.[25]

Most evidence does not support survival advantage of extended resections including wide resections of the para-aortic lymph nodes and nerve plexus, multi-visceral resections routinely.[26-28] Such extended resections are associated with compromised quality of life because of intractable diarrhea. Although in highly selected patients, with preserved performance status and stable or non-progressive disease on neoadjuvant treatment, such extended resection can provide survival advantage over palliative treatments.[29] Radical surgeries in presence of oligo-metastatic disease have also been reported, prolonging survival in highly selected patients.[30]

To improve margin negative resections especially in borderline resectable tumors, SMA first approach (6 different approaches) was proposed as a new modification of standard pancreaticoduodenectomy.[31] In a systematic review, SMA first approach was shown to be associated with better perioperative outcomes, such as blood loss, transfusion requirements, pancreatic fistula, delayed gastric emptying and lower local and metastatic recurrence rate.[32,33]

Mortality, complications, length of hospital stay, margin status, survival, and overall cost after pancreaticoduodenectomy have been reported to be related to hospital volume.[7,34-36] The complications and mortality largely depends on pancreatic anastomotic leak, and consistent practice of any standardized technique of anastomosis by an experienced surgeon may decrease the rate of clinically relevant postoperative pancreatic fistula.[25,37] Results of 1,200 pancreaticoduodenectomies from Tata Memorial Hospital (unpublished data) also indicate the same (Table 1). Therefore, it is recommended that pancreaticoduodenectomy should be done in specialized centers with experienced teams that perform a large number (>15-20) of pancreatic resections annually.

Locally Advanced Tumors

Most patients with locally advanced pancreatic cancer (LAPC) are treated with initial chemotherapy instead of immediate radiotherapy or chemo-

Table 1: Postoperative outcomes following 1200 whipple resections [Tata Memorial Hospital (unpublished data)].

Parameter	Period A (n = 500)	Period B (n = 700)	Total (n = 1200)
CR-POPF	55 (11%)	115 (16.4%)	170 (14.2%)
DGE	16 (3.2%)	56 (8%)	72 (6%)
PPH	29 (5.8%)	21 (3%)	50 (4.2%)
Bile leak	17 (3.4%)	9 (1.3%)	26 (2.1%)
Morbidity	165 (33%)	209 (30%)	374 (31.2%)
Mortality	27 (5.4%)	21 (3%)	48 (4%)

As per ISGPS definition:
- CR-POPF, clinically relevant postoperative pancreatic fistula
- DGE, delayed gastric emptying
- PPH, post-pancreatectomy hemorrhage

Note: Period A: Standardization of pancreatic resections and anastomosis, unit developing into a high volume centre for pancreatic surgery; Period B: Increased complexity of surgery (extended/vascular resection), use of neoadjuvant treatment, early experience with minimally invasive surgery.

radiotherapy.[11] The optimum chemotherapy regimen is still to be established and participation in clinical trials is preferred.

Chemotherapy Regimens for Locally Advanced Pancreatic Cancer

- *Gemcitabine monotherapy:* Trials evaluating different chemotherapy combinations in mixed populations of patients with locally advanced and metastatic pancreatic cancer have shown that gemcitabine-based chemotherapy offers similar survival outcomes in LAPC as compared to chemoradiotherapy.[38,40] Hence, gemcitabine monotherapy or a gemcitabine-based combination regimen (gemcitabine plus nanoparticle albumin-bound paclitaxel [nab-paclitaxel]) is considered as standard approach.
- *FOLFIRINOX:* Although toxicities are higher, FOLFIRINOX is presently preferred choice of chemotherapy in LAPC when patients have good performance status and normal bilirubin levels. It offers good objective response rates and in some patients it achieves significant downsizing in order to permit an R0 resection.[40,41]

Radiotherapy

Definitive chemoradiation therapy for locally advanced pancreatic cancer has been intensively studied. However, there have been long-lasting debates about the survival benefits of chemoradiation therapy.[42] The Eastern Cooperative Oncology Group (ECOG) 4201 trial compared chemoradiotherapy with chemotherapy in patients with locally advanced pancreatic cancer and median survival was 9.2 months for chemotherapy with gemcitabine and 11.1 months for chemoradiotherapy. However, the number of recruited patients were too small to draw any definitive conclusions.[43] Findings from a randomized study comparing chemoradiation therapy and chemotherapy after 4 months of gemcitabine with or without erlotinib (LAP 07) showed that administering chemoradiation therapy was not superior to continuing chemotherapy in patients with locally advanced pancreatic cancer.[44] Further investigations are needed to validate the potential survival advantages of chemoradiation therapy in these locally advanced tumors.

Chemoradiotherapy after Initial Chemotherapy

It was hoped that reserving chemoradiotherapy for patients who did not progress after initial chemotherapy would improve survival. However, data from the LAP-07 trial did not show any survival benefit from chemoradiotherapy as compared with continued systemic chemotherapy alone. Hence, chemoradiotherapy cannot be recommended for all patients who do not have a progressive disease after initial chemotherapy. However, it may be worthwhile to add radiotherapy when sufficient downsizing is achieved after chemotherapy and surgery is planned, in order to facilitate R0 resection.

Stereotactic Body Radiation Therapy

Stereotactic body radiation therapy (SBRT) and intensity-modulated radiation therapy (IMRT) have been shown to be safe and effective in neoadjuvant[45] and palliative situations. SBRT has been evaluated in a number of clinical studies as an alternative approach to conventionally fractionated EBRT with concurrent chemotherapy for the management of LAPC. However, the benefit of SBRT remains uncertain, since it is not clear that median survival is better than would be expected with other forms of therapy, and toxicity has been worse in some studies.[46]

Surgery for Locally Advanced Pancreatic Cancer

The possibility of complete resection and long-term survival is low for patients who initially are classified as unresectable tumors. However, all patients with LAPC who have good response with chemotherapy or chemoradiotherapy and have good performance status should be offered exploration and trial of resection. As per reports, approximately one-third of initially unresectable tumors can become potentially resectable, after neoadjuvant therapy.[1,47]

Supportive Care for Progressive Disease including Specific Palliative Measures

Palliative care is as important as other therapies, because patients with pancreatic cancer require palliation at some point. Obstructive jaundice and obstruction of the duodenum in patients with pancreatic cancer require surgical, endoscopic, or radiological interventions. With technical advances in endoscopic intervention during the past decade, percutaneous biliary drainage has been replaced by endoscopic stenting in most cases. The use of a large diameter metal stent is preferred to that of a small caliber plastic stent because of the longer patency time and lower incidence of cholangitis.[48] For gastric outlet obstruction, both surgical gastrojejunostomy and endoscopic duodenal stents are used. Endoscopic duodenal stents are preferred in patients with a short life expectancy, poor performance status, or both.

Pain can be a significant feature of advanced pancreatic cancer, and all patients should have a charting on the level of pain and degree of pain relief from analgesics addressed at every clinic visit. The mainstay of pain management is typically opioid medication, and palliation of pain can often be successfully achieved by opioid analgesics alone. For patients with persistent nausea and vomiting, for whom taking oral medications is difficult, pain control may be achieved using transdermal patches, provided they have sufficient adipose tissue for transdermal absorption. In cases with intractable pain refractory to other medication, pain may be relieved by inhibiting synaptic pathways within the celiac plexus without nerve destruction (i.e. celiac plexus block using a bolus injection of local anesthetic) or chemical destruction of the pathways and ganglia using dehydrated alcohol (celiac plexus neurolysis).[49]

The knowledge of the aggressive nature of locally advanced and metastatic pancreatic cancer may lead to depression and anxiety in patients. Patients with depression experience a significant worsening of their quality of life and have more intense pain compared with those who are not depressed. These patients can benefit from a discussion of their psychosocial concerns with the palliative care team and some may warrant treatment with antidepressants or anxiolytics.

Pancreatic cancer has a high risk of venous thromboembolism (VTE). Treatment with chemotherapy further increases this risk. The presence of thromboembolism significantly increases the risk of short-term as well as long-term mortality.[50] All patients should be educated as to the warning signs and symptoms of VTE. All non-ambulatory patients should receive low molecular weight heparins (LMWHs) as a preventive measure.

Anorexia, weight loss and cachexia are common in advanced pancreatic cancer. All patients should be referred to a nutritionist and/or dietician. Some patients develop exocrine pancreatic insufficiency and require pancreatic enzyme replacement, which can help improve digestion and absorption of nutrients.

Addressing all these issues offers best form of supportive care and leads to improvement in quality of life.

PROGNOSIS

If R0 resection is achieved, the survival of borderline resectable tumors equals that of the resectable tumors. The most important prognostic factors for completely resected patients is nodal involvement and margin status. 5-year survival after surgery is approximately 10% for node positive disease,[51] while it is approximately 30% for node negative disease.[52] The median survival for patients with untreated, locally advanced, unresectable pancreatic cancer is 8–12 months and only 3–6 months for those with metastatic disease at presentation. With current chemotherapy regimens such as FOLFIRINOX, the median survival can be extended in the range of 12 months in advanced disease.[41,42]

REFERENCES

1. Gillen S, Schuster T, ZumBüschenfelde CM, et al. Preoperative/neoadjuvant therapy in pancreatic cancer: a systematic review and meta-analysis of response and resection percentages. PLoS Med. 2010;7(4):e1000267.
2. Maisey NR, Norman AR, Hill A, et al. CA19-9 as a prognostic factor in inoperable pancreatic cancer: the implication for clinical trials. Br J Cancer. 2005;93(7):740.
3. Berger AC, Garcia Jr M, Hoffman JP, et al. Postresection CA 19-9 predicts overall survival in patients with pancreatic cancer treated with adjuvant chemoradiation: a prospective validation by RTOG 9704. J Clin Oncol. 2008;26(36):5918.
4. Zhang Y, Huang J, Chen M, et al. Preoperative vascular evaluation with computed tomography and magnetic resonance imaging for pancreatic cancer: a meta-analysis. Pancreatology. 2012;12(3):227-33.
5. Ahn SS, Kim MJ, Choi JY, et al. Indicative findings of pancreatic cancer in prediagnostic CT. Eur Radiol. 2009;19(10):2448-55.
6. Diehl SJ, Lehmann KJ, Sadick M, et al. Pancreatic cancer: value of dual-phase helical CT in assessing resectability. Radiology. 1998;206(2):373-8.
7. Lu DS, Reber HA, KraSny RM, et al. Local staging of pancreatic cancer: criteria for unresectability of major vessels as revealed by pancreatic-phase, thin-section helical CT. Am J Roentgenol. 1997;168(6):1439-43.
8. Park HS, Lee JM, Choi HK, et al. Preoperative evaluation of pancreatic cancer: comparison of gadolinium-enhanced dynamic MRI with MR cholangio-pancreatography versus MDCT. J Magn Reson Imaging. 2009;30(3):586-95.
9. Wang Z, Chen JQ, Liu JL, et al. FDG-PET in diagnosis, staging and prognosis of pancreatic carcinoma: a meta-analysis. World J Gastroenterol. 2013;19(29):4808.
10. Shrikhande SV, Barreto SG, Goel M, et al. Multimodality imaging of pancreatic ductal adenocarcinoma: a review of the literature. HPB (Oxford). 2012;14(10):658-68.
11. National Comprehensive Cancer Network (2017). NCCN clinical practice guidelines in oncology. Pancreatic adenocarcinoma. NCCN Guidelines version 3. 2017. [online] Available from *https://www.nccn.org/professionals/physician_gls/f_guidelines.asp* [Accessed December 2018].

12. Hayasaki A, Isaji S, Kishiwada M, et al. Survival Analysis in Patients with Pancreatic Ductal Adenocarcinoma Undergoing Chemoradiotherapy Followed by Surgery According to the International Consensus on the 2017 Definition of Borderline Resectable Cancer. Cancers (Basel). 2018;10(3):65.
13. Balaban EP, Mangu PB, Khorana AA, et al. Locally Advanced, Unresectable Pancreatic Cancer: American Society of Clinical Oncology Clinical Practice Guideline. J Clin Oncol. 2016;34:2654.
14. Kim SS, Nakakura EK, Wang ZJ, et al. Is neoadjuvant chemoradiation important in borderline resectable pancreatic cancer (BRPC)? Clinical and surgical outcomes associated with preoperative FOLFIRINOX alone in BRPC. J Clin Oncol. 2016; 34(4);351.
15. Katz MH, Shi Q, Ahmad SA, et al. Preoperative modified FOLFIRINOX treatment followed by capecitabine-based chemoradiation for borderline resectable pancreatic cancer: alliance for clinical trials in oncology trial A021101. JAMA Surg. 2016;151(8):e161137.
16. Shrikhande SV, Barreto SG, Somashekar BA, et al. Evolution of pancreatoduodenectomy in a tertiary cancer center in India: improved results from service reconfiguration. Pancreatology. 2013;13(1):63-71.
17. Tang K, Lu W, Qin W, et al. Neoadjuvant therapy for patients with borderline resectable pancreatic cancer: a systematic review and meta-analysis of response and resection percentages. Pancreatology. 2016;16(1):28-37.
18. Jang JY, Han Y, Lee H, et al. Oncological benefits of neoadjuvant chemoradiation with gemcitabine versus upfront surgery in patients with borderline resectable pancreatic cancer: a prospective, randomized, open-label, multicenter phase 2/3 trial. Ann Surg. 2018;268(2):215-22.
19. Katz MH, Ou FS, Herman JM, et al. Alliance for clinical trials in oncology (ALLIANCE) trial A021501: preoperative extended chemotherapy vs. chemotherapy plus hypofractionated radiation therapy for borderline resectable adenocarcinoma of the head of the pancreas. BMC Cancer. 2017;17(1):505.
20. Tempero MA, Malafa MP, Al-Hawary M, et al. Pancreatic adenocarcinoma, version 2.2017, NCCN clinical practice guidelines in oncology. J Natl Compr Cancer Netw. 2017;15:1028-61.
21. Bockhorn M, Uzunoglu FG, Adham M, et al. Borderline resectable pancreatic cancer: a consensus statement by the International Study Group of Pancreatic Surgery (ISGPS). Surgery. 2014;155(6):977-88.
22. Ouaissi M, Hubert C, Verhelst R, et al. Vascular reconstruction during pancreatoduodenectomy for ductal adenocarcinoma of the pancreas improves resectability but does not achieve cure. World J Surg. 2010;34(11):2648-61.
23. Mollberg N, Rahbari NN, Koch M, et al. Arterial resection during pancreatectomy for pancreatic cancer: a systematic review and meta-analysis. Ann Surg. 2011;254(6):882-93.
24. Tol JA, Gouma DJ, Bassi C, et al. Definition of a standard lymphadenectomy in surgery for pancreatic ductal adenocarcinoma: a consensus statement by the International Study Group on Pancreatic Surgery (ISGPS). Surgery. 2014;156(3): 591-600.

25. Shrikhande SV, Sivasanker M, Vollmer CM, et al. Pancreatic anastomosis after pancreatoduodenectomy: a position statement by the International Study Group of Pancreatic Surgery (ISGPS). Surgery. 2017;161(5):1221-34.
26. Evans DB, Farnell MB, Lillemoe KD, et al. Surgical treatment of resectable and borderline resectable pancreas cancer: expert consensus statement. Ann Surg Oncol. 2009;16(7):1736-44.
27. Nimura Y, Nagino M, Takao S, et al. Standard versus extended lymphadenectomy in radical pancreatoduodenectomy for ductal adenocarcinoma of the head of the pancreas: long-term results of a Japanese multicenter randomized controlled trial. J Hepatobiliary Pancreat Sci. 2012;19(3):230-41.
28. Jang JY, Kang MJ, Heo JS,. A prospective randomized controlled study comparing outcomes of standard resection and extended resection, including dissection of the nerve plexus and various lymph nodes, in patients with pancreatic head cancer. Ann Surg. 2014 ;259(4):656-64.
29. Mitra A, Pai E, Dusane R, et al. Extended pancreatectomy as defined by the ISGPS: useful in selected cases of pancreatic cancer but invaluable in other complex pancreatic tumors. Langenbecks Arch Surg. 2018;403(2):203-12.
30. Hackert T, Niesen W, Hinz U, et al. Radical surgery of oligometastatic pancreatic cancer. Eur J Surg Oncol. 2017;43(2):358-63.
31. Sanjay P, Takaori K, Govil S, et al. 'Artery-first' approaches to pancreatoduodenectomy. Br J Surg. 2012;99(8):1027-35.
32. Negoi I, Hostiuc S, Runcanu A, et al. Superior mesenteric artery first approach versus standard pancreaticoduodenectomy: a systematic review and meta-analysis. Hepatobiliary Pancreat Dis Int. 2017;16(2):127-38.
33. Ironside N, Barreto SG, Loveday B, et al. Meta-analysis of an artery-first approach versus standard pancreatoduodenectomy on perioperative outcomes and survival. Br J Surg. 2018;105(6):628-36.
34. Begg CB, Cramer LD, Hoskins WJ, et al. Impact of hospital volume on operative mortality for major cancer surgery. JAMA. 1998;280(20):1747-51.
35. Vincent A, Herman J, Schulick R, et al. Pancreatic cancer. Lancet. 2011; 378(9791):607-20.
36. Basavaiah G, Rent PD, Rent EG, et al. Financial Impact of Complex Cancer Surgery in India: A Study of Pancreatic Cancer. J Glob Oncol. 2018;4:1-9.
37. Shrikhande SV, Barreto G, Shukla PJ. Pancreatic fistula after pancreaticoduodenectomy: the impact of a standardized technique of pancreaticojejunostomy. Langenbeck's Arch Surg. 2008;393(1):87-91.
38. Louvet C, Labianca R, Hammel P, et al. Gemcitabine in combination with oxaliplatin compared with gemcitabine alone in locally advanced or metastatic pancreatic cancer: results of a GERCOR and GISCAD phase III trial. J Clin Oncol. 2005;23(15):3509-16.
39. Ishii H, Furuse J, Boku N, et al. Phase II study of gemcitabine chemotherapy alone for locally advanced pancreatic carcinoma: JCOG0506. Jpn J Clin Oncol. 2010;40(6):573-9.
40. Marthey L, Sa-Cunha A, Blanc JF, et al. FOLFIRINOX for locally advanced pancreatic adenocarcinoma: results of an AGEO multicenter prospective observational cohort. AnnSurg Oncol. 2015;22(1):295-301.

41. Suker M, Beumer BR, Sadot E, et al. FOLFIRINOX for locally advanced pancreatic cancer: a systematic review and patient-level meta-analysis. Lancet Oncol. 2016;17(6):801-10.
42. Huguet F, Girard N, Guerche CS, et al. Chemoradiotherapy in the management of locally advanced pancreatic carcinoma: a qualitative systematic review. J Clin Oncol. 2009;27(13):2269-77.
43. Loehrer PJ Sr, Feng Y, Cardenes H, et al. Gemcitabine alone versus gemcitabine plus radiotherapy in patients with locally advanced pancreatic cancer: an Eastern Cooperative Oncology Group trial. J Clin Oncol. 2011;29(31):4105.
44. Hammel P, Huguet F, Van Laethem JL, et al. Comparison of chemoradiotherapy (CRT) and chemotherapy (CT) in patients with a locally advanced pancreatic cancer (LAPC) controlled after 4 months of gemcitabine with or without erlotinib: Final results of the international phase III LAP 07 study. Pancreatology. 2013;S89.
45. Chapman BC, Gleisner A, Rigg D, et al. Perioperative outcomes and survival following neoadjuvant stereotactic body radiation therapy (SBRT) versus intensity-modulated radiation therapy (IMRT) in pancreatic adenocarcinoma. J Surg Oncol. 2018;117(5):1073-83.
46. Mahadevan A, Jain S, Goldstein M, et al. Stereotactic body radiotherapy and gemcitabine for locally advanced pancreatic cancer. Int J Radiat Oncol Bio Phys. 2010;78(3):735-42.
47. Andriulli A, Festa V, Botteri E, et al. Neoadjuvant/preoperative gemcitabine for patients with localized pancreatic cancer: a meta-analysis of prospective studies. Ann Surg Oncol. 2012;19(5):1644-62.
48. Soderlund C, Linder S. Covered metal versus plastic stents for malignant common bile duct stenosis: a prospective, randomized, controlled trial. Gastrointest Endosc. 2006;63(7):986-95.
49. Arcidiacono PG, Calori G, Carrara S, et al. Celiac plexus block for pancreatic cancer pain in adults. Cochrane Database of Systematic Reviews. 2011(3):CD007519.
50. Epstein AS, Soff GA, Capanu M, et al. Analysis of incidence and clinical outcomes in patients with thromboembolic events and invasive exocrine pancreatic cancer. Cancer. 2012;118(12):3053-61.
51. Kang MJ, Jang JY, Chang YR, et al. Revisiting the concept of lymph node metastases of pancreatic head cancer: number of metastatic lymph nodes and lymph node ratio according to N stage. Ann Surg Oncol. 2014;21(5):1545-51.
52. Allen PJ, Kuk D, Castillo CF, et al. Multi-institutional Validation Study of the American Joint Commission on Cancer Changes for T and N Staging in Patients With Pancreatic Adenocarcinoma. Ann Surg. 2017;265(1):185-91.

Chapter 8

Minimally Invasive Thoracic Surgery

Belal Bin Asaf, Harsh Vardhan Puri, Arvind Kumar

INTRODUCTION

Since the advent of thoracoscopy by Jacobeous in early 1900s, thoracic surgery has travelled a long way from large thoracotomies to a point where today even resectional lung surgery can now be performed in spontaneously breathing nonintubated patients using a single incision in a minimally invasive fashion. The adoption of newer minimally invasive techniques has revolutionized general thoracic surgery.

Concerns about the feasibility, safety, efficacy, maintenance of oncologic principles of resection and cost have all been cited by critics. But since last two decades of its inception, minimally invasive thoracic surgery (MITS) has been demonstrated to significantly reduce pain, hasten recovery, minimize complications, and improve postoperative quality of life for patients requiring thoracic surgery when compared to open thoracotomy.[1,2] There is more and more evidence growing in favor of oncological equivalence particularly for early stage lung cancer, so much, so that video-assisted thoracic surgery (VATS) lobectomy has now become the preferred technique for early stage lung cancer and is no longer considered an emerging technique rather, it is the standard of care for selected patients. The National Comprehensive Cancer Network (NCCN) guidelines for non-small cell lung cancer (NSCLC) calls for the "strong consideration" of VATS lobectomy for early stage lung cancer.[3] Even the American College of Chest Physicians (ACCP) in its guidelines recommends that VATS should be the preferred means of resection for early stage lung cancer.[4] While VATS for lung cancer surgery is the most talked about procedure, the scope of MITS is not limited to resectional lung surgery. Minimally invasive surgery is being used more and more these days for various diagnostic and therapeutic procedures involving the pleura, mediastinum, esophagus, lung and diaphragm.

Before we proceed into the applications, it is imperative that we understand the various terms prevalent for MITS which are often used interchangeably such as MITS, VATS or thoracoscopic surgery. While there are no standardized definitions used for MITS, it is largely a consensus that to qualify as a MITS or VATS, the following prerequisites should be fulfilled:
- No rib spreading
- Single or multi-port <6 cm
- Operating while looking at the vision on the monitor provided by the endovision system
- It is important here to realize that more than the length of the incision, it is the rib spreading that is more traumatic to the patient and its avoidance goes a long way in reducing postoperative pain and morbidity and is an essential prerequisite for any procedures to be classified as a minimally invasive thoracic surgery.

DIFFERENCE BETWEEN THORACOSCOPIC SURGERY AND VIDEO-ASSISTED THORACIC SURGERY

By and large, when the entire surgery is done in a completely portal fashion (Fig. 1) without the utility or access incision, it is called thoracoscopic surgery whereas VATS involves the use of a utility incision or access port: a minithoracotomy incision without rib spreading (Fig. 2).

Thus, MITS can be considered as the broad family under which all these minimally invasive surgical procedures such as VATS, thoracoscopic surgery and mediastinoscopic surgery can be included.

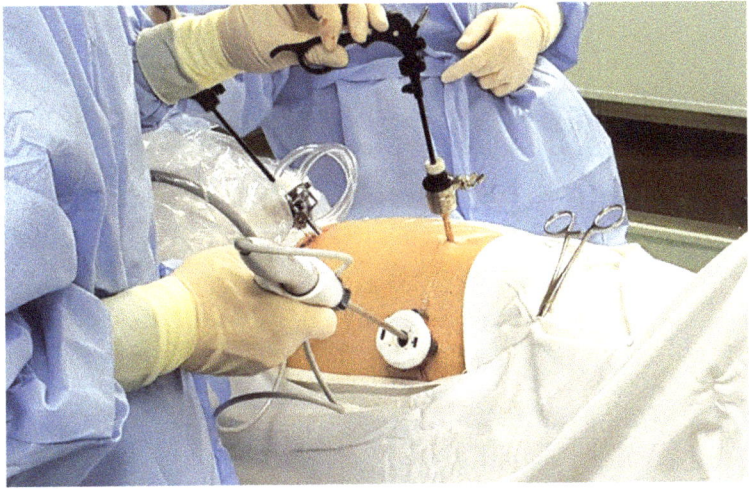

Fig. 1: Photograph showing ports for thoracoscopic surgery.

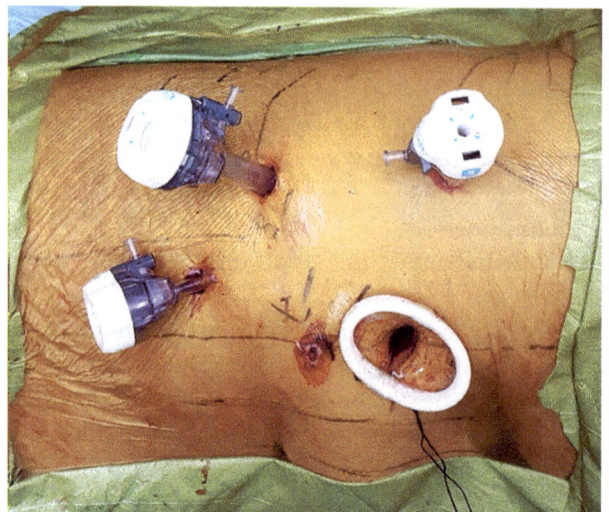

Fig. 2: Photograph of VATS ports with utility incision and wound protector.

Equipment for Thoracoscopic surgery

> **Box 1:** Equipment required for thoracoscopic surgery.
> - A camera system
> - Rigid endoscope: 5 or 10
> - High-definition TV monitor
> - Light source and light cable
> - Tower (cart), and high-flow CO_2 insufflator, as well as various trocar cannula units
> - VATS/thoracoscopy instruments (Fig. 3)

(VATS: video-assisted thoracic surgery)

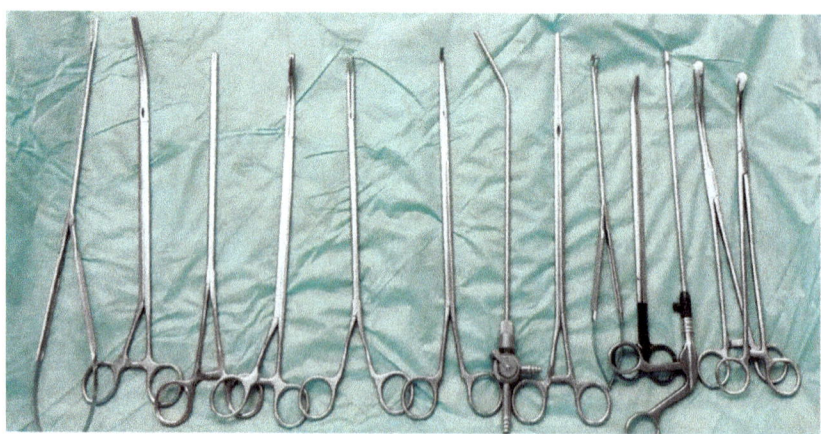

Fig. 3: VATS instruments.

INDICATIONS FOR MINIMALLY INVASIVE THORACIC SURGERY

Early thoracoscopic procedures were limited to diagnostic procedures or management of early empyema or effusions and were performed under local anesthesia with the patient spontaneously ventilating or with mask-assisted ventilation and ether drip anesthesia. Exposure and visualization were quite limited. It was not until the introduction of endotracheal intubation and improved anesthetic technique for cardiopulmonary support that surgeons began to embrace a thoracoscopic approach towards diagnosis and treatment of diseases of the chest. The development of double lumen endotracheal tube (enabling single lung ventilation) and refinement in the anesthetic techniques allowed for both excellent exposure and superior visualization of the thoracic cavity pushing enthusiastic thoracic surgeons to perform a variety of diagnostic and therapeutic procedures without requiring open thoracotomy.

The indications for MITS can be divided broadly into:
- Diagnostic procedures
- Therapeutic procedures.

Indications for Diagnostic Minimally Invasive Thoracic Surgery

- Undiagnosed recurrent pleural effusion
- Pleural biopsy
- Wedge resection of a lung nodule for tissue diagnosis
- Mediastinal lymph node biopsy.

Indications for Therapeutic Minimally Invasive Thoracic Surgery

- *Lung*: Early stage lung cancer, nonanatomical wedge resection, segmentectomy, lobectomy, pneumonectomy, blebectomy for pneumothorax, bullectomy, lung volume reduction surgery
- *Mediastinum*: Thymectomy for myasthenia gravis, surgery for anterior mediastinal masses such as thymoma, posterior mediastinal tumors, various cysts such as bronchogenic cyst and esophageal duplication cyst
- *Esophagus*: Esophagectomy, esophageal leiomyoma enucleation
- *Pleura*: Decortication, pleurodesis
- *Diaphragm*: Diaphragmatic plication
- *Miscellaneous*: Thoracoscopic pericardial window, thoracoscopic sympathectomy for hyperhidrosis.

Thus, virtually any thoracic surgical procedure can be performed using VATS, if proper expertise is available.

CONTRAINDICATIONS

There is no absolute contraindication that is specific to MITS. However, some relative contraindications are:
- Chest wall invasion
- Coagulopathy
- Hemodynamically unstable patient
- Inability to maintain one-lung ventilation.

PRINCIPLES OF MINIMALLY INVASIVE THORACIC SURGERY

While the scope of MITS is very wide now and various procedures have specific requirements, certain general considerations are helpful for understanding MITS.

Anesthesia

Barring a few, almost all MITS procedures will require general anesthesia and some form of lung isolation technique to deflate the lung on the side of which surgery has to be performed. This can be achieved with either controlled pneumothorax, thereby slightly depressing the lung volume, or by purposely deflating one lung on the side of surgery. This is most commonly achieved by using a double lumen endotracheal tube or bronchial blocker. Wherever possible a double lumen tube is preferred over the bronchial blocker because it offers wider channel allowing better deflation and confers the ability to do endobronchial suction. Under ideal circumstances, a right-sided tube is needed for left-sided procedure and vice versa.

A 5- or 10-mm 30° telescopes (Box 1) are used most commonly for MITS. The 5-mm scope is preferred wherever possible because it causes less torque leading to better movement during surgery and also reduces postoperative pain.

Benefits of Video-assisted Thoracic Surgery versus Open Thoracotomy

Reduction in the postoperative complications is cited as one of the most significant benefit of MITS (Box 2). Numerous studies have documented with a decrease in overall complication rates.[5-9] On the other hand, a recent multicenter randomized control trial of 425 patients (215 VATS vs 210 open lobectomy) was published by Long et al. in which no significant difference in postoperative complications, such as length of stay, chest tube duration or number of lymph nodes sampled[10] was found. However, VATS was associated with less intraoperative blood loss (p = 0.001). The authors concluded that

> **Box 2:** Benefits of MITS.
> - Less postoperative pain
> - Lesser blood loss
> - Less pulmonary complications
> - Faster recovery and return to work
> - Less need for ICU stay
> - Cosmetically superior

(MITS: Minimally invasive thoracic surgery; ICU: intensive care unit)

VATS lobectomy is safe and reliable to treat NSCLCs, and it may be superior to thoracotomy in terms of operation time and intraoperative blood loss.

The most important benefit of MITS appears to be the reduction in postoperative pain. Sakuraba M et al.[11] in their study demonstrated that pain occurred in up to 50–70% of patients at 2 months or more after thoracotomy procedures using a retractor and over 40% of the patients still complained of pain at 1 year after surgery with 5% of patients experiencing significant levels of pain. Pain can cause a number of peri- and postoperative complications both immediately and long after the surgery. It is interesting to note that according to some reports there are no significant differences between the intensity and duration of pain following VATS lobectomy and open thoracotomy. In a study by Scott et al. the percentage of patients experiencing intense postoperative pain at 4, 8, and 12 months after VATS and open thoracotomy was comparable.[12] However, postoperative respiratory parameters [forced expiratory volume in 1 sec (FEV1) and forced vital capacity (FVC)] were demonstrated to be significantly higher after VATS as compared to open thoracotomy in several studies.

Amongst the other reported benefits of VATS are reduced chest tube durations and shorter lengths of stay and recovery period. In a study by Sakuraba et al.[11] statistically significant differences were demonstrated in 752 patients who underwent either VATS or open lobectomy with VATS group showing a shorter median operative time, lower chest tubes drainage and shorter length of stay. Studies have also shown VATS to be associated with a statistically significant difference in perioperative blood loss.[6]

Few of the recent studies investigate the patterns of postoperative immunosuppression. VATS was associated with a less significant reduction in lymphocyte T (CD4), C-reactive protein (CRP), and interleukin 6 counts. These data may be indicative of a lower degree of invasiveness of VATS, which is helpful in achieving a shorter post-surgery recovery.[13]

Limitations of Video-assisted Thoracic Surgery

However, despite its obvious advantages, the general thoracic surgical community has been relatively slow in adapting VATS more widely. Recent reviews have shown that over 70% of stage I lung cancers are still being performed by open technique.[14] Even in the USA, Society of Thoracic Surgeon's database show that only 45% of lobectomies are being performed by VATS.[15] The reasons for this slow adaptation of VATS include 2-D vision with lack of depth perception and the use of long rigid instruments in a counter-intuitive manner. The lack of maneuverability, with ribs acting as fulcrum points, limits accessibility and ease of movement in difficult to access areas, prevents fine dissection and makes dealing with large and fragile pulmonary vessels really demanding. These concerns about the VATS approach make it difficult to adopt and increase the learning curve. These findings suggest that surgeons are still struggling with the VATS platform and the outcomes claimed by expert VATS groups may not be replicated uniformly across the general thoracic surgical community.

Minimally Invasive Thoracic Surgery for Benign Indications

By far the most common benign indication for MITS is empyema thoracis. There has been significant debate regarding the appropriateness of the use of MITS for management of empyema. While, there is a consensus amongst thoracic surgeons regarding its usefulness in early stage empyema, its efficacy for stage III and tubercular empyema has been a topic of debate. We started our program of VATS empyema surgery nearly a decade back. In our experience, we found that the initial phase of our program, i.e. the first 30 or so cases, had higher conversion rates close to 50% and was quite frustrating. However, the desire to reduce the morbidity of the procedure pushed us and with perseverance, we were able to achieve outstanding results. After about 50 cases, our conversion rates dropped and in our published report on surgical outcomes of Stage III tuberculous empyema 90% of the cases were successfully completed by VATS.[16] Thoracoscopic decortication of advanced tuberculous empyema is thus feasible, safe, and effective with good short- and long-term results in selected patients. VATS does require careful and meticulous surgical execution to avoid lung injury and reduce resultant prolonged air leak which is the most common cause of morbidity after decortication.

Use minimally invasive thoracic surgery for benign lung resection, although a less well-established indication is nevertheless feasible and safe. The fear of pleural symphysis deters most thoracic surgeons from attempting thoracoscopic surgery. However, in our experience, this fear while true for some cases was usually not a problem in most. In our own retrospective analysis on 41 patients operated for pulmonary aspergilloma, 56% of patients were managed by VATS (23/41) and 44% by thoracotomy. Proper case selection is very vital for good outcomes. VATS for pulmonary aspergilloma, if applicable, may be a safe and efficacious option in experienced hands. Simple aspergilloma, in particular, is considered to be a good indication for VATS. Some cases of complex aspergilloma may also be amenable to VATS.

However, the long-term results need to be further analyzed. Sympathectomy for hyperhidrosis, blebectomy/bullectomy with or without pleurodesis/pleurectomy for spontaneous pneumothorax, palliation of recurrent pleural effusion, lung volume reduction surgery and diaphragmatic plication for eventration are some of the other established applications for MITS.

Oncological Aspect of Minimally Invasive Thoracic Surgery

MITS is being applied more and more commonly in oncological resections. In fact majority of recent research and publication are focusing on the application of MITS in various oncological procedures, the most prominent ones being lung resection for lung cancer, thymectomy for thymoma and esophagectomy in esophageal cancer. Detailed description of thoracolaparoscopic esophagectomy is outside the purview of this chapter.

Video-assisted Thoracic Surgery in Lung Cancer Surgery

There is a lot of debate regarding the oncological adequacy of VATS in Lung Cancer Surgery. Proponents of open approach are skeptical regarding radicality of resection being performed in VATS and hence believe that it may lead to poorer long-term outcomes as compared to open thoracotomy. While surgeons propagating VATS claim that the basic surgical oncological principles are not violated during VATS and that the patients with only early stage lung cancers are carefully selected for surgery. Multiple studies have evaluated both locoregional recurrence and survival after VATS lobectomy. Shiriashi et al. in their study on the impact of VATS lobectomy for cT1N0M0 lung cancer on locoregional control, found no difference in disease-free or locoregional recurrence-free survival between VATS or thoracotomy.[17] In a prospective randomized study of 100 consecutive patients with clinical stage IA non-small cell lung cancer treated with VATS or thoracotomy, Sugi et al. detected no difference in recurrence or 5-year survival.[18] There are studies that report similar, stage for stage 5-year survival, even for more advanced stage malignancies.[19,20] These studies are however retrospective and possibly have a selection bias. Recent meta-analyses have pooled the results from thousands of patients and suggest not only oncologic equivalency, but in some studies even superiority in terms of 5-year survival rates.[21,22]

The extent of the lymph node dissection has always been the most important concern raised by the critics of VATS approach. There are many publications that suggest equivalence in term of lymph node yield. Watanabe et al. in their comparison between 191 patients undergoing VATS versus 159 patients receiving thoracotomy reported no difference in adverse outcomes or the number of nodes removed.[23] The NCCN oncology outcome database, in a multi-institutional study, analyzed the adequacy of mediastinal lymph node dissection based on the number of N2 stations and the total number of nodes removed in patients undergoing either VATS or thoracotomy. In this study, the minimally invasive approach resulted in at least three N2 lymph node stations being dissected in 66% of the patients undergoing VATS lobectomy versus 58% in the thoracotomy group. Additionally, no difference was observed in the median number of N1 and N2 nodes resected in each group. In one of the latest studies, the findings seem to support the arguments in favor of open thoracotomy.[24] The mean number of nodes dissected in the VATS group was significantly lower (9.9/patient) as compared to the open group (P value 0.003). The differences were particularly more significant for N2 group (P value 0.002). In the open lobectomy group, 24.6% of patients were upstaged from N0 to N1 and from N1 to N2 compared with 10% in the VATS group. These findings actually fuel the controversy further. Despite the noted difference in lymph node yield and nodal upstaging, the 3-year survival was similar between the groups (89.9% for VATS versus 84.7% for open lobectomy).

On the other hand, several papers report comparable efficacy of both the methods. Merritt et al. demonstrated equivalence in lymph node yield when they compared VATS with open approach.[25] In a study by Whitson et al. 5-year survival rate in VATS patients of 75% was comparable to lobectomy with thoracotomy.[6] The 5-year overall survival rate in the VATS patients of 95% was found to be higher than in the open group in a study by Palade et al. wherein they compared open vs. VATS lymphadenectomy for stage I non-small cell lung cancer in a prospective randomized trial.

The rate of recurrences following VATS treatment is also an issue of concern. Of particular concerns are local recurrences and access port or utility incision site recurrences associated with the very narrow access space. Walker et al. demonstrated a lower recurrence rate in VATS versus open thoracotomy group of 18% and 29%, respectively.[26] The percentage of distant metastases was higher in patients after thoracotomy as compared to VATS (63% versus 32% in VATS). The risk of surgical access site recurrences could not be confirmed in a number of studies, which is possibly due to the current prevention measures such as surgical field protection by wound protectors in VATS as shown in Figure 2 and mandatory use of retrieval bags for specimen removal.

While it is quite clear from the available literature that though the answer of superiority of VATS over thoracotomy has not been conclusively answered, there is enough to suggest equivalence, and hence the recommendations from bodies such as ACCP to consider VATS strongly for early stage lung cancer. It is imperative to understand here that VATS lobectomy is an advanced procedure and has a learning curve which can affect the lymph node yield and radicality of surgery, particularly in centers where individual surgeons are progressing to VATS from thoracotomy. Also, one has to realize that studies describing equivalent or better outcomes are mostly from high volume centers and the excellent results may not be replicated uniformly by centers with lesser volumes.

Oncological Aspects of Minimally Invasive Thoracic Surgery in Surgery for Thymoma

Thymoma is the most common primary mediastinal neoplasm in adults, with an estimated incidence of 0.15 cases per 100,000.[27] The single most important prognostic marker for thymoma is complete resection with clear and adequate margins.[28] Median sternotomy is currently considered to be the gold standard for thymoma resection.[29,30] The desire to reduce the morbidity of a sternotomy and improve quality of life has led to emergence of significant interest in minimally invasive thymectomy both for myasthenia gravis as well as thymoma. Several authors demonstrated the decreased invasiveness of thoracoscopic thymectomy for thymoma with significantly shorter postoperative hospital stay, decreased intraoperative blood loss, and fewer complications compared to open trans-sternal thymectomy.[31-34]

There have been significant concerns raised about the risk of possible capsule rupture and of pleural dissemination by the thoracoscopic approach. But these concerns have not been substantiated by available literature.[35] The reported recurrences after thoracoscopic thymectomy are not so different from that after open thymectomy and the oncological outcomes are similar.[34,36-38] Sakamaki Y et al. in their study showed that though the overall 5-year survival was different between the two groups the 5-year disease or recurrence free survival was comparable between the VATS and open groups and concluded that the oncologic outcomes of VATS for early stage thymoma is as favorable as for open surgery. Several reports demonstrated that there was no significant difference in the disease-free survival between the groups.[39]

No definitive guidelines have yet been established regarding the appropriate size of the thymoma that can be considered an indicator for thoracoscopic surgery. Minimal invasive surgery for a relatively large-sized thymoma remains controversial. There is presently no consensus on the appropriate size of the thymoma for which thoracoscopic thymectomy can be performed. Most investigators accept that thoracoscopic thymectomy is technically safe and feasible for thymomas with a diameter of less than 5 cm. The optimal treatment for thymoma should be performed according to the Masaoka stage and World Health Organization (WHO) type classification. Like conventional VATS, a significant literature is available on Robotic-assisted thymectomy for myasthenia gravis and thymoma as well. We believe that the robotic platform is an advancement of thoracoscopic approach and should not be considered separate from MITS. Significant concerns are raised by critics regarding the cost efficiency of the robotic system for use in thoracic surgical cases. Despite the lack of randomized trial level evidence, we strongly believe that the robotic system provides unparalleled dexterity particularly in the narrow mediastinal space for thymic surgery. The improved vision and the intuitive dexterity allow for a more precise dissection and decreased risk of capsular rupture. Also, the articulated movements offer far superior dissection in the region of brachiocephalic vein and the thymic horns. In our experience of over 150 robotic thymectomies for various indications, the surgical robot has helped us in performing a more radical thymectomy when compared with the conventional thoracoscopic techniques by enhancing the dissection. The only disadvantage that we can perceive at this moment, taking into consideration the available experience in the literature, is the higher cost involved in robotic-assisted procedures when compared with the thoracoscopic thymectomy.[40]

There are very few studies that directly compare robotic approach with conventional approach. Most revealed similar surgical results, except for the increased operative time and hospitalization costs (increased for robotic approach). Rückert et al. showed a better outcome for myasthenic patients after robotic thymectomy.[41] For early stage thymomas, Qian and colleagues in their comparison between VATS, robotic approach and sternotomy, showed better postoperative outcome, particularly in terms of duration of hospital stay and postoperative pleural drainage volume, in patients treated through the robotic approach when compared to median sternotomy and also to VATS group.[42]

However, there are no randomized controlled trials available comparing the outcomes of the various surgical approaches and it is going to be extremely difficult to perform such a trial in future. However, till such time that results from such trials is available, the choice of technique will be based on a surgeon's experience and preference. While there is not much to debate regarding the advantages of MITS, the question regarding ultimate long-term results remain to be answered and at this point all the minimally invasive approaches including robotic appear to be equivalent, if not superior.

FUTURE PROSPECTS IN MINIMALLY INVASIVE THORACIC SURGERY

Reduction in the morbidity and improvement in the postoperative quality of life after a thoracic surgical procedure continues to possess surgeons across the world and to achieve this target various technical and technological advances have been made. Few of the most prominent ones have been discussed briefly here.

Uniportal Video-assisted Thoracic Surgery

Uniportal VATS which involves performing a surgical procedure using a single utility incision has developed over the last decade or so. The technique, popularized by Spanish surgeon Diego Gonzales Rivas, is now being utilized by increasing number of thoracic surgeons for performing complex thoracic surgical procedures. The proponents of uniportal VATS claims reduced access trauma, less pain paresthesia, morbidity, better cosmesis[43-45] and faster recovery[46] as the main advantages over multiportal thoracoscopic surgery. It is supposed to offer a better visualization ergonomics leading to superior hand eye coordination.[47]

However, opponents of the approach do not agree. They argue that it is unnecessary to make an already demanding surgery more challenging one by using a single port to insert all the instruments including endostaplers. This may leads to poor ergonomics and decreased dexterity and may therefore lead to rise of concern about oncological adequacy and patient safety. Also, long-term data regarding survival benefits are lacking for uniportal VATS as it is the new kid on the block, and there is simply no long-term data available when compared to multiportal VATS. There are nevertheless a significant number of case reports and case series ranging from lobectomies, segmentectomies to sleeve and double sleeve resections.[48-51] Nearly all of them proclaim safety and feasibility. There are very few comparative data, but whatever data is available, it does not prove the superiority of one over the other. So, while uniportal VATS is not superior as per the current evidence, it is also not proven to be inferior and further studies in future may definitively answer the question of superiority. In words of Alan DL Sihoe, another prominent promoter of Uniportal VATS, the future appears to be headed in a direction that may be favorable to uniportal VATS, as in the coming years and given the number of high volume centers adopting the technique, the proponents of uniportal VATS will have ample time and volume to prove its worth through generation of clinical evidence of increasingly better quality.[52]

Non-intubated Thoracic Surgery

Non-intubated minor and major thoracic surgeries are now being performed by experienced uniportal VATS surgeon. It involves performance of thoracoscopic procedures under regional anesthetic techniques including local anesthesia, intercostal nerve blocks, interpleural block, paravertebral blocks or thoracic epidural anesthesia along with sedation in spontaneously breathing patients.[53-57]

The proposed benefits of non-intubated VATS include enhanced recovery, better postoperative respiratory parameters, an attenuated stress response, reduced inflammation as measured by lower postoperative white blood cell counts and tumor necrosis factor-α and C-reactive protein levels,[58-60] improved analgesia, reduced chest drainage, early oral intake, early ambulation, and shortened recovery time.[61,62]

The current applications of non-intubated thoracoscopic surgery are:
- *Minor procedures*:
  - Management of pleural effusions or talc pleurodesis
  - Pulmonary biopsies
  - Mediastinal biopsies
  - Spontaneous pneumothorax
  - Early empyema thoracis
  - Hyperhidrosis.
- Resection of pulmonary nodules
- Thymectomy in myasthenic patients
- Emphysema and lung volume reduction surgery
- Major anatomic pulmonary resections by conventional video-assisted thoracoscopic surgery.

Limitations of Non-intubated Thoracoscopic Surgery

Patients may experience inadequate analgesia, panic attacks. The spontaneous ventilation and respiratory movement of the lung and mediastinum may make bronchovascular dissection and resection, difficult. Hypoxia, hypercapnia, and the conversion to general anesthesia (GA) are other known complications. There is also a risk of loss of airway and aspiration of gastric contents. It is not a suitable modality for prolonged operations as the dependent lung is not adequately protected thus limiting its use to less complex operations. Also, in the event of a vascular bleed the conversion to thoracotomy will require conversion to intubated VATS with general anesthesia which may be difficult, time consuming and potentially life-threatening. Further advancement in surgical technique and technology that might in future help circumvent these limitations and we will have to closely observe its development further. It does appear to be very encouraging for patients in whom general anesthesia and lung isolation is difficult due to poor cardiopulmonary reserve. Long-term studies need to be done to establish safety and survival benefits.

TECHNOLOGICAL ADVANCES IN MINIMALLY INVASIVE THORACIC SURGERY

Three-dimensional Video-assisted Thoracic Surgery

One of the major limitations of conventional thoracoscopic surgery was the two-dimensional (2D) vision wherein depth perception was difficult resulting in image distortion, impaired hand-eye coordination and decreased ability to estimate size and to assess spatial orientation. The robotic platform offered a solution to this problem by providing a high definition three-dimensional (3D) stereoscopic vision. However, the robotic platform's availability is an issue due to significant cost involved. Use of 3D technology in conventional endovision system has the potential to combine the advantages of robotic-assisted thoracic surgery (RATS) and VATS. Despite the perceived benefits, early experiences with 3D endoscopic surgery was fraught with problems of headaches and ocular fatigue due to the requirement of 3D glasses. Improvement in technology has led to reduction in these problems to some extent. Despite the significant advantages, it is unclear whether 3D-VATS is superior to the 2D-VATS systems. In an era of drastic cuts in healthcare costs, 3D is definitely more attractive than the much more expensive robotic technology. However, results of 3D VATS need to be confirmed and compared in larger, prospective and multi-institutional databases.

Augmented Reality in Video-assisted Thoracic Surgery

In the preoperative phase, surgeons draw a mental map of target lesion and do a mental simulation of the surgery. This technology enables superimposition of target structures or lesions on live video camera images allowing the surgeon to simultaneously visualize the surgical site and the overlaid graphic images, creating a so-called augmented reality (AR). Its application in surgery is being experimented and applied in various specialties, particularly neurosurgery, otolaryngology, and maxillofacial surgery. Also, its role in thoracic surgery for localization of lung nodules is already being considered.[63]

Infrared thoracoscopy (IRT) with indocyanine green (ICG) is another example of use of AR which allows for assessment of lung perfusion and has been used to identify the intersegmental border during segmentectomies. The technology has also been used to identify the location of phrenic nerve during minimally invasive thymectomy. Technology is already available in the form of prototype for integration of radiological imaging with live surgical endoscopic view thereby guiding the surgeon to the location of lesion and other important anatomical structures.

Robotic Thoracic Surgery

The robotic surgical system is the next development in the field of minimally invasive chest surgery. It offers the advantages of true stereoscopic 3D vision along with articulated endowristed movement of the surgical instruments in a very intuitive manner. This along with the 7 degrees of freedom of movements together with tremor filtration offers unparalleled dexterity which helps the surgeon to perform complex surgical maneuvers including endosuturing with much ease and comfort. The robot has been extensively used for lung resection including lobectomies and segmentectomies, thymectomies, esophagectomies and for posterior mediastinal tumors and diaphragmatic plication. Despite the benefits, the robot also has certain disadvantages.

The most commonly quoted limitation is the cost of the system in the form of a significant initial investment and a recurring cost of the instruments, drapes and maintenance of the system. Current robotic system also does not have any haptic feedback. Despite these limitations, the robotic system is undoubtedly an advancement of MITS and has a shorter learning curve and is ergonomically superior. With further research and development and more use, the cost will eventually come down. The available literature is abounding[64] with reports which suggest at least equivalency to open and thoracoscopic surgery. It has the potential to expand the use of minimally invasive surgery to a larger patient base by enabling more surgeons to adopt the difficult technique of advanced MITS.

CONCLUSION

Minimally invasive thoracic surgery has revolutionized the field of general thoracic surgery and is well positioned to eventually become the standard of care particularly in thoracic oncology for early stage lung cancers and mediastinal tumors. Its role in benign lung surgery is not very clearly defined but numerous reports suggest safety and feasibility. While its use has expanded significantly, it is unlikely to completely replace open thoracic surgery, particularly in countries like India, where a significant proportion of thoracic surgery is for benign indications and these may not be ideal candidates for thoracoscopic surgery. Further studies exploring long-term outcomes are required to establish superiority, but with the available evidence at least equivalence is less debatable. Minimally invasive thoracic surgery is slated to become the preferred approach, wherever possible. Future studies will give us more proof regarding its long-term outcomes and benefits.

REFERENCES

1. Li WW, Lee TW, Lam SS, et al. Quality of life following lung cancer resection: video-assisted thoracic surgery vs thoracotomy. Chest. 2002;122:584-9.
2. Sihoe AD. The Evolution of VATS Lobectomy. In: Cardoso P (Ed). Topics in Thoracic Surgery. Rijeka: Intech; 2011. pp. 181-210.
3. Ettinger DS, Wood DE, Aisner DL, et al. Non-Small Cell Lung Cancer, Version 5. 2017, NCCN Clinical Practice Guidelines in Oncology. J Natl Compr Canc Netw. 2017;15(4):504-35.
4. Howington JA, Blum MG, Chang AC, et al. Treatment of stage I and II non-small cell lung cancer: Diagnosis and management of lung cancer. 3rd edition: American College of Chest Physicians evidence-based clinical practice guidelines. Chest. 2013;143(5):e278S-e313S.
5. Paul S, Altorki NK, Sheng S, et al. Thoracoscopic lobectomy is associated with lower morbidity than open lobectomy: a propensity-matched analysis from the STS database. J Thorac Cardiovasc Surg. 2010;139(2):366-78.

6. Whitson BA, Groth SS, Duval SJ, et al. Surgery for early stage non-small cell lung cancer: a systematic review of the video-assisted thoracoscopic surgery versus thoracotomy approaches to lobectomy. Ann Thorac Surg. 2008;86(6):2008-18.
7. Flores RM, Park BJ, Dycoco J, et al. Lobectomy by video-assisted thoracic surgery (VATS) versus thoracotomy for lung cancer. J Thorac Cardiovasc Surg. 2009;138(1):11-8.
8. Cajipe MD, Chu D, Bakaeen FG, et al. Video-assisted thoracoscopic lobectomy is associated with better perioperative outcomes than open lobectomy in a veteran population. Am J Surg. 2012;204(5):607-12.
9. Nwogu CE, D'Cunha J, Pang H, et al. VATS lobectomy has better perioperative outcomes than open lobectomy: CALGB 31001, an ancillary analysis of CALGB 140202 (Alliance). Ann Thorac Surg. 2015;99(2):399-405.
10. Long H, Tan Q, Luo Q, et al. Thoracoscopic surgery versus thoracotomy for lung cancer: short-term outcomes of a randomized trial. Ann Thorac Surg. 2018;105(2):386-92.
11. Sakuraba M, Miyamoto H, Oh S, et al. Video-assisted thoracoscopic lobectomy vs. conventional lobectomy via open thoracotomy in patients with clinical stage IA non-small cell lung carcinoma. Interact Cardiovasc Thorac Surg. 2007;6(5):614-7.
12. Scott WJ, Allen MS, Darling G, et al. Video-assisted thoracic surgery versus open lobectomy for lung cancer: a secondary analysis of data from the American College of Surgeons Oncology Group Z0030 randomized clinical trial. J Thorac Cardiovasc Surg. 2010;139(4):976-81.
13. Rizk NP, Ghanie A, Hsu M, et al. A prospective trial comparing pain and quality of life measures after anatomic lung resection using thoracoscopy or thoracotomy. Annals of Thorac Surg. 2014;98(4):1160-6.
14. Boffa DJ, Kosinski AS, Paul S, et al. Lymph node evaluation by open or video-assisted approaches in 11,500 anatomic lung cancer resections. Ann Thorac Surg. 2012;94:347-53.
15. Ceppa DP, Kosinski AS, Berry MF, et al. Thoracoscopic lobectomy has increasing benefit in patients with poor pulmonary function: A Society of Thoracic Surgeons database analysis. Ann Surg. 2012;256:487-93.
16. Kumar A, Asaf BB, Lingaraju VC, et al. Thoracoscopic decortication of stage III tuberculous empyema is effective and safe in selected cases. Ann Thorac Surg. 2017;104(5):1688-94.
17. Shiraishi T, Shirakusa T, Hiratsuka M, et al. Video-assisted thoracoscopic surgery lobectomy for c-T1N0M0 primary lung cancer: its impact on locoregional control. Ann Thorac Surg. 2006;82:1021-6.
18. Sugi K, Kaneda Y, Esato K. Video-assisted thoracoscopic lobectomy achieves a satisfactory long-term prognosis in patients with clinical stage IA lung cancer. World J Surg. 2000;24:27-31.
19. Yamamoto K, Ohsumi A, Kojima F, et al. Long-term survival after video-assisted thoracic surgery lobectomy for primary lung cancer. Ann Thorac Surg. 2010;89:353-9.

20. Yang X, Wang S, Qu J. Video-assisted thoracic surgery (VATS) compares favorably with thoracotomy for the treatment of lung cancer: a five-year outcome comparison. World J Surg. 2009;33:1857-61.
21. Taioli E, Lee D, Lesser, M, et al. Long-term survival in video-assisted thoracoscopic lobectomy vs open lobectomy in lung-cancer patients: a meta-analysis. Eur J Cardiothorac Surg. 2013;44:591-7.
22. Yan T, Black D, Bannon P, et al. Systematic review and meta-analysis of randomized and nonrandomized trials on safety and efficacy of video-assisted thoracic surgery lobectomy for early-stage non-small-cell lung cancer. J Clin Oncol. 2009;27:2553-62.
23. Watanabe A, Koyanagi T, Ohsawa H, et al. Systematic node dissection by VATS is not inferior to that through an open thoracotomy: a comparative clinicopathologic retrospective study. Surgery. 2005;138:510-7.
24. Leaver HA, Craig SR, Yap PL, et al. Lymphocyte responses following open and minimally invasive thoracic surgery. European Journal of Clinical Investigation. 2000;30(3):230-8.
25. Merritt RE, Hoang CD, Shrager JB. Lymph node evaluation achieved by open lobectomy compared with thoracoscopic lobectomy for N0 lung cancer. Annals of Thorac Surg. 2013;96(4):1171-6.
26. Palade E, Passlick B, Osei-Agyemang T, et al. Video-assisted vs open mediastinal lymphadenectomy for Stage I non-small-cell lung cancer: results of a prospective randomized trial. Euro J Cardiothorac Surg. 2013;44(2):244-9.
27. Walker WS, Codispoti M, Soon SY, et al. Long-term outcomes following VATS lobectomy for non-small cell bronchogenic carcinoma. Euro J Cardiothorac Surg. 2003;23(3):397-402.
28. Davenport E, Malthaner RA. The role of surgery in the management of thymoma: a systematic review. Ann Thorac Surg. 2008;86(2):673-84.
29. Regnard JF, Magdeleinat P, Dromer C, et al. Prognostic factors and long-term results after thymoma resection: a series of 307 patients. J Thorac Cardiovasc Surg. 1996;112:376-84.
30. Zahid I, Sharif S, Routledge T, et al. Video-assisted thoracoscopic surgery or trans-sternal thymectomy in the treatment of myasthenia gravis? Interact Cardiovasc Thorac Surg. 2011;12:40-6.
31. Kondo K. Therapy for thymic epithelial tumors. Gen Thorac Cardiovasc Surg. 2014;62:468-74.
32. Liu TJ, Lin MW, Hsieh MS, et al. Video-assisted thoracoscopic surgical thymectomy to treat early thymoma: a comparison with the conventional transsternal approach. Ann Surg Oncol. 2014;21:322-8.
33. Chao YK, Liu YH, Hsieh MJ, et al. Long-term outcomes after thoracoscopic resection of stage I and II thymoma: a propensity-matched study. Ann Surg Oncol. 2015;22:1371-6.
34. He Z, Zhu Q, Wen W, et al. Surgical approaches for stage I and II thymoma-associated myasthenia gravis: feasibility of complete video-assisted thoracoscopic surgery (VATS) thymectomy in comparison with trans-sternal resection. J Biomed Res. 2013;27:62-70.

35. Ye B, Tantai JC, Ge XX, et al. Surgical techniques for early-stage thymoma: video-assisted thoracoscopic thymectomy versus transsternal thymectomy. J Thorac Cardiovasc Surg. 2014;147:1599-603.
36. Raza A, Woo E. Video-assisted thoracoscopic surgery versus sternotomy in thymectomy for thymoma and myasthenia gravis. Ann Cardiothorac Surg. 2016;5:33-7.
37. Kimura T, Inoue M, Kadota Y, et al. The oncological feasibility and limitations of video-assisted thoracoscopic thymectomy for early-stage thymomas. Eur J Cardiothorac Surg. 2013;44:e214-8.
38. Lucchi M, Davini F, Ricciardi R, et al. Management of pleural recurrence after curative resection of thymoma. J Thorac Cardiovasc Surg. 2009;137:1185-9.
39. Manoly I, Whistance RN, Sreekumar R, et al. Early and mid-term outcomes of trans-sternal and video-assisted thoracoscopic surgery for thymoma. Eur J Cardiothorac Surg. 2014;45:e187-93.
40. Sakamaki Y, Oda T, Kanazawa G, et al. Intermediate-term oncologic outcomes after video-assisted thoracoscopic thymectomy for early-stage thymoma. J Thorac Cardiovasc Surg. 2014;148:1230-7.
41. Kumar A, Goyal V, Asaf BB, et al. Robotic thymectomy for myasthenia gravis with or without thymoma–surgical and neurological outcomes. Neurol India. 2017;65:58-63.
42. Rückert JC, Swierzy M, Ismail M. Comparison of robotic and nonrobotic thoracoscopic thymectomy: a cohort study. J Thorac Cardiovasc Surg. 2011;141:673-7.
43. Qian L, Chen X, Huang J, et al. A comparison of three approaches for the treatment of early-stage thymomas: robot-assisted thoracic surgery, video-assisted thoracic surgery, and median sternotomy. J Thorac Dis. 2017;9:1997-2005.
44. Gonzalez-Rivas D, Paradela M, Fernandez R, et al. Uniportal video-assisted thoracoscopic lobectomy: two years of experience. Ann Thorac Surg. 2013;95:426-32.
45. Jutley RS, Khalil MW, Rocco G. Uniportal vs standard three-port VATS technique for spontaneous pneumothorax: comparison of post-operative pain and residual paresthesia. Eur J Cardiothorac Surg. 2005;28:43-6.
46. Tam JK, Lim KS. Total muscle-sparing uniportal video-assisted thoracoscopic surgery lobectomy. Ann Thorac Surg. 2013;96:1982-6.
47. Sihoe AD. The evolution of minimally invasive thoracic surgery: implications for the practice of uniportal thoracoscopic surgery. J Thorac Dis. 2014;6:S604-17.
48. Bertolaccini L, Rocco G, Viti A, et al. Geometrical characteristics of uniportal VATS. J Thorac Dis. 2013;5(3):S214-6.
49. Gonzalez D, Paradela M, Garcia J, et al. Single-port video-assisted thoracoscopic lobectomy. Interact Cardiovasc Thorac Surg. 2011;12:514-5.
50. Gonzalez-Rivas D, Fieira E, Mendez L, et al. Single-port video-assisted thoracoscopic anatomic segmentectomy and right upper lobectomy. Eur J Cardiothorac Surg. 2012;42:e169-71.
51. Gonzalez-Rivas D, Fernandez R, Fieira E, et al. Uniportal video-assisted thoracoscopic bronchial sleeve lobectomy: first report. J Thorac Cardiovasc Surg. 2013;145:1676-7.

52. Gonzalez-Rivas D, Fieira E, Delgado M, et al. Is uniportal thoracoscopic surgery a feasible approach for advanced stages of non-small cell lung cancer? J Thorac Dis. 2014;6:641-8.
53. Sihoe AD. Reasons not to perform uniportal VATS lobectomy. J Thorac Dis. 2016;8(3):S333-43.
54. Pompeo E, Mineo TC. Awake operative videothoracoscopic pulmonary resections. Thorac Surg Clin. 2008;18:311-20.
55. Katlic MR. Video-assisted thoracic surgery utilizing local anesthesia and sedation. Eur J Cardiothorac Surg. 2006;30:529-32.
56. Piccioni F, Langer M, Fumagalli L, et al. Thoracic paravertebral anesthesia for awake video-assisted thoracoscopic surgery daily. Anesthesia. 2010;65:1221-4.
57. Rocco G, La Rocca A, Martucci N, et al. Awake single-access (uniportal) video-assisted thoracoscopic surgery for spontaneous pneumothorax. J Thorac Cardiovasc Surg. 2011;142:944-5.
58. Inoue K, Moriyama K, Takeda J. Remifentanil for awake thoracoscopic bullectomy. J Cardiothorac Vasc Anesth. 2010;24:386-7.
59. Liu J, Cui F, Li S, et al. Non-intubated video-assisted thoracoscopic surgery under epidural anesthesia compared with conventional anesthetic option: a randomized control study. Surg Innov. 2015;22:123-30.
60. Tacconi F, Pompeo E, Sellitri F, et al. Surgical stress hormones response is reduced after awake video thoracoscopy. Interact Cardiovasc Thorac Surg. 2010;10:666-71.
61. Mineo TC, Tacconi F. Systemic inflammation and pulmonary metastasectomy: ideas for further development. Interact Cardiovasc Thorac Surg. 2015;21:623.
62. Liu J, Cui F, Pompeo E, et al. The impact of non-intubated versus intubated anesthesia on early outcomes of video-assisted thoracoscopic anatomical resection in non-small-cell lung cancer: a propensity score matching analysis. Eur J Cardiothorac Surg. 2016;50:920-5.
63. Tacconi F, Pompeo E. Non-intubated video-assisted thoracic surgery: where does evidence stand? J Thorac Dis. 2016;8:S364-75.
64. Miller AP, Peine WJ, Son JS, et al. Tactile imaging system for localizing lung nodules during video assisted thoracoscopic surgery. proceedings 2007 ieee International Conference on Robotics and Automation, Roma, Italy. 2007, pp. 2996-3001.

9
Chapter

Abdominal Tuberculosis

Rahul, Richa Sinha, Puneet

INTRODUCTION

Tuberculosis (TB) is a chronic granulomatous ailment caused by microaerophilic bacteria. It is an important health issue worldwide, especially in developing countries. Primary description similar to TB is evident in ancient literature. It was referred to as "Yakshma" in "The Vedas", meaning an illness that leads to wasting. Similar descriptions could be traced in Chinese and Arabic literature.[1] The word "Tuberculosis" originates from the Latin word "tubercula", which means a small lump.[2] Tuberculosis was considered a contagious disease from time immemorial. According to the Hindu texts dated 1500 BC, the sufferers of "Yakshma" were considered impure and marriage in the affected family was prohibited for Brahmins. The patients suffering from the disease were nursed in isolation. However, it was not until 24th March 1882, when Robert Koch introduced the "tubercle bacillus" to the world, that the causative agent of TB became known. Same day is commemorated as the "World TB Day" since 1982. Tuberculosis remained incurable till the 4th decade of the 20th century. Streptomycin followed by para-aminosalicylic acid (PAS) and isoniazid was discovered in the 1940s. They emerged as an effective treatment for the formidable ailment. With the addition of rifampicin and ethambutol, a short course regimen was introduced which could affect cure. This was a ray of hope to the healthcare providers and heralded the era of modern chemotherapy.[1] In the 1970s, developed countries became optimistic regarding the containment of the disease. This optimism was put to an end in the 1980s with the dawn of human immunodeficiency virus (HIV) infection and the emergence of multidrug resistance (MDR). World Health Organization (WHO) declared tuberculosis as a "global emergency" in 1993.[2]

Tuberculosis is endemic in South-East Asian countries. India accounts for the largest share (26%) of TB cases in the world, followed by China and South Africa.[3] Tuberculosis primarily affects the lungs. Extrapulmonary disease accounts for 15-20% of all cases in immunocompetent patients and 50% in HIV positive patients.[4] Poor hygiene, low socioeconomic status, use of immune suppressants and immune modulators, poor nutritional status and uncontrolled diabetes are other factors associated with the increase in the risk of extrapulmonary tuberculosis (EPTB).[5] Abdominal TB (ATB) ranks sixth among the list of EPTB only after lymphatic, genitourinary, skeletal, miliary and meningeal disease. It comprises of nearly 11% of all EPTB.[4,6] Abdominal TB presents with nonspecific symptoms and signs, especially in the immunocompromised. It requires a high degree of suspicion to diagnose the disease in time and administer appropriate treatment. Delayed recognition entails high morbidity and mortality.

PATHOPHYSIOLOGY

Abdominal TB can develop primarily due to ingestion of infected milk or food. This mode of transmission is now rare after the introduction of methods of pasteurization of milk. Usually, abdomen is involved secondary to a tubercular infection elsewhere in the body. The routes of spread are as follows:[3,7]

- *Hematogenous* dissemination from an active pulmonary infection or miliary TB. The bacilli spread through the portal circulation or abdominal arteries. This mainly affects the solid organs like spleen, liver, pancreas, kidneys and peritoneum.
- *Ingestion* of infected sputum in an active pulmonary disease. The mucosal layer of the gastrointestinal tract (GIT) is infected by the bacilli in areas of stasis. They lodge in the submucosal lymphoid tissue, form epithelioid tubercles and embark a granulomatous inflammation. It is characterized by coagulative and liquefactive necrosis, presenting as cheesy material (caseous necrosis). It bursts out leading to ulceration of the overlying mucosa as well as spreads into the deeper layers. The bacilli can later affect the mesenteric lymph nodes and peritoneum. Hematogenous dissemination through the portal circulation from peritoneum into the solid organs like liver, spleen and pancreas is also possible.
- *Direct spread* from the adjacent organs like fallopian tubes, vertebrae or psoas muscle. This mainly affects the peritoneum and mesenteric nodes.
- The tubercle bacilli can also spread through *lymphatic route* to involve the mesenteric lymph nodes, followed by the intestine.

SITES OF INVOLVEMENT OF ABDOMINAL TUBERCULOSIS

Abdominal tuberculosis commonly involves GIT, peritoneum, lymph nodes and rarely the solid organs (Table 1). It usually presents as a chronic disease.

Table 1: Clinical presentation of abdominal tuberculosis.

Type	Distribution	Clinical presentation	Differential diagnosis
Intestinal—ulcerative	80% of intestinal tuberculosis (ITB)	Chronic diarrhea, anemia, malabsorption. Rarely lower gastrointestinal bleed	Inflammatory bowel disease (IBD) (Crohn's), Celiac disease
Intestinal—hypertrophic		Abdominal lump, pain, acute intestinal obstruction	Lymphoma, intestinal/ileocecal carcinoma
Intestinal—stricturous		Chronic form—recurrent subacute intestinal obstruction, abdominal pain, loss of weight Acute form—abdominal distension, vomiting, obstipation, perforation peritonitis	Intestinal malignancy, ischemic strictures, inflammatory bowel disease (IBD)
Esophageal	<1% of ITB	Dysphagia, retrosternal pain	Esophageal malignancy, esophageal motility disorder
Gastroduodenal	2–3% of ITB	Dyspepsia, upper abdominal pain, weight loss and may present with gastric outlet obstruction with recurrent vomiting	Peptic ulcer disease, gastroduodenal malignancy, lymphoma
Colonic	10–12% ITB	Diarrhea, loss of weight, occasionally bleeding per rectum and late in course can present with obstruction due to stricture	IBD, malignancy
Anorectal	<1% of intestinal TB	Ulcers, per rectal bleeding and multiple fistulas in anorectum especially in acquired immunodeficiency syndrome (AIDS)	Immunodeficiency syndromes, anorectal malignancy
Peritoneal—wet type	60% of ATB	Abdominal distension, weakness, early satiety	Chronic liver disease with decompensation, malnutrition, peritoneal carcinomatosis
Peritoneal—dry type	More common in children.	Recurrent abdominal pain and subacute intestinal obstruction	Small bowel congenital bands, malignancy, volvulus
Tubercular lymphadenitis	20–25% of ATB	Pain abdomen, lump in case of matted lymph nodes, weight loss, low-grade fever	Lymphoma, HIV with AIDS
Solid organ tuberculosis	15–20% of ATB	Liver—pain, fever, weight loss and rise in hepatic enzymes Pancreas—fever, gastric outlet obstruction and obstructive jaundice	Liver-abscess, metastatic lesion Pancreas—malignancy, pancreatic abscess

Acute manifestations in the form of acute abdominal pain, intestinal obstruction or peritonitis are common in intestinal and nodal variant, especially in South-East Asian countries. In the chronic form, the common complains include low grade fever (40-70%), abdominal pain (80-90%), altered bowel habits (40%), anorexia, generalized weakness and weight loss (40-90%).[3] Peritoneum is most commonly affected in ATB (58%), followed by GIT in 40%.[8] Mesenteric lymph nodes are affected in 25% of cases.

Gastrointestinal Tuberculosis

Abdominal tuberculosis can affect the whole gastrointestinal tract (GIT) from esophagus to anus, but most commonly the ileocecal region.

Esophageal Tuberculosis

Esophagus is rarely involved in immunocompetent patients. It constitutes 0.2-1% of all cases of ATB.[3] The involvement of esophagus is usually the result of lymphatic spread from the adjacent mediastinal lymph nodes or hematogenous spread from endobronchial disease. It presents with low grade fever, retrosternal discomfort and dysphagia. Extraluminal disease is usually not overt. The symptoms mimic those of malignancy. Mid-esophagus is the most commonly affected region due to proximity to the mediastinal nodes. It manifests in the form of an ulcer, mass or a traction diverticulum. Later, it may develop fistula or strictures, especially in immunocompromised patients.[9]

Gastroduodenal Tuberculosis

Stomach and duodenum constitute 2-3% of all cases of ATB. The presence of acidic juice, thick mucosa, less number of lymph nodes and rapid transition of the food prevents primary involvement of these organs.[10] Distal stomach and third part of duodenum (Fig. 1) are most commonly affected. Intrinsic form presents as gastric ulcer with symptoms of dyspepsia and weight loss. Extrinsic form involves the perigastric and periduodenal lymph nodes, which present as gastric outlet obstruction due to external compression and strictures. The largest series on duodenal TB from India describes 30 patients; with extrinsic involvement in majority and gastric outlet obstruction (GOO) as the presenting complain in three-fourth of the patients. Rest one-fourth presented with dyspepsia. Hematemesis was present in 7%.[11]

Jejunal and Ileocecal Tuberculosis

Ileocecal region is the most common site of gastrointestinal TB. It is involved in 44-93% of cases. The factors that predispose this region for the bacillary infection are:

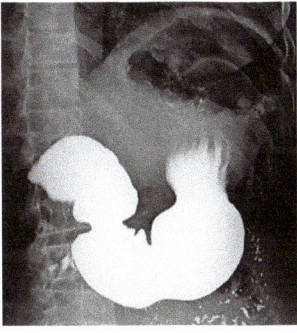
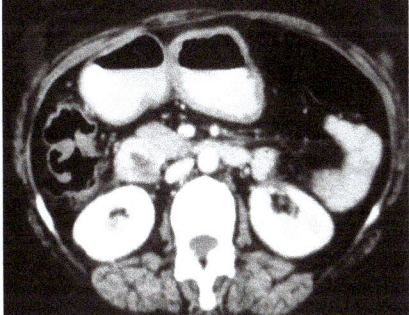

Fig. 1: Barium meal followthorough shows abrupt cut-off in the 2nd part of the duodenum. Contrast-enhanced CT (CECT) images show mild asymmetrical thickening of duodenum. Endoscopic biopsy was suggestive of tuberculosis.

- Stasis of food due to ileocecal valve and relatively narrow lumen
- Abundant lymphatic tissue in the region
- Favorable pH of the food
- High absorption rate of the food material in distal ileum as well as close contact of the mucosa with the causative agent.[5]

Isolated or primary involvement of jejunum is rare due to relatively acidic environment and quick transit of intestinal contents. It can be involved synchronously with ileocecal disease, presenting as single or multiple strictures. This may be secondary to the stasis of intestinal contents proximal to the ileocecal stricture. Intestinal TB can exist in three forms:[12]

- *Ulcerative variety*—ulcers are evident in the early phase of the disease caused by rupture of the submucosal caseous lymph nodes. The ulcers can be linear, transverse or circumferential. It may present with pain, diarrhea and rarely bleeding.
- *Hypertrophic or ulcerohypertrophic variety*—this is the result of robust immune response of the host against the tubercle bacilli resulting in enlarged lymph nodes and hypertrophic mucosa. It presents as a lump and is common in primary tuberculosis involving the ileocecal region.
- *Fibrous stricture*—in the late phase, the ulcers heal by cicatrization in response to antitubercular treatment (ATT) or host immunity, resulting in strictures (Fig. 2). Such patients present with features of obstruction—colicky abdominal pain, distension abdomen and recurrent vomiting resulting in weight loss.

Intestinal TB usually runs a chronic course with nonspecific features. Pain in abdomen (70-90%) and fever (40-70%) are the most common presenting features. Other symptoms include altered bowel habits, diarrhea and generalized weakness. Clinical and radiological features have a considerable overlap with Crohn's disease. Subtle differences between the two entities are enlisted in Table 2.

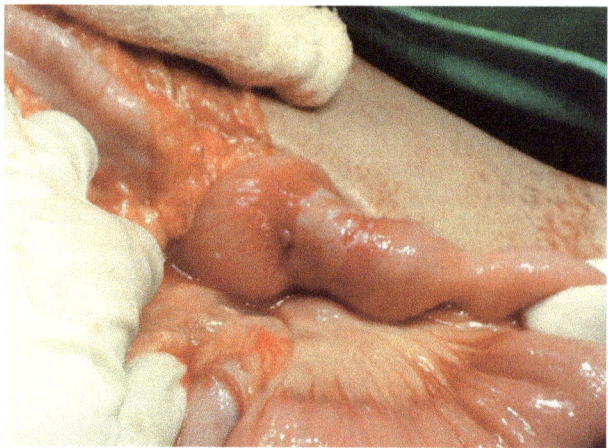

Fig. 2: Operative photograph showing stricture in terminal ileum. Segmental resection of bowel revealed tuberculosis on histology.

Table 2: Differentiation of abdominal tuberculosis from Crohn's disease.

Characteristics	Abdominal tuberculosis	Crohn's disease
Symptoms	Altered bowel habits, recurrent obstruction is more common	Diarrhea is common with per rectal bleed, obstruction in late phase in 10%
	Perianal involvement is uncommon	Perianal involvement in ~20%
	Skin and joint involvement rare	Extraintestinal manifestation in one-third
Radiological features	Mild mural thickening of bowel	Mural thickening marked with stratification
	Hypodense LNs with central necrosis and calcification	Nodes are discrete and few
	Dense ascites	Abscesses are common
Intraoperative findings	Mesentery is normal	Mesentery is hypervascular
	No creeping of fat	Fibro-fatty proliferation onto the bowel wall
	Strictures are concentric	Strictures are eccentric

One-third of TB patients present as acute abdomen. The most common complications are intestinal obstruction and perforation peritonitis.[3] Around 5–9% of all intestinal perforations presenting in India are tubercular, second only to typhoid fever. These perforations occur in the dilated bowel loop proximal to a stricture. Intestinal obstruction due to TB is common in India and accounts for nearly 20% of all the causes.[13]

Colorectal Tuberculosis

Colon is the second most common site of involvement after ileocecal region in the gut. Sigmoid is the most common site of involvement after the cecum. Colonic lesions are more common in immunocompromised individuals. They are multifocal in nearly one-third of the cases and present with pain abdomen, abdominal fullness, weight loss, anorexia, anemia and altered bowel habits. Linear or transverse ulcers are commonly evident on colonoscopy with features of narrowing in the involved segment.[3,14]

Peritoneal Tuberculosis

Peritoneum is most commonly affected in the abdominal cavity, accounting for 1-6% of all EPTB. It is more frequent in the third and the fourth decade of life.[15] Women are more commonly affected due to direct spread from the infected fallopian tubes. The other modes of transmission of infection to the peritoneal cavity include hematogenous and lymphatic route.[16] The peritoneal involvement can manifest in three ways:[16,17]

- *Gross ascites or wet type:* This is associated with moderate to large amount of free fluid in the peritoneal cavity. Occasionally, the fluid collection can be loculated or encysted. The patient presents with abdominal pain, distension, discomfort, low grade fever and anorexia. The fluid examination may reveal increased protein content with lymphocytosis. Coexisting liver disease and cirrhosis, which presents with low density ascites can obscure the picture on fluid analysis.
- *Fixed fibrotic or plastic type:* This form of TB involves the mesentery or the omentum resulting in bands and matted bowel loops. The bands may cause intestinal obstruction. Sclerosing encapsulating peritonitis (Fig. 3) or abdominal cocoon is an uncommon presentation, wherein a membranous sac covers the small intestine (partial) and sometimes the large intestine and solid organs as well (complete). It presents as abdominal lump, recurrent intestinal obstruction and abdominal pain.

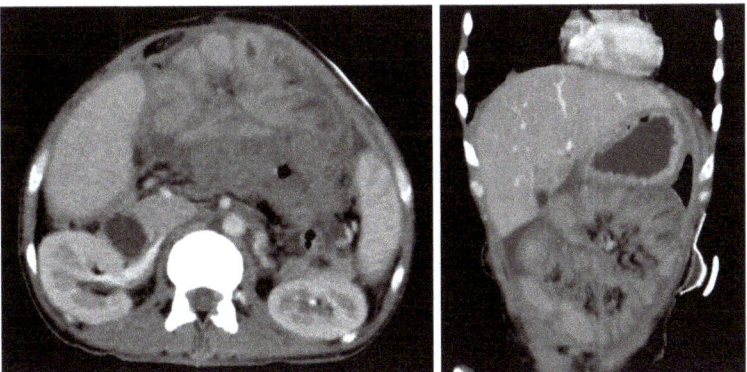

Fig. 3: Contrast-enhanced CT (CECT)—abdomen reveals encapsulation of small bowel loops within fibrous capsule in the central abdomen region with moderate interloop fluid collection, omental and mesenteric thickening with fat stranding, minimal ascitis with pneumoperitoneum.

Diagnosis can be established by cross-sectional imaging. At times, it is discovered on exploratory laparotomy when the patient lands in acute intestinal obstruction.
- *Purulent form:* Purulent ascites or loculated fluid collection is more common in females due to bacterial translocation from the genital tract. These patients present with persistent abdominal distension, pain, fever and paralytic ileus.

SOLID ORGAN TUBERCULOSIS

Involvement of solid viscera is reported in 15–20% patients with ATB. The affected organs include liver, spleen and pancreas. The disease usually spreads by hematogenous route. Pancreas can be affected secondarily by adjacent infected lymph nodes as well. Hepatic disease is commonly evident in the form of focal granulomatous lesions (tuberculous hepatitis). It can present as fever, weight loss, jaundice and hepatomegaly. The diagnosis is confirmed by liver biopsy. Pancreas is a highly vascular organ. It is seldom affected by the disease. It may present as pancreatic abscess or pancreatic mass mimicking a malignancy. The diagnosis can be established by biopsy from the mass or the adjacent lymph nodes. At times it is diagnosed postoperatively after pancreaticoduodenectomy.[12,18]

LYMPH NODE TUBERCULOSIS

Tubercular lymphadenitis mainly affects the mesenteric (tabes mesenterica), omental and the retroperitoneal lymph nodes (LNs). This is the most common manifestation of ATB in children and young. The incidence in adults is increasing due to the insurgence of acquired immunodeficiency syndrome (AIDS). Nodal involvement usually follows the organ affected. Presentation can vary from increase in the number of nodes to increase in size of nodes and formation of a conglomerate mass. The latter represents a cluster of inflamed lymphatic tissue and may present as a mass in children. Common symptoms include unexplained fever, weight loss, abdominal pain and at times abdominal lump. The nodes also get calcified and can be detected on radiographs.[12,19]

LABORATORY DIAGNOSIS

Abdominal TB often presents with nonspecific clinical features. A high index of suspicion is necessary to direct the correct set of investigations. Definitive diagnosis of TB can be established only on demonstration of *Mycobacterium tuberculosis (acid-fast bacilli or AFB)* by microbiologic, histologic or molecular methods. These tests often require fluid (ascitic fluid, pus) or tissues

(peritoneal/endoscopic/surgical biopsy) for diagnosis. Sample collection and handling should be done as per protocol to avoid contamination. Laboratory investigations, which are helpful for the establishment of diagnosis of TB, include:
- All cases of EPTB should be screened for HIV.
- *Mantoux test:* Tuberculin test was first described by Koch in 1890. Later in 1912, it was modified to intradermal injection of the antigen by Charles Mantoux. Purified protein derivative (PPD) is extracted from the cultures of *M. tuberculosis*. Five TU (Tuberculin unit) of the PPD is intradermally injected on the volar surface of the left forearm. Results are interpreted 48–72 hours later based on the size of induration measured in millimeters.[20]

Area of induration is not related to the disease activity, rather is affected by the medical risk factors. In immunosuppressed patients, induration of more than or equal to 5 mm, while in immunocompetent patients; that of more than or equal to 10 mm is considered significant. However, the specificity and positive predictive value of the test is poor.[21] Previous Bacillus Calmette-Guérin (BCG) vaccination can produce false positive results. Similarly, false-negative results can be seen with wrong technique, elderly patients and immunocompromised individuals. Moreover, the compliance is poor as it requires multiple visits. It is of little or no diagnostic value for abdominal tuberculosis and stands obsolete.
- *Interferon-gamma release assay (IGRA) (QuantiFERON-TB Gold):* It detects interferon gamma (IFN-γ) response produced by T lymphocytes, when stimulated by specific proteins such as ESAT-6 (Early secreted antigenic target of 6 kDa) and CFP-10 (culture filtrate protein 10) encoded by a genomic sequence unique to *M. tuberculosis*. The absence of cross-reactivity with other mycobacteria including BCG increases the specificity, when compared to Mantoux test. Additional advantage is that the results appear within 24 hours. However, it carries little significance in endemic areas as it does not differentiate between latent and active disease.[22]
- *Mycobacterial culture:* This remains the gold standard for diagnosis especially in peritoneal and solid organ tuberculosis. However, the time required for definitive results and frequent false negative results in paucibacillary specimens are important limitations. Various methods are available for the culture and drug sensitivity test (DST) as shown in Table 3.
- *Molecular methods:* A major development towards diagnosis of EPTB is the introduction of nucleic acid amplification tests (NAAT) such as polymerase chain reaction (PCR). This detects the nucleotide sequences specific to *M. tuberculosis* in ascitic fluid or tissue directly. The results are available within hours.

Table 3: Current diagnostic methods for *Mycobacteria* detection, culture and drug sensitivity.[23-29]

Diagnostic method	Time taken for final outcome	Detection time for drug resistance	Special features
Interferon-gamma release assay (IGRA)	24 hours	–	*Highly specific*: Can be performed on body fluids including ascitic fluid and serum. Little value in endemic region
Ziehl-Neelsen (ZN) staining	30 minutes	–	Classically used for pulmonary tuberculosis for detection of the bacilli in the sputum, but can be positive in biopsy specimens obtained after definitive surgery or endoscopy, peritoneal fluid or pus from abscesses in solid organs. Sensitivity is as low as 15–20% in biopsy specimens and below 5% in ascitic fluid
Lowenstein-Jensen (LJ) culture	6–8 weeks	8–12 weeks	Gold standard. Sample is incubated at 35–37°C in 5–10% CO_2 in the dark for 8 weeks. It facilitates drug sensitivity test (DST) as well. LJ culture in ascitic fluid is positive in ~20% of TB cases, but the sensitivity increases to nearly 90% in histopathologic specimens when combined with pathological evaluation
Liquid culture (BACTEC-TB460)	5–12 days	5–10 days	Based on the radiometric system that detects radioactive $^{14}CO_2$ liberated by live TB bacilli in the sample. Radioactivity can be used for quantitative assessment of the bacterial load. Addition of the inhibitory substances can help to assess DST. Can detect as low as 100 bacilli/mL of the infected fluid
New methods			
Nitrate reductase assay (NRA)	14–18 days	10 days	Works on the principle of detection of nitrite in the solution. *Mycobacteria* can convert nitrate to nitrite. NRA is run on the mycobacteria grown in the LJ medium. Sensitivity and specificity similar to BACTEC in detection of the drug resistant strains
Thin layer agar culture	14–18 days	10 days	Allows early detection of mycobacterial growth based on morphology and subsequent inoculation on Middlebrook medium. Sensitivity and specificity–similar to LJ culture
Calorimetric redox indicator assay	–	8 days	Based on the detection of metabolic activity (redox reactions with indicators like Resazurin) of mycobacteria. Very useful to detect MDR tuberculosis in nonresponders with an accuracy of over 90%

- *Polymerase chain reaction (PCR):* This technique involves three steps:
  - Shock treatment (acute temperature changes)—breaks the bacterial cell wall
  - Chemical lysis
  - DNA purification.

  The pathogen's DNA specific region is then amplified (IS6110 in *M. tuberculosis*) and detected by agarose gel electrophoresis. PCR confers high sensitivity. It is effective in paucibacillary samples with viable bacilli count as low as 10 bacilli/mL.[23] When combined with mycobacterial culture, accuracy is further enhanced and time to diagnosis is reduced significantly as well.
- *Reverse transcriptase PCR (RT PCR):* This is based on detection of specific mRNA in a sample after amplification. This can differentiate between viable and nonviable *M. tuberculosis*, as mRNA decomposes very fast in a dead cell. It is used for both the diagnosis of EPTB and monitoring drug resistance.
- *Fluorescence in-situ hybridization (FISH):* This uses an oligonucleotide probe labeled with fluorophore. It involves direct fluorescent microscopy and differentiates *M. tuberculosis* from other species. Studies have shown that FISH is more sensitive than PCR.[30]
- *Xpert M. tuberculosis or detection of rifampicin resistance (MTB/RIF):* It was initially developed for pulmonary tuberculosis to evaluate the sputum samples. Recently, it has been shown to be useful in EPTB as well. High degree of specificity is ensured by the use of 3 specific primers and 5 unique molecular probes. It targets the *rpoB* gene, critical in identifying the mycobacteria along with mutations related to rifampicin resistance. Results can be obtained within hours. In EPTB specimens (ascitic fluid and tissue biopsy), sensitivity and specificity is 81% and 99%, respectively.[27]
- *Immuno-PCR:* It is an ultrasensitive assay that detects protein antigens. It combines the versatility of ELISA with the sensitivity of NAA by PCR. This improves the sensitivity by 10^3–10^4 times as compared to an analogous ELISA. It uses MTB-specific RD1 and RD2 antigens and their antibodies in biological specimens of both pulmonary as well as extrapulmonary tuberculosis.[31] The accuracy improves many-fold, but the only deterrent to its use in developing countries is the cost.

Radiologic Investigations

Clinical presentation of ATB can be acute, subacute or chronic. Traditionally, X-ray abdomen and barium studies were used frequently for the evaluation of intestinal tuberculosis. Plain X-ray may show dilated small bowel loops and multiple air fluid levels depending on the severity of obstruction. In cases of intestinal perforation, air under the diaphragm is a confirmatory sign.

> **Box 1:** Diagnosis of intestinal TB based on barium studies.[33]
>
> *Group 1: Highly suggestive of TB:* If one or more is seen:
> - Deformed ileocecal valve with dilated ileum
> - Contracted cecum with abnormal ileocecal valve or terminal ileum
> - Stricture of ascending colon with shortening or involvement of ileocecal region
>
> *Group 2: Suggestive of intestinal TB:* If one or more characteristic is evident
> - Contracted cecum
> - Ulceration or narrowing of terminal ileum
> - Multiple sites of narrowing of small bowel
> - Stricture of ascending colon
>
> *Group 3:* Nonspecific changes
>
> *Group 4:* Normal study.

Barium studies are very informative. Barium meal followthrough is a dynamic study and is the best investigation to evaluate the ileal strictures. However, it does not give any information regarding the extraluminal disease. Few specific signs on barium are described in intestinal TB (Box 1):

- *Chicken intestine:* Hypersegmentation of the barium column due to increased peristalsis in the intestinal segment with ulceration and inflammation.
- *Hour-glass stenosis:* Multiple strictures with intermittent dilated bowel loops present with such a picture on barium studies.
- *Fleischner or inverted umbrella sign:* This is evident when there is a wide open ileocecal valve with thickened lips and narrowed terminal ileum.
- *Goose neck deformity:* Retracted, fibrosed cecum with dilated terminal ileum and loss of normal ileocecal angle.
- *Purse-string stenosis:* It is a localized stenosis near the ileocecal valve of the terminal ileum with a smooth cecum and distended distal ileum.
- *Stierlin sign:* This is seen in a case of acute inflammation superimposed on chronically diseased segment of bowel. On barium contrast study, the inflamed segment (ileocecal region) does not retain the contrast with normal appearance of barium column in the bowel on either side.
- *String sign:* This signifies a strictured segment, which appears as a string on barium contrast study.
- Stierlin and string signs are not specific to tuberculosis as they can be seen in Crohn's disease as well.[32]

Computed Tomographic (CT) Scan

It has an advantage over barium studies in demonstrating both the intraluminal and extraluminal pathologies, though it may not be very accurate for early strictures. Nowadays, they are being commonly used. Typical features are circumferential wall thickening (Fig. 4) of the bowel, omental

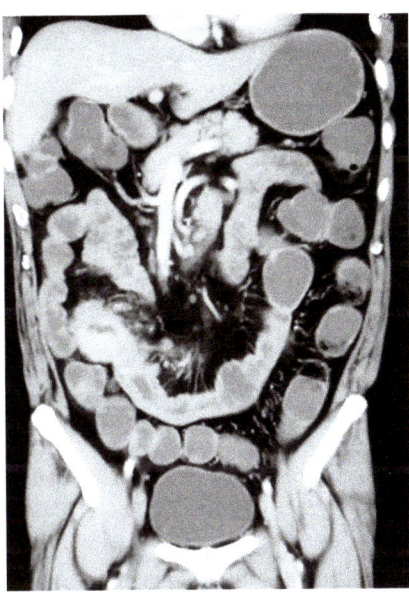

Fig. 4: Contrast-enhanced CT (CECT) abdomen showing multiple strictures in the small bowel with circumferential thickening of the wall.

soft tissue densities, high density ascites and lymphadenopathy (caseation/calcification). The wall thickness may go up to 3 cm. Contrast-enhanced CT (CECT) is better than plain CT. Peripheral rim enhancement of lymph nodes is typical of ATB. Involvement of mesenteric, omental and upper para-aortic LNs is common in TB, while lower para-aortic LN involvement suggests lymphoma. In ileocecal tuberculosis, asymmetrically thickened cecum and ileum with adjacent lymphadenopathy is evident (Fig. 5). CT enteroclysis is more informative with respect to strictures and it is located by the point of abrupt tapering in the bowel.

Contrast-enhanced CT can be used to differentiate peritoneal carcinomatosis from TB. The peritoneum in ATB appears smooth and mildly thickened, while in malignancy, it appears nodular with irregular thickening. Tuberculosis of solid organs is best evaluated by CECT. Hepatosplenomegaly with areas of calcification and multiple small round lesions with peripheral enhancement in the parenchyma are suggestive of granulomatous inflammation. CT-guided biopsy is useful to establish the diagnosis in deep seated lesions. Pancreas involvement can present with hypodense areas in and around the organ.[34]

Ultrasonography (USG)

It is useful in peritoneal and lymph node tuberculosis. The following features may be evident, usually in combination:

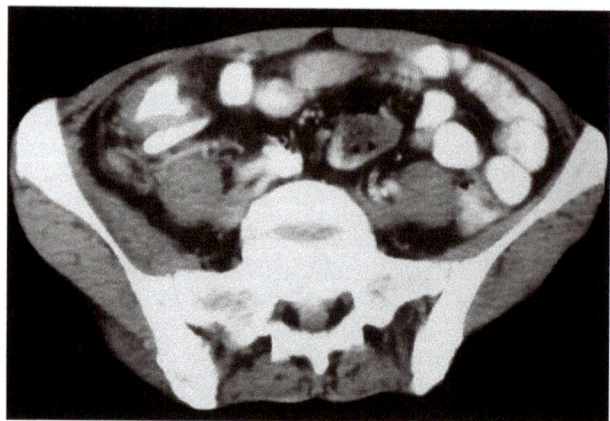

Fig. 5: Contrast-enhanced CT (CECT) axial image shows mild asymmetrical thickening of the ileocecal region. Adjacent few lymph nodes are also noted. Findings typical but not pathognomonic of tuberculosis.

- Intra-abdominal free fluid or loculated ascites. Septae can be appreciated on USG.
- Lymph node involvement—discrete or matted nodes can be detected with heteroechoic features in case of central necrosis or caseation. Calcification can be seen in healing lesions as reflective lines. This distinguishes TB from lymphoma and malignancy.
- Bowel wall thickening can be easily appreciated on sonogram.
- Pseudo-kidney sign—pulled up ileocecal complex in subhepatic region appears as a pseudo-kidney.

Endoscopy

Morphologically, on colonoscopy, the lesions can be ulcerative or ulceroproliferative. The right colon (ascending colon and cecum) may appear thickened and shortened. The ileocecal valve is often narrowed and deformed. At times, the valve may appear wide open with stricture in the distal ileum. It may become difficult to distinguish TB from malignancy and Crohn's disease, but for the histology. Presence of caseation with granuloma forms the hallmark of tuberculosis. The granulomas are not present in the intestinal wall, instead are found in the lymph nodes, unlike the Crohn's disease.[13] In case of gastric TB, upper GI endoscopy may reveal ulcers in the distal stomach. In cases of gastric outlet obstruction, stomach will be full of food materials. After lavage, concentric stricture may be evident at pylorus or the third part of the duodenum. In esophagus, traction diverticulae are evident in the mid esophagus. Tubercular ulceration in the esophagus is very rare.

Double balloon enteroscopy (DBE) and capsule endoscopy (CE) are novel techniques used to evaluate the small intestine. Insertion depth for DBE when put per oral is up to 270 cm beyond ligament of Treitz and up to 150 cm per anal. Capsule endoscope traverses through the length of the bowel and keeps on taking pictures. The typical characteristics of a tubercular ulcer are: multiple 1-2 cm transverse or oblique mucosal ulcers with necrotic base. It is difficult to distinguish from ulcers in inflammatory bowel disease (IBD). DBE scores over capsule endoscopy (CE) from the fact that it can be used for taking biopsies. Studies comparing both the techniques including a meta-analysis has found no statistical difference in the diagnostic yield. However, high retention rate of capsules (~2%) which entails surgery remains a matter of concern.[35]

Other Supportive Tests in Tuberculosis

Diagnosis of tuberculosis is usually made by relevant radiological studies and histopathological correlation obtained by endoscopic [(colonoscopic, endoscopic or endoscopic ultrasound- fine-needle aspiration (EUS FNA)] or image guided biopsies (USG/CT). Caseation in granulomas is the hallmark of TB. Suri et al. reported 58% sensitivity of USG-guided fine-needle aspiration cytology (FNAC) in abdominal lymphadenopathy. EUS-FNA was studied by Puri et al. as a tool for diagnosing abdominal lymphadenopathy of unknown etiology. It was found to be effective in 76% of cases in establishing TB.[36]

Hematological parameters (raised erythrocyte sedimentation rate, low hemoglobin or hypoalbuminemia) are nonspecific for TB.[3] Ascitic fluid analysis in peritoneal TB usually shows lymphocytosis with low SAAG (serum ascitic albumin gradient <1.1 g/L). Acid-fast bacilli detection on staining of ascitic fluid smear is productive in less than 3% cases and culture of the same yields positive results in around one-fifth of the cases. Adenosine deaminase (ADA) levels are increased in tubercular ascites. Level above 36 IU/L is suggestive of a positive diagnosis.[37] Gupta et al. documented sensitivity and specificity of 100% and 94% respectively with cut-off level of 30 IU/L.[38] American Diabetes Association (ADA) measurement is misleading in certain circumstances like HIV, where the levels are falsely low and in malignancies where they can be falsely high. Thus, the overall diagnostic yield remains low. Analysis of ascitic fluid interferon-γ assay adds to the sensitivity and specificity when used in combination with ADA. Recently, various molecular and immunological tests have been proposed for the abdominal tuberculosis (described in Laboratory Diagnosis). These tests can be performed on ascitic fluid, lymph node biopsies, sampled omentum or mesentery after diagnostic laparoscopy. In one study, which used real time assay by FISH (Fluorescence Resonance Energy Transfer) improved the detection rate by 36% in patients with suspicion of TB on clinical examination and radiologic studies, but with an unyielding smear test and fluid culture for AFB.[39] The target antigen for polymerase chain reaction (PCR) is IS6110. Multiplex PCRs (using IS6110 and MPB64) have further improved the diagnostic yield to around 70% in suspected cases of gastrointestinal tuberculosis. The sensitivity and specificity is 90% and 100% respectively in histologically or microbiologically proven cases of tuberculosis.[40]

Role of Diagnostic Laparoscopy

Clinical features of abdominal tuberculosis are nonspecific. Therapeutic trial with antitubercular treatment is not warranted. Thus, histological evidence holds great importance. This makes laparoscopy valuable in the diagnosis of ATB. Features on diagnostic laparoscopy: small whitish tubercles over peritoneum (Fig. 6); inflammatory adhesions; thickening, hyperemia and retraction of the greater omentum and fibrous bands extending from the parietal to the visceral peritoneum termed "*stalactic*" are highly suggestive of tubercular pathology.[41] These should be supported by histological examination. Early laparoscopy is safe and avoids expensive, time consuming and at times fruitless investigations.

Histopathology in Tuberculosis

Specimens in the setting of TB are characterized by:[42]
- Central caseous necrosis
- Granulomatous inflammation (>400 μm) containing macrophages, lymphocytes and Langhans giant cells (50–80%)
- An acid-fast bacilli staining is occasionally positive (5–10%).

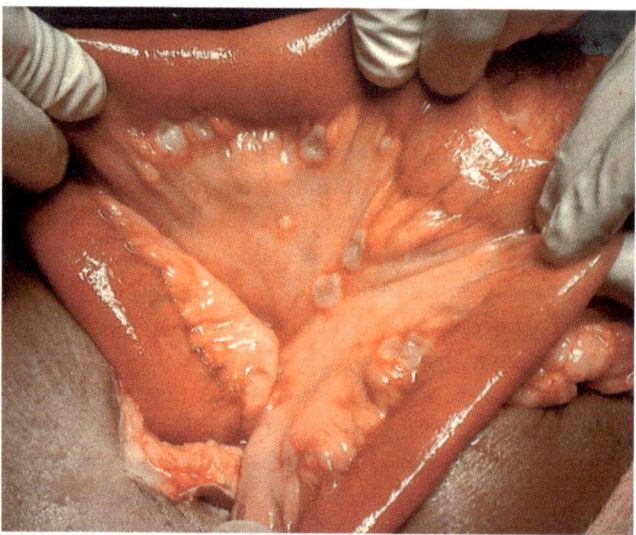

Fig. 6: Intraoperative photograph of multiple mesenteric tubercles with caseation.

Granulomas may be seen in CD as well, but they are noncaseating, nonconfluent and less than 200 μm in diameter.

Criteria for the Diagnosis of Abdominal Tuberculosis

Paustian's Criteria

It consists of four criteria. Any of the criteria if positive, establishes the diagnosis:
1. Histology of specimen obtained by surgery or endoscopy shows tubercles with caseation
2. Operative findings suggestive of TB and the mesenteric lymph nodes with caseation or calcification
3. Tissue positive for AFB staining
4. Tissue culture reveals Mycobacteria.

Logan modified the Paustian's criteria and uses response to ATT as a criterion to establish diagnosis. These criteria hold true in present time. New investigative modalities have enabled to establish the diagnosis in almost all the patients except few.[43]

Management of Abdominal Tuberculosis

Abdominal TB responds well to antitubercular drugs. Early diagnosis and proper treatment can avoid surgical intervention in most of the patients.[44] Anand BS et al. (1988) concluded in their study on 34 patients that most of the tubercular strictures can be safely treated with antitubercular drugs. In this study, 90% patients became asymptomatic and 70% strictures resolved by the end of the treatment. They also concluded that the strictures unlikely to respond are long strictures (> 12 cm in length) and the disease involving multiple segments. Surgery should be the last resort in the management of ATB.[45]

Some of the reports have shown that healing after ATT can lead to strictures. Use of rifampicin has been subjected to the increased incidence of fibrosis and cicatrisation.[46] Few authors have recommended that once bowel obstruction is evident, ATT is of little help and surgery becomes imperative. Surgery becomes unavoidable in perforation peritonitis, nonresolving intestinal obstruction, enterocutaneous fistula and abscess as well.

Diagnosed cases of abdominal TB must be administered at least 6 months of ATT. This comprises of two months of four drug regimen (Rifampicin, Isoniazid, Pyrazinamide and Ethambutol), followed by two drugs (Rifampicin and Isoniazid) for 4 months. It is effective in peritoneal tuberculosis and nodal disease. Perianal fistulae and intestinal ulcers usually resolve on appropriate treatment. Some clinicians do extend the therapy for 9-12 months, but it has been established that there is no added benefit of long-term treatment.

In fact, the compliance is affected and complications increase on extending the duration of therapy.[47] In patients coinfected with HIV, WHO recommends antiretroviral therapy (ART) irrespective of CD4 cell count. The ART should be introduced after ATT by the earliest. Efavirenz is the preferred non-nucleoside reverse transcriptase inhibitor in such patients.[48]

One of the dreaded complications of ATT is fulminant hepatitis. It usually presents in the 2nd week of therapy. It is more common when Isoniazid (H) and Rifampicin (R) are given in combination. The primary drugs [H, R and Pyrazinamide (Z)] are stopped and liver function test (LFT) is monitored regularly. Meanwhile patient is started on second line therapy. Second line drugs include: fluoroquinolones, amikacin along with ethambutol and streptomycin. Once the transaminases become normal, isoniazid is reintroduced in an escalating dose with continuous monitoring of the liver enzymes. Three reintroduction regimens proposed in literature are:

1. Three drug regimen (HRZ) at maximum dosage from day 1.[49]
2. R at maximum dosage from day 1, H at maximum dosage from day 8, and Z at maximum dosage from day 15 (American Thoracic Society).[50]
3. H at dosage of 100 mg/day from day 1, maximum dosage from day 4; R at dosage of 150 mg/day from day 8, maximum dosage from day 11; and Z at dosage of 500 mg/day from day 15, maximum dosage from day 18 (British Thoracic Society)[51] *(Maximum dosage was determined according to body weight, as follows: H-5 mg/kg; R-10 mg/kg; and Z-25 mg/kg.)*[49,50] Sharma et al.[50] in his comparative study on the three regimens documented that all the drugs can be reintroduced at the same time with equal safety. This enables timely treatment in adequate doses.

Role of Surgery

Surgery is considered as the last resort in the management of ATB.

Gastroduodenal Tuberculosis[11]

These patients present with GOO or upper gastrointestinal bleed. Patients presenting with GOO should undergo gastrojejunostomy rather than pyloroplasty. Biopsy should be taken from prominent node or the stomach or duodenal wall. Stomach ulcer with intractable bleed requires truncal vagotomy with antrectomy. Duodenal ulcers with bleed can be managed by segmental resection.

Ileocecal and Small Bowel Tuberculosis

Three types of surgeries have been described depending on the radicality:[3]
1. *First* is bypass surgery, usually performed in emergency settings, where the dissection of the bowel segment, especially the ileocecal region is not possible or the patient is not very stable to prolong the procedure.

It is usually avoided due to the likely chances of blind loop syndrome, development of a fistula and persistence of the diseased segment.
2. *Second* type of procedure includes conservative approach–stricturoplasty. It is possible till 50% of luminal narrowing and is useful in cases with multiple strictures or single short length stricture. The type of surgery is decided by the length of stricture. Short stricture can be managed by Heineke-Mikulicz technique, which includes longitudinal opening of the affected segment and transverse closure of the same to restore the lumen size. Disadvantages of stricturoplasty are: inadequate tissue sampling and persistence of diseased segment. In case of longer strictures (>10 cm) or multiple short strictures over a small segment of bowel, resection anastomosis is warranted. Rarely, when there is a risk of short bowel syndrome, Jabuolay's or Finney's strictureplasty (commonly described for Crohn's disease) can be done.
3. Finally, the *third* type of surgery is radical and curative. Involved small bowel is resected and anastomosed. For the ileocecal region, right hemicolectomy eradicates the disease completely. Such surgeries are increasingly being performed in elective setting with the advent of effective ATT.[52]

Earlier, right hemicolectomy and intestinal resection required large abdominal incisions, compelling prolonged use of analgesics and increased hospital stay. Laparoscopy assisted procedure decreases the size of incision, thus cutting on the postoperative morbidity and early return to work for the patients doing manual labor. These are the patients who often are affected by tuberculosis in developing countries. Moreover, such a procedure is cosmetically superior for young adults.[53] The advantage of minimally invasive technique has decreased the threshold for intervention as well. Peritoneal bands causing obstruction can be easily divided laparoscopically.

Other indications for surgery include acute abdomen with intestinal obstruction or perforation peritonitis. The perforation usually occurs in the ileum proximal to the stricture. The perforated segment with the strictured bowel is resected and primarily anastomosed or is exteriorized as a two-staged procedure. Restoration of bowel continuity can be safely done after 8–12 weeks of primary surgery.

Enterocutaneous Fistula[54,55]

Enterocutaneous fistula can be spontaneous or postoperative. The management remains similar. Usual presentation postoperative is in the 2nd week. The major risk factors include poor nutritional status, gross intra-abdominal contamination, hemodynamic instability and immunosuppressed status. Initial issues with a new fistula include sepsis, electrolyte imbalance and poor nutrition. The patient should be resuscitated and started on broad spectrum antibiotics. Commonly lost electrolytes (sodium, potassium) should be replaced and monitored regularly. Enterostomal nurse should be involved to affect adequate peri-incisional skin care. Once the patient is stabilized, he or she should be started on parenteral nutrition and ATT. Use of somatostatin analogs to decrease the fistula output and hasten the closure remains a matter of debate.

After 7–10 days, assessment of fistula anatomy is done by fistulography. Low output fistulae (<200 mL/day) without evidence of sepsis usually respond to ATT with progressive decrease in output. Most of them close by 6–8 weeks. High output fistula (> 500 mL/day) with no decreasing trend are unlikely to close spontaneously. The waiting period for the definitive surgery in such cases should preferably be 6 weeks post sepsis.

In patients with evidence of ongoing infection and sepsis, CECT helps to detect any missed enterotomy, intra-abdominal collection and can direct drainage of the same. Those who do not respond to conservative trial are taken up for reexploration with the intent to drain pus pockets, perform peritoneal lavage and fashion a formal enterostomy.

Perianal Fistula

The perianal fistula in TB is common in immunocompromised individuals. They should be screened for HIV and enquired about the use of immunosuppressant. Low anal fistula is usually diagnosed after excision biopsy. They should receive ATT for 6 months as there is a high chance of recurrence. It is common to find complex and high fistula in association with TB. The management is usually conservative. Some patients may require diversion of stool by a colostomy. Biopsy becomes very important to direct medical therapy, which is usually effective. Video-assisted fistula therapy can be used safely for residual disease as the chances of sphincter injury are minimal with this technique.

Enterovesical Fistula[56]

This is a rare entity with ATB. The pathophysiology remains transmural inflammation of the bowel wall involving the bladder. Secondly, a contained perforation resulting in localized abscess may rupture into the bladder. The patient presents with pneumaturia, cystitis and fecaluria. Best investigation to demonstrate the pathology is CECT abdomen with pelvis. These patients are initially started on ATT. Those who do not respond to medical management or there is severe cystitis, resection of the bowel segment with closure of the bladder defect results in cure.

VISCERAL ORGAN TUBERCULOSIS

Liver abscess may be managed by diagnostic aspirate followed by ATT. If the lesions do not resolve, get secondarily infected or get ruptured, then may

Table 4: New modalities in management of TB.

Newer drugs	Mode of action	Dose	Effectiveness
Delamanid (OPC-67683)[59]	A nitro-dihydro-imidazooxazole derivative–inhibits mycolic acid synthesis against MDR strains	100–200 mg twice daily in combination × 8 weeks	Patients with MDR-TB 45–50% culture conversion. Effective against MDR-TB
Bedaquiline (TMC207)[60]	A diarylquinoline–targets protons pump of adenosine triphosphate (ATP) synthase Leads to inadequate synthesis of ATP	400 mg once daily for 2 weeks then 200 mg thrice daily in combination with other drugs × 8–24 weeks	Seroconversion and culture conversion rate after 24 weeks is ~80% in MDR-TB
PA-824[61]	The nitroimidazole-oxazine PA-824- derivative of metronidazole Inhibits synthesis of ketomycolates–essential component of cell wall of *Mycobacteria* Paralyses respiratory apparatus of the bacilli by donating nitric oxide during enzymatic nitroreduction	150 mg/200 mg daily for 14 days is safe and efficacious in combination with other drugs	PA-824 in combination with other drugs such as pyrazinamide and moxifloxacin is more effective than bedaquiline in treating MDR-TB and sensitive strains as well
Oxazolidinones (Cycloserine and Linezolid) (New drug is sutezolid and posizolid)[62]	Competitive inhibition of translation of the messenger RNA by binding to specific transfer proteins	Sutezolid–well tolerated in doses 600–1,200 mg per day for 14 days Posizolid—being evaluated in phase II studies–500 mg once and twice daily for 14 days	Efficacy being evaluated in studies

New Drug Delivery Systems

Nanotechnology[63]	"Nanoparticle" refers to a colloidal particle with a size of <1 μm		
Nanodispersion	Nanosuspensions are submicron colloidal dispersions of pure drugs stabilized with surfactants. Reduction of size of solid drug particles facilitates solubility of drugs and thus bioavailability		
Nanosuspension	Nanoemulsions are thermodynamically stable oil-in-water dispersions. They are generated spontaneously and easily produced on a large scale		
Niosomes	Niosomes are thermodynamically stable liposome-like vesicles. Can host hydrophilic drugs within the core. Oral delivery of nanoparticle encapsulated anti-TB drugs is advantageous–increases the efficacy, reduces degradation in the bowel, and increasing uptake and bioavailability. This is effective in parental and inhalational drugs as well[64]		

require image guided drainage or laparoscopic lavage. Splenic abscess is rare and can be easily managed by splenectomy. Pancreatic involvement mimics pancreatic carcinoma. At times, caseous LNs detected at the time of surgery may suggest TB. Such nodes should be sent for frozen section. Later, they can be managed well with ATT.

Emerging Newer, Repurposed Drugs against Tuberculosis

Development of better and more effective vaccines as well as drugs is required to achieve the WHO goal of eliminating the disease by 2,050.[57,58] Several new drugs against TB are in various stages of development. Delamanid (OPC-67683), Bedaquiline (TMC-207) and the nitroimidazole-oxazine PA-824 are effective against both drug-sensitive and drug-resistant strains (Table 4). Bedaquiline (TMC-207) has been approved for use by the United States Food and Drug Administration (US FDA). Indian government has plans to regulate the introduction and use of these new drugs in a streamlined way.

CONCLUSION

Abdominal TB remains a diagnostic challenge. Early diagnosis avoids complications and unnecessary surgical interventions. Laparoscopy is of great help in diagnostic dilemma. Abdominal disease usually responds well to medical treatment. Surgery is reserved for nonresponders and in case of complication. Resection of the diseased segment is preferred over conservative approach. Decline in number of TB cases worldwide since 2006 is encouraging. With new drugs, improving technology, political will and effective policies, the goal of TB elimination by 2,050 appears to be achievable.

REFERENCES

1. Rosenblatt MB. Pulmonary tuberculosis: evolution of modern therapy. Bull NY Acad Med. 1973;49(3):163-96.
2. Sharma SK, Mohan A. Tuberculosis: From an incurable scourge to a curable disease–journey over a millennium. Indian J Med Res. 2013;137(3):455-93.
3. Sharma MP, Bhatia V. Abdominal tuberculosis. Indian J Med Res. 2004;120(4):305-15.
4. Shaikh MS, Dholia KR, Jalbani MA. Prevalence of intestinal tuberculosis in cases of acute abdomen. Pakistan J Surg. 2007;23:52-6.
5. Choi EH, Coyle WJ. Gastrointestinal tuberculosis. Microbiol Spectr. 2016;4(6):10.
6. Paustian FF, Marshall JB. Intestinal tuberculosis. In: Berk JE (Ed). Bokus Gastroenterology, 4th edition. Philadelphia: WB Saunders; 1985. pp. 2018-36.
7. Gondal KM, Khan AF. Changing pattern of abdominal tuberculosis. Pak J Surg. 1995;11:109-13.
8. Donoghue HD, Holton J. Intestinal tuberculosis. Curr Opin Infect Dis. 2009;22(5):490-6.

9. DiFebo G, Calabrese C, Areni A, et al. Oesophageal tuberculosis mimicking secondary oesophageal involvement by mediastinal neoplasm. Ital J Gastroenterol Hepatol. 1997;29(6):564-8.
10. Ali W, Sikora SS, Banerjee D, et al. Gastroduodenal tuberculosis. Aust NZ J Surg. 1993;63(6):466-7.
11. Gupta SK, Jain AK, Gupta JP, et al. Duodenal tuberculosis. Clin Radiol. 1998;39(2):159-61.
12. Khan IA, Khattak IU, Asif S, et al. Abdominal tuberculosis an experience at Ayub Teaching Hospital Abbottabad. J Ayub Med Coll Abbottabad. 2008;20(4):115-8.
13. Sharma R. Abdominal Tuberculosis. Imaging Science Today. 2009;146.
14. Sharma SK, Mohan A. Extrapulmonary tuberculosis. Indian J Med Res. 2004;120(4):316-53.
15. Guirat A, Koubaa M, Mzali R, et al. Peritoneal tuberculosis. Clini Res Hepatol Gastroenterol. 2011;35(1):60-9.
16. Vaid U, Kane GC. Tuberculous peritonitis. Microbiol Spectr. 2017;5(1):10.
17. Skopin MS, Batyrov FA, Kornilova Z. The prevalence of abdominal tuberculosis and the specific features of its detection. Probl Tuberk Bolezn Legk. 2007;(1):22-6.
18. Sharma V, Rana SS, Kumar A, et al. Pancreatic tuberculosis. J Gastroenterol Hepatol. 2016;31(2):310-8.
19. Debi U, Ravisankar V, Prasad KK et al. Abdominal tuberculosis of the gastrointestinal tract: Revisited. World J Gastroenterol. 2014;20(40):14831-40.
20. American Thoracic Society. The tuberculin skin test. Am Rev Respir Dis. 1981;124:346-51.
21. Al Zahrani K, Al Jahdali H, Menzies D. Does size matter? Utility of size of tuberculin reactions for the diagnosis of mycobacterial disease. Am J Resp Crit Care Med. 2000;162(4 Pt 1):1419-22.
22. Dosanjh DP, Hinks TS, Innes JA, et al. Improved diagnostic evaluation of suspected tuberculosis. Ann Intern Med. 2008;148(5):325-36.
23. Negi SS, Khan SF, Gupta S, et al. Comparison of the conventional diagnostic modalities, bactec culture and polymerase chain reaction test for diagnosis of tuberculosis. Indian J Med Microbiol. 2005;23(1):29-33.
24. Palomino JC. Current developments and future perspectives for TB diagnostics. Future Microbiol. 2012;7(1):59-71.
25. Brossier F, Veziris N, Aubry A, et al. Detection by Geno Type MTBDRsl test of complex mechanisms of resistance to second-line drugs and ethambutol in multidrug-resistant *Mycobacterium tuberculosis* complex isolates. J Clin Microbiol. 2010;48(5):1683-9.
26. Martin A, Portaels F, Palomino JC. Colorimetric redox-indicator methods for the rapid detection of multidrug resistance in *Mycobacterium tuberculosis*: A systematic review and meta-analysis. J Antimicrob Chemother. 2007;59(2):175-83.
27. Lawn SD, Nicol MP. Xpert MTB/RIF assay: development, evaluation and implementation of a new rapid molecular diagnostic for tuberculosis and rifampicin resistance. Future Microbiol. 2011;6(9):1067-82.
28. Ling DI, Zwerling AA, Pai M. GenoType MTBDR assays for the diagnosis of multidrug-resistant tuberculosis: A meta-analysis. Eur Respir J. 2008;32(5):1165-74.

29. Martin A, Panaiotov S, Portaels F, et al. The nitrate reductase assay for the rapid detection of isoniazid and rifampicin resistance in Mycobacterium tuberculosis: A systematic review and meta-analysis. J Antimicrob Chemother. 2008;62(1): 56-64.
30. Fenhalls G, Stevens L, Moses L, et al. In situ detection of *Mycobacterium tuberculosis* transcripts in human lung granulomas reveals differential gene expression in necrotic lesions. Infect Immun. 2002;70(11):6330-8.
31. Mehta PK, Raj A, Singh N, et al. Diagnosis of extrapulmonary tuberculosis by PCR. FEMS Immunol Med Microbiol. 2012;66(1):20-36
32. Harisinghani MG, McLoud TC, Shepard JA, et al. Tuberculosis from head to toe. Radiographics. 2000;20(2):449-70.
33. Kumar N, Aggarwal R. Abdominal tuberculosis. In: API Textbook of Medicine, 7th edition. Mumbai: National Book Depot (Distributor); 2003. pp. 562.
34. Nagi B, Kochhar R, Bhasin DK, et al. Colorectal tuberculosis. Eur Radiol. 2003;13(8):1907-12.
35. Chen WG, Shan GD, Zhang H, et al. Double-balloon enteroscopy in small bowel diseases: Eight years single-center experience in China. Medicine (Baltimore). 2016;95(42):e5104.
36. Puri R, Mangla R, Eloubeidi M, et al. Diagnostic yield of EUS-guided FNA and cytology in suspected tubercular intra-abdominal lymphadenopathy. Gastrointest Endosc. 2012;75(5):1005-10.
37. Bhargava DK, Gupta M, Nijhawan S, et al. Adenosine deaminase (ADA) in peritoneal tuberculosis: Diagnostic value in ascitic fluid and serum. Tubercle. 1990;71(2):121-6.
38. Gupta VK, Mukherjee S, Dutta SK, et al. Diagnostic evaluation of ascetic adenosine deaminase activity in tuberculosis peritonitis. J Assoc Physicians India. 1992;40(6):387-9.
39. Mishra PK, Bhargava A, Punde RP, et al. Diagnosis of gastrointestinal tuberculosis: Using cytomorphological, microbiological, immunological and molecular techniques: A study from Central India. Indian J Clin Biochem. 2010;25(2):158-63.
40. Sharma K, Sinha SK, Sharma A, et al. Multiplex PCR for rapid diagnosis of gastrointestinal tuberculosis. J Glob Infect Dis. 2013;5(2):49-53.
41. Safarpor F, Aghajanzade M, Kohsari MR, et al. Role of laparoscopy in the diagnosis of abdominal tuberculosis. Saudi J Gastroenterol. 2007;13(3):133-5.
42. Alvares JF, Devarbhavi H, Makhija P, et al. Clinical, colonoscopic and histological profile of colonic tuberculosis in a tertiary hospital. Endoscopy. 2005;37(4): 351-6.
43. Paustian FF. Tuberculosis of the intestine. In: Bockus HL (Ed). Gastroenterology, 2nd edition. Philadelphia: WB Saunders Co; 1964.
44. Logan VS. Anorectal tuberculosis. Proc R Soc Med. 1969;62(12):1227-30.
45. Anand BS, Nanda R, Sachdev GK. Response of tuberculous stricture to antituberculous treatment. Gut, 1988;29(1):62-9.
46. Uzunkoy A, Harma M, Harma M. Diagnosis of abdominal tuberculosis: experience from 11 cases and review of the literature. World J Gastroenterol. 2004;10(24):3647-9.

47. Pimparkar BD. Abdominal tuberculosis. J Assoc Physicians India. 1977;25(11): 801-11.
48. Das HS, Rathi P, Sawant P, et al. Colonic tuberculosis: Colonoscopic appearance and clinico-pathologic analysis. J Assoc Physicians India. 2000;48(7):708-10.
49. Antiretroviral therapy for HIV infection in adults and adolescents. Recommendations for a public health approach: 2010 revision. Geneva: World Health Organization; 2010.
50. Sharma SK, Singla R, Sarda P, et al. Safety of 3 Different reintroduction regimens of antituberculosis drugs after development of antituberculosis treatment-induced hepatotoxicity. Clin Infect Dis. 2010;50(6):833-9.
51. Saukkonen JJ, Cohn DL, Jasmer RM, et al. on the behalf of ATS Hepatotoxicity of Antituberculosis Therapy Subcommittee. An official ATS statement: Hepatotoxicity of Antituberculosis Therapy. Am J Respir Crit Care Med. 2006;174(8):935-52.
52. Joint Tuberculosis Committee of the British Thoracic Society. Chemotherapy and management of tuberculosis in the United Kingdom. Thorax. 1998;53(7):536-48.
53. Pujari BD. Modified surgical procedures in intestinal tuberculosis. Br J Surg. 1979;66(3):180-1
54. Balsara KP, Shah CR, Maru S, et al. Laparoscopic-assisted ileo-colectomy for tuberculosis. Surg Endosc. 2005;19(7):986-89.
55. Machoki SM, Saidi H, Ahmed M. Conservative management of a high output enterocutaneous fistula in abdominal tuberculosis. BMJ Case Rep. 2011;2011.
56. Schecter WP, Hirshberg A, Chang DS, et al. Enteric fistulas: Principles of management. J Am Coll Surg. 2009;209(4):484-91.
57. Balachandra D, Nag HH, Sakhuja P, et al. Tuberculosis of intestine with concurrent complex enterovesical and enterocutaneous fistula. J Clin Diagnosis Res. 2018;12(7):PD03-05.
58. Zumla A, Hafner R, Lienhardt C, et al. Advancing the development of tuberculosis therapy. Nat Rev Drug Discov. 2012;11(3):171-2.
59. Sachdeva KS, Kumar A, Dewan P, et al. New vision for Revised National Tuberculosis Control Program (RNTCP): Universal access—"Reaching the unreached." Indian J Med Res. 2012;135:690-4.
60. Gler MT, Skripconoka V, Sanchez-Garavito E, et al. Delamanid for multidrug-resistant pulmonary tuberculosis. N Engl J Med. 2012;366(23):2151-60.
61. Deoghare S. Bedaquiline: a new drug approved for treatment of multidrug-resistant tuberculosis. Indian J Pharmacol. 2013;45(5):536-7.
62. Diacon AH, Dawson R, Hanekom M, et al. Early bactericidal activity and pharmacokinetics of PA-824 in smear-positive tuberculosis patients. Antimicrob Agents Chemother. 2010;54(8):3402-7.
63. Villemagne B, Crauste C, Flipo M, et al. Tuberculosis: the drug development pipeline at a glance. Eur J Med Chem. 2012;51:1-16.
64. Smith JP. Nanoparticle delivery of anti-tuberculosis chemotherapy as a potential mediator against drug-resistant tuberculosis. Yale J Biol Med. 2011;84(4):361-9.

10
Chapter

Recent Advances in Renal Cell Carcinoma

Sameer Trivedi, Manish Pandey

INTRODUCTION

Renal cell carcinoma (RCC), considered to be the most deadly of all urologic cancers, epitomizes a significant health challenge. The Worldwide incidence of RCC is 5% of all cancers in men and 3% in women, making it the sixth most common malignancy in men and the 10th most common malignancy in women.[1] The incidence of RCC is increasing, in part due to the earlier detection of asymptomatic renal masses found incidentally on abdominal imaging for nonrelated symptoms, but also due to an actual rise in the occurrence, presumably as a result of increased penetration of various genetic and epigenetic factors which are hitherto not fully characterized.[2] Although most RCCs in contemporary era are small incidental tumors at diagnosis, yet locally advanced lesions are still seen in a significant number of patients and up to 17% patients are reported to carry distant metastases at the time of diagnosis.[3]

Recent research into the pathogenesis of inheritable variants of RCC has imparted important understanding of the genetic mechanisms with the characterization of precise genetic alterations that play a key role in the origin of RCC.[4] This insight has resulted in the advent of novel therapeutic agents that target specific molecular pathways vital in pathogenesis of RCC, creating new avenues for better disease control and improved outcomes.

Likewise, many new developments in the imaging, pathological characterization and surgical therapy have significantly altered the management of RCC in recent times. Currently, the focus of therapy in RCC is on minimally invasive and noninvasive techniques to achieve oncological control similar to the conventional open surgical approaches.

In this chapter, we review the recent advancements in the diagnosis and treatment of RCC with special emphasis on the role of minimally invasive surgery and targeted therapy in the management.

EPIDEMIOLOGY

Incidence

Renal cell carcinoma comprises 85–90% of all primary renal neoplasms and 3–5% of all malignant neoplasms. As per the recent data from World Health Organization, RCC is the 13th most common cause of cancer death worldwide with over 140,000 RCC-related deaths annually.[5] The incidence of RCC varies widely from region to region, with the highest rates observed in the Czech Republic and North America.[6] In general, the incidence is higher in developed nations as compared to the developing countries. The estimated incidence of RCC in India is 2/100,000 population in males and about 1/100,000 population in females.[7]

Gender and Age

The incidence of RCC is higher in males with a male-to-female ratio of 3:2. Historically, RCC has been a disease of the elderly with peak incidence between 50 years and 70 years of age.[8] However, in recent times the demographic profile of RCC is shifting toward younger age and many cases are now diagnosed at an earlier age.[9]

The incidence of RCC in childhood is low with a reported rate of only 2.3–6.6% of all renal tumors in children.[10] The mean age at presentation in children is 8–9 years, and there is no difference in incidence between boys and girls. Wilms tumor is the most common primary renal malignancy in younger children. However, the incidence of RCC and Wilms tumor is identical during the second decade of life. The clinical presentation of childhood RCCs is characterized by locally advanced, high grade, aggressive lesions, which are more likely to be symptomatic and of unfavorable histologic subtypes.[11]

ETIOLOGY

A wide array of factors has been correlated with origin of RCC according to the epidemiological studies. However, the inferences drawn from most of these studies about the role of etiological factors are prone to errors on account of the confounding variables that make it difficult to draw convincing deductions about the real role of these factors. On the other hand, recent studies into the heritable variants of RCC have furnished important understanding about the genetic pathways involved in pathogenesis of RCC and isolation of genetic alterations.[4] There is a growing body of evidence which suggests that RCC is a heterogeneous constellation of lesions with distinct genetic mutations with complex pathogenetic pathways rather than a discrete entity.

Modifiable Risk Factors

Tobacco

The risk of RCC increases with tobacco use in a dose dependent manner. The relative risk has a linear relation to the duration of smoking and is believed to have a cause- and effect relationship as evidenced by the decrease in risk after cessation of smoking.[12] Overall, tobacco consumption is believed to be related to RCC in 20–30% males and 10–20% females.

Obesity

The higher incidence of RCC in developed countries is believed to be partly on account of the increased prevalence of obesity, and this causal association is estimated to be present in more than 40% of cases of RCC in the United States.[13] Some of the postulated mechanisms linking obesity to RCC include increased insulin-like growth factor 1 expression, local inflammation, increased arteriolar nephrosclerosis, and increased circulating estrogen levels.[14]

Hypertension

A weak association of RCC and hypertension has been proposed and the suggested mechanisms include inflammation or metabolic or functional changes in renal tubules that may increase susceptibility to carcinogens and hypertension induced renal injury.

Others

A host of other potential etiologic factors have been recognized in animal models including viruses, lead containing substances, and numerous other chemical compounds like aromatic hydrocarbons. However, a direct causal relationship with RCC in humans has not been conclusively verified. Likewise, workers in the metal, chemical, rubber, and printing industries, particularly those exposed to asbestos or cadmium, have been reported to carry a marginally higher relative risk for developing RCC, but the evidence is weak and inconclusive.[15] There are a number of iatrogenic factors, which have been implicated in the etiopathogenesis of RCC, although the reported relative risks are low.[16] These include analgesic abuse, radiation to the retroperitoneum, as for Wilms tumor or testicular cancer, and patients on hemodialysis for end-stage renal disease.

FAMILIAL RENAL CELL CARCINOMA AND ROLE OF GENETIC FACTORS

There is a distinct association between RCC and certain familial syndromes such as von Hippel–Lindau disease and tuberous sclerosis.[4] Recent advances in molecular genetics have paved the way for identifying novel familial syndromes of RCC and characterizing the oncogenes and tumor suppressor genes responsible for promoting the development of both sporadic and familial forms of RCC. As a result of these advances in molecular genetics, the various subtypes of RCC are now distinctly characterized, which has paved the way for a substantial amendment in the existing histological categorization of RCC (Table 1).

PATHOLOGY

Histologically, RCCs are adenocarcinomas originating from different parts of renal tubules. The majority of RCCs including clear cell and papillary variants are believed to originate from proximal tubular cells of the nephron as shown by the similarity in ultra-structural features. However, collecting duct carcinoma and renal medullary carcinoma are two poor prognosis variants of RCC, which are derived from the collecting ducts.

On gross appearance, most RCCs are oval in shape initially and lack a real histological capsule. Rather, the lesion compresses the surrounding renal parenchyma to form a pseudocapsule. Except for the aggressive variants like sarcomatoid tumors and collecting duct carcinomas, most of the RCCs are not obviously infiltrative. The size of lesion has been used as a criterion to distinguish benign adenomas from RCCs because there is paucity of dependable histologic or ultrastructural differentiating factors. On cut section, RCCs grossly appear as yellow, tan, or brown tumor sprinkled with areas of necrosis, hemorrhage and fibrosis. Stippled or rim like calcification is seen in 10-20% while cystic degeneration is evident in 10-25% of RCCs.

Sporadic forms of RCCs are usually unilateral and unifocal as opposed to the familial forms where bilaterality and multicentricity are much more common as in von Hippel-Lindau disease. Similarly, multicentricity is seen more commonly in association with papillary variant and familial forms of RCC.[17]

Based on the recent advances in histopathological studies like electron microscopy, immunohistochemistry, molecular genetics, and cytogenetics, a revised and restructured classification of renal malignant epithelial tumors was introduced by the World Health Organization in 2004 and is currently accepted worldwide(Table 2). This WHO system is in resonance with the contemporary concepts of considering RCC as a group of many diverse tumors with distinct genetic origin and distinctive clinical features.

Morphological features of nuclei play an important role in the prognosis of RCC and Fuhrman's nuclear grading system has been shown to be an independent prognostic factor, especially for clear cell and papillary variants but not so much for the chromophobe subtype.[18,19] The Fuhrman's grading system takes into account nuclear size and shape and the presence or

Table 1: Renal cell carcinoma: Familial subtypes.

Syndrome	Mode of inheritance	Gene/Chromosome/ Mutation/Mechanism	Risk of RCC	Histological subtype	Other manifestations
Von Hippel–Lindau disease	AD	VHL(3p); Activation of hypoxic response pathways	70%	Clear cell RCC	Retinal angiomas, CNS hemangioblastomas Pheochromocytoma
Birt-Hogg-Dubé syndrome	AD	FLCN, Folliculin (17p11), BHD 1 gene, Activation of mTOR Pathway TSP	25%	Chromophobe RCC	Hybrid oncocytic tumor, oncocytomas Facial fibrofolliculomas Lung cysts Spontaneous pneumothorax
Familial leiomyomatosis and RCC	AD	Fumarate hydratase (FH), 1q, Activation of hypoxic response pathways, DNA methylation	15%	Type 2 papillary RCC, CD carcinoma	Leiomyomas of skin or uterine leiomyosarcomas
Hereditary type papillary RCC	AD	MET, Proto-oncogene, MET signaling pathway activation		Type 1 papillary RCC, multiple, bilateral	
Succinate dehydrogenase RCC	AD	SDHB(1p), SDHD*, SDHC(11q), SDHA DNA methylation	More with SDHB	Chromophobe, clear cell, type 2 papillary RCC	Oncocytoma, paragangliomas (benign and malignant) Papillary thyroid carcinoma

Contd...

Contd...

Syndrome	Mode of inheritance	Gene/Chromosome/ Mutation/Mechanism	Risk of RCC	Histological subtype	Other manifestations
PTEN hamartoma tumor syndrome, COWDEN syndrome	AD	PTEN, 10q	Up to 35%	Papillary RCC	Breast tumors (malignant and benign) Epithelial thyroid carcinoma
Hereditary BAP1 tumor syndrome	AD	BAP 1		Clear cell	
Tuberous sclerosis	AD	TSC1 (9q34) or TSC2 (16p13)		Clear cell RCC (occasionally)	Multiple renal AMLs, Renal cysts/ polycystic kidney disease, Cutaneous angiofibromas, Pulmonary lymphangiomyomatosis
Chromosome 3 translocations		Chromosome 3			Loss of translocated chromosome 3p and somatic mutation of VHL leads to activation of hypoxic response pathways

Source: Table adapted and modified from:
1. Menko FH, Mahere ER. Diagnosis and management of hereditary renal cell cancer. Recent Results Cancer Res. 2016;205:85-104.
2. Linehan WM. Molecular targeting of the VHL gene pathway in clear cell kidney cancer. J Urol. 2003;170:593-4.
3. Linehan WM. The genetic basis of kidney cancer: implications for management and use of targeted therapeutic approaches. Eur Urol. 2012;61:896-8.
4. Linehan WM, Ricketts CJ. The metabolic basis of kidney cancer. Semin Cancer Biol. 2013;23:46-55.

Table 2: Histological subtypes of renal cell carcinoma.

Histologic subtype	Percentage of RCC	Genetic defect	Origin	Dominant gross features	Microscopic	Prognosis	Others
Clear cell RCC	70–85%	Mutation or hypermethylation of VHL gene; Loss of 3p; Tumor suppressor genes SETD2, BAP1, and PBRM1	PCT	Pale Yellow, distinct, with/without areas of hemorrhage and necrosis	Abundant clear cytoplasm due to deposition of lipid and glycogen	Poor prognosis Aggressive tumors	Hypervascular, coagulative tumor necrosis; Renal vein, perinephric fat, and/or renal sinus invasion common
Papillary RCC	10–16%	Type 1: activation of MET Type 2: activation of the NRF2-ARE pathway.	PCT	Yellow/tan well defined, pseudocapsule, soft/firm/a mixed cystic/solid consistency.	Papillary/tubulopapillary structure Calcification, necrosis, and foamy macrophage infiltration **Papillary type 1:** Thin papillae, tumor cells with pale cytoplasm and smaller nuclei, appear basophilic on H&E staining **Papillary type 2:** Thicker papillae lined by tumor cells with abundant, granular cytoplasm and larger, pleomorphic nuclei	Type 1 better prognosis than type 2.	Synchronous bilateral and multifocal- ~ 10% cases CT—hypodense central area surrounded by vital tumor tissue - contrast-enhancing margin on CT. Common in acquired renal cystic disease.
Chromophobe RCC	5%	Loss of chromosomes Y, 1, 2, 6, 10, 13, 17 and 21 hereditary RCC syndrome Birt-Hogg-Dubé (BHD)	Collecting ducts	Pale brown, homogeneous distinct mass, no capsule	Abundant cytoplasm; Two variants: Clear/classic and eosinophilic. Nuclei show perinuclear halos, binucleation, irregular wrinkled nuclear membrane	Good prognosis except when sarcomatoid transformation	Grading by Fuhrman system not possible due to nuclear atypia WHO/ISUP Grading system utilized

Contd...

Contd...

Histologic sub type	Percentage of RCC	Genetic defect	Origin	Dominant gross features	Microscopic	Prognosis	Others
Collecting duct RCC	<0.5%	Mostly unknown; Loss of 8p, 16p, 1p, and 9p, and gain of 13q	Collecting ducts, rarely from renal medulla	Partly cystic, white-gray appearance	Tubulopapillary architecture, desmoplastic stroma Anaplastic tumor cells often take on a columnar pattern with a hobnail appearance	Extremely aggressive with poor prognosis	Local invasion into renal sinus and/or renal vein common Commonly have metastases at presentation
Medullary RCC	<200 cases reported in the literature	Not known	Renal papillae or calyceal epithelium (attributed to chronic medullary hypoxia due to hemoglobinopathy)	Usually pale/ brown/ white, lack of capsule, commonly has extensive hemorrhage and necrosis	Poorly differentiated eosinophilic cells Abundant neutrophils infiltrating the tumor and adjacent desmoplastic stroma	Very poor prognosis with advanced disease at presentation	Common in young black patients with sickle cell trait/ disease More common in right for unclear reasons
Microphthalmia transcription factor family translocation RCC	Only 30 confirmed cases reported	Translocations of transcription factors of MiT family		Identical to clear cell RCC, hemorrhage and necrosis are common	Papillary/nested pattern Calcification common Cells granular and eosinophilic with abundant clear cytoplasm	Aggressive lesions	More common in women, recipients of cytotoxic chemotherapy during childhood, adolescents and young adults

Source: Modified from:
1. Eble JN, Sauter G, Epstein JI, et al. Pathology and Genetics of Tumours of the Urinary System and Male Genital Organs, 3rd edition. WHO Classification of Tumours. Lyon (France): IARC Press; 2004.
2. Srigley JR, Delahunt B, Eble JN, et al. ISUP Renal Tumor Panel. The International Society of Urological Pathology (ISUP) Vancouver Classification of Renal Neoplasia. Am J Surg Pathol. 2013;37:1469-89.

Table 3: Renal cell carcinoma grading systems.

Grade	Fuhrman's grading	ISUP grading
1	Absent or inconspicuous	Tumor cell nucleoli invisible or small and basophilic at X 400 magnification
2	Small (visible at 400X magnification)	Tumor cell nucleoli conspicuous at X 400 magnification but inconspicuous at X 100 magnification
3	Prominent	Tumor cell nucleoli eosinophilic and clearly visible at X 100 magnification
4	Prominent, heavy chromatin clumps present	Tumors showing extreme nuclear pleomorphism and/or containing tumor giant cells and/or the presence of any proportion of tumor showing sarcomatoid and/or rhabdoid dedifferentiation

(ISUP: International Society of Urological Pathology)

absence of prominent nucleoli. Although the Fuhrman grading system is well established, its prognostic value has been debated in the recent times owing to the subjective nature and interobserver variability in the results. This has resulted in a new grading system from the International Society of Urological Pathology (ISUP). As per the ISUP grading system, first three grades are based on degree of nucleolar prominence while grade four comprises tumor cells with sarcomatoid and/or rhabdoid morphology and/or tumors containing tumor giant cells or showing extreme nuclear pleomorphism. A comparison of old Fuhrman's grading with the new ISUP grading system is shown in Table 3.

Renal cell carcinomas can spread locally into the renal sinus, renal capsule and collecting system (approximately 20%), into the venous system including inferior vena cava as a tumor thrombus (approximately 10%), via lymphatics into the hilar, para-aortic, paracaval, and interaortocaval lymph nodes according to the side of the tumor, and hematogenous spread to lungs, liver, bones, brain, etc.

CLINICAL FEATURES

The clinical presentation of RCC has undergone a sea change over the last few decades. As the use of abdominal imaging like ultrasonography for unrelated indications has increased, more than 50% of RCCs are currently detected incidentally on noninvasive imaging for other indications.[20] The historically described "classic triad" of flank pain, visible hematuria, and palpable abdominal mass is rarely seen (6–10%) in current era and denotes an advanced disease with poor prognosis, leading to the coining of term "too late triad".[21]

The clinical manifestations of RCC can be diverse, thus earning the name "the internist's tumor". It has been suggested that a more apt description would be "Radiologist's tumor" because of the high incidence of detection of asymptomatic lesions by the radiologists. The clinical features of RCC can arise from local disease, bleeding, metastatic lesions and paraneoplastic syndromes. The symptoms due to local disease include flank mass, pain, and hematuria. Bleeding can produce hematuria with clot colic and at times spontaneous perirenal bleed can lead to formation of perirenal hematomas. The involvement of inferior vena cava by tumor thrombus can produce edema over both lower limbs as well as nonreducing varicocele. Likewise, enlarged retroperitoneal lymph nodes can lead to lower extremity edema. The symptoms of metastatic disease include constitutional symptoms like anorexia, weight loss, malaise, fatigue, and low-grade fever; cough, dyspnea, hemoptysis, jaundice, skeletal pain, and palpable cervical and supraclavicular lymphadenopathy.

A wide variety of paraneoplastic syndromes have been demonstrated in approximately 30% of patients with symptomatic RCCs.[22] These include raised erythrocyte sedimentation rate (ESR) (55%), hypertension (37%), anemia (36%), cachexia (34%), pyrexia (17%), Stauffer's syndrome with nonmetastatic hepatic dysfunction (14%), hypercalcemia (5-13%), polycythemia (3.5%), and amyloidosis (2%). Hypercalcemia can be due to either paraneoplastic phenomenon by secretion of parathyroid hormone-like peptides, tumor-derived 1,25-dihydroxycholecalciferol and prostaglandins or due to osteolytic metastatic bone involvement.[23]

The RCC-associated hypertension is suggested to be on account of renin produced by the tumor itself or due to the compression of renal artery or its branches, or formation of abnormal arteriovenous fistulae within the lesion, and less frequently on account of polycythemia, hypercalcemia, ureteral obstruction, and increased intracranial pressure associated with cerebral metastases. Polycythemia in RCC is believed to be because of the increased erythropoietin secretion, either by the tumor tissue itself or by the normal renal parenchyma in response to the hypoxia produced by the tumor compression.

Stauffer syndrome is characterized by nonmetastatic reversible hepatic dysfunction seen in association with RCC in about 3-20% cases.[24] The most common components include raised alkaline phosphatase levels, increased prothrombin time, reduced albumin levels, and elevated serum bilirubin and transaminase levels. It is vital to rule out presence of hepatic metastases in presence of these clinical manifestations. In over two-thirds patients, the hepatic function recovers after the definitive management of RCC. Failure of normalization of hepatic function portrays a poor prognosis and signifies presence of residual disease.

Physical Examination

The role of physical examination in the diagnosis of RCC has diminished in the recent years as more cases are being diagnosed radiologically at an earlier stage before manifestation of clinical signs. However, a thorough clinical examination forms an essential component of evaluation and can reveal important findings keeping in mind the myriad presentations of RCC. Moreover, the presence of physical findings usually indicates an advanced disease and portrays poor outcomes. The common findings, which may be apparent on physical examination, include presence of a palpable renal mass with its distinctive features, palpable cervical or supraclavicular lymphadenopathy, nonreducing varicocele, bilateral lower extremity edema, and signs of systemic involvement according to the site of metastases.

Laboratory Findings

Serum biochemistry in advanced RCC often demonstrates anemia, elevated ESR, hypercalcemia, deranged liver function parameters, or elevated serum alkaline phosphatase and lactate dehydrogenase (LDH) levels. Serum LDH levels are often used in prognostic scoring systems designed for predicting outcomes of RCC. Renal function assessment using biochemical tests is mandatory prior to therapy. In cases with deranged renal function, split renal function needs to be estimated using nuclear scintigraphy. Likewise, renal function estimation is important for RCC in solitary kidneys or with bilateral RCCs. For hilar renal masses adjacent to the collecting system, urinary cytology and if required, endoscopic evaluation should be considered in order to exclude urothelial cancer.

Imaging

Ultrasonography is an excellent screening study, which can detect majority of renal masses and can also differentiate between solid and cystic masses. Most renal tumors in the contemporary era are in fact diagnosed by abdominal USG performed for other medical reasons. However, ultrasonography findings are not reliable enough to confirm the diagnosis of RCC, nor accurately stage the disease. A useful role for USG is during the follow-up owing to its wide availability, noninvasive nature, and relatively lower cost.

Computed Tomography

Contrast-enhanced computed tomography (CT) is the most preferred modality for characterization of renal masses. The postcontrast enhancement in renal masses as reflected by change in Hounsfield units (HUs) of 15 HU or more is strongly suggestive of RCC. The valuable information obtained from abdominal CT scan includes characterization of the lesion in terms of size, location, extent, local spread, vascularity and calcification, anatomy and function of the opposite kidney, presence and level of tumor venous thrombus, regional lymphadenopathy, and possible involvement of other

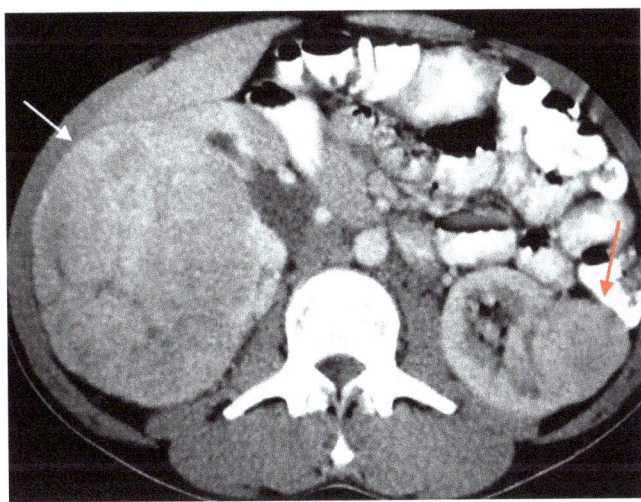

Fig. 1: Computed tomography scan showing bilateral renal cell carcinoma (RCC): A large lesion involving the right kidney (white arrow) and a smaller lesion (red arrow) in the left kidney.

abdominal organs such as liver, spleen, and adrenals (Fig. 1). Despite being an excellent imaging modality for diagnosis of RCC, CT scan is limited in certain scenarios such as oncocytomas and fat-free angiomyolipoma (AML) which are difficult to distinguish from RCC. Moreover, CT angiography furnishes valuable information about renal vasculature, which is critical when considering nephron sparing surgery as a treatment modality for RCC.

Magnetic Resonance Imaging

Magnetic resonance imaging (MRI) is equivalent to CT scan in characterization of renal masses and may be superior in certain aspects like differentiation between histological subtypes of RCC. It is indicated in situations where CT scan cannot be performed as in patients with history of anaphylactic reactions to intravenous contrast media, in pregnancy, and in patients with deranged renal function. Newer MRI techniques like diffusion-weighted and perfusion-weighted imaging can be superior to conventional MRI imaging for evaluation of renal masses and their role is under investigation.

On T2-weighted MRI images, clear cell RCC is characterized by heterogeneously high signal intensity on account of areas of hemorrhage, necrosis, and cystic degeneration. Likewise, chemical shift MRI sequences can differentiate clear cell and other subtypes by identifying intracytoplasmic lipids. On the other hand, papillary renal cell carcinoma demonstrates homogeneously low signal intensity on T2-weighted images, due to the deposition of histiocytes (containing hemosiderin) within the lesion. Likewise, demonstration of enhancing walls of hemorrhagic cysts and low signal intensity hypoattenuating solid mass on T2 sequences can differentiate papillary RCC from other variants with a sensitivity of 80% and a specificity of 94%.[25]

Another aspect in which MRI is considered superior to CT scan is in the evaluation of venous tumor thrombus, particularly for determining the level of an inferior vena cava tumor thrombus.[26]

Other Investigations

Renal arteriography and inferior vena cavography, which were used traditionally, have a limited role in the current era in the work-up of RCC. At times, vena cavography may be useful in patients with ambiguous MRI or CT findings or in patients unsuitable for cross-sectional imaging. Nuclear scintigraphy by means of a radioisotope renogram is indicated in poorly functioning kidneys for GFR estimation in order to decide the correct management options.

The role of positron-emission tomography (PET) scanning in the workup of RCC is controversial. It can be useful in situations where the findings of conventional cross-sectional imaging are confusing and likelihood of metastatic lesions on PET scan can affect the management decisions.[27] Although transesophageal echocardiography has been described for evaluation of tumor thrombus within the inferior vena cava, it does not have any additional benefit over the conventional imaging and is also invasive in nature.[28]

All cases of RCC require workup including imaging of likely metastatic sites. This includes a chest radiograph, liver function tests and a comprehensive appraisal of cross-sectional abdominal and pelvic imaging. Radioisotope bone scan is performed only in patients with suspected bony involvement as evidenced by abnormally raised serum alkaline phosphatase levels and/or presence of skeletal pain. Likewise, a CT scan of the chest is only indicated in patients with pulmonary symptoms and/or presence of any abnormal lesion on chest radiograph (Figs. 2A and B).

STAGING

Currently, the most accepted staging system for RCC is the eighth TNM classification system (2017) that is used for all histologic variants of renal carcinoma. This staging system is adopted by both the American Joint Committee on Cancer (AJCC) and the International Union for Cancer Control (UICC).[29]

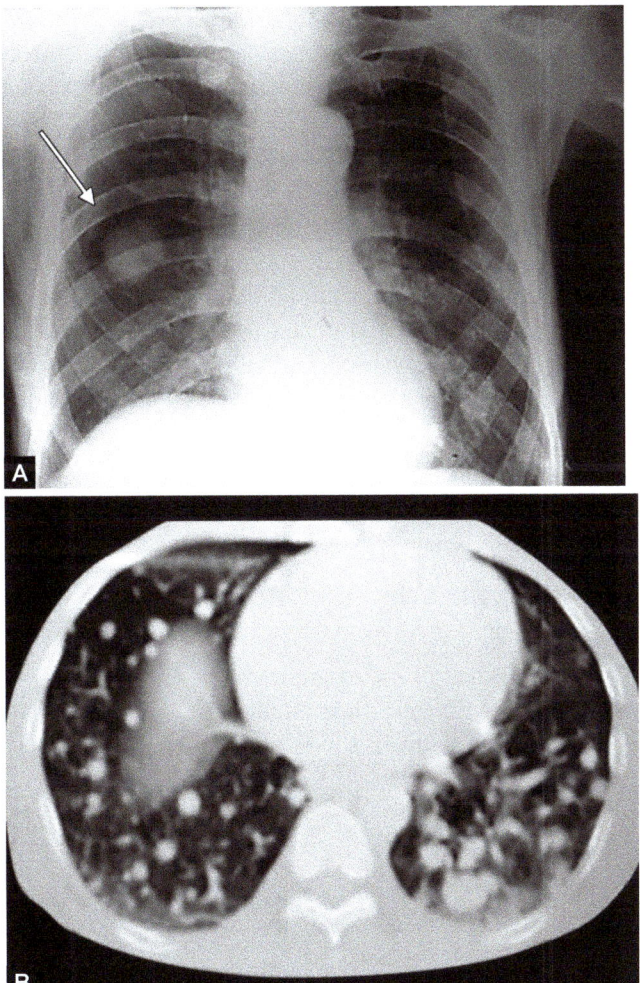

Figs. 2A and B: Pulmonary metastases in renal cell carcinoma (RCC): (A) Chest radiograph (white arrow); (B) Chest CT scan.

Renal Cell Carcinoma TNM Staging AJCC UICC 2017

Primary Tumor (T)

T category	T criteria
Tx:	Primary tumor cannot be assessed
T0:	No evidence of primary tumor
T1:	Tumor ≤ 7 cm in greatest dimension, limited to the kidney
T1a:	Tumor ≤ 4 cm in greatest dimension, limited to the kidney
T1b:	Tumor > 4 cm but ≤ 7 cm in greatest dimension, limited to kidney

T category	T criteria
T2:	Tumor > 7 cm in greatest dimension, limited to the kidney
T2a:	Tumor > 7 cm but ≤ 10 cm in greatest dimension, limited to kidney
T2b:	Tumor > 10 cm, limited to the kidney
T3:	Tumor extends into major veins or perinepheric tissues, but not into ipsilateral adrenal gland and not beyond Gerota's fascia
T3a:	Tumor extends into the renal vein or its segmental branches, or invades pelvicalyceal system/perirenal and/or renal sinus fat but not beyond Gerota's fascia
T3b:	Tumor extends into the vena cava below the diaphragm
T3c:	Tumor extends into vena cava above diaphragm or invades the wall of the vena cava
T4:	Tumor invades beyond Gerota's fascia (including contiguous extension into the Ipsilateral adrenal gland).

Regional Lymph Nodes (N)

N category	N criteria
Nx:	Regional lymph nodes cannot be assessed
N0:	No regional lymph node metastasis
N1:	Metastasis in regional lymph node(s).

Distant Metastasis (M)

M category	M criteria
M0:	No distant metastasis
M1:	Distant metastasis.

MANAGEMENT

The management options available across all stages for RCC include:
- Surveillance
- *Surgery*:
  - *Radical nephrectomy*: Open/laparoscopic/robotic
  - *Nephron sparing surgery*: Open/laparoscopic/robotic
- Ablative therapy: Cryoablation/radiofrequency ablation
- Chemotherapy
- Immunotherapy
- Targeted therapy
- Radiotherapy
- Palliative interventions
  - Angioembolization
  - Metastasectomy.

Treatment of Localized Renal Cell Cancer

Active Surveillance

The concept of active surveillance involves serial monitoring of the tumor by periodic imaging and intervention is held in abeyance till it is necessitated on account of tumor progression in serial imaging modalities during monitored follow-up (USG, CT, or MRI). This concept is in contrast to watchful waiting which is utilized in patients who harbor comorbidities which preclude any intervention and routine serial follow-up imaging is not practiced unless clinically necessary. Active surveillance is a suitable therapeutic option for elderly and poor surgical risk patients who are diagnosed as having small incidentally detected renal masses where the morbidity and mortality of interventions clearly outweighs the cancer specific mortality.[30]

Surgical Treatment

Surgery is the mainstay for definitive treatment of RCC. The surgical treatment aims to resect the complete tumor along with a suitable margin of adjacent healthy tissue. Historically, the treatment of choice has been radical nephrectomy, which entails complete removal of the involved kidney with its Gerota's fascia, perinephric fat, ipsilateral adrenal gland, and upper one-third of the ureter and an extended lymph node dissection from the crus of the diaphragm to the aortic bifurcation (Figs. 3A to D). Ever since Robson described the classical radical nephrectomy procedure in 1963, the concept has been universally accepted and adopted over the last few decades.[31] However, the advances in minimally invasive surgery including advent of laparoscopic techniques along with better understanding of surgical and oncological principles and concerns about long-term renal insufficiency following radical nephrectomy have significantly altered the current surgical management of RCC. The classical radical nephrectomy procedure has been modified in the recent years as findings from several large studies with long-term follow-up have been incorporated into the contemporary guidelines. It is now widely accepted that removal of the ipsilateral adrenal gland is not necessary unless indicated on account of radiographic adrenal enlargement, large upper pole tumors or locally advanced lesions.[32]

Likewise, the utility of routinely performing an extensive lymphadenectomy in all patients as a part of radical nephrectomy has been challenged and several studies have highlighted the lack of any survival benefit with standard lymphadenectomy.[33] Overall, the therapeutic benefit of standard lymph node dissection is evident only in a minor fraction of patients (<2–3%) who are likely to harbor micrometastatic disease. Thus, the current indications of lymphadenectomy in RCC are based on imaging findings, patient age, tumor characteristics, and coexisting morbidities.[34]

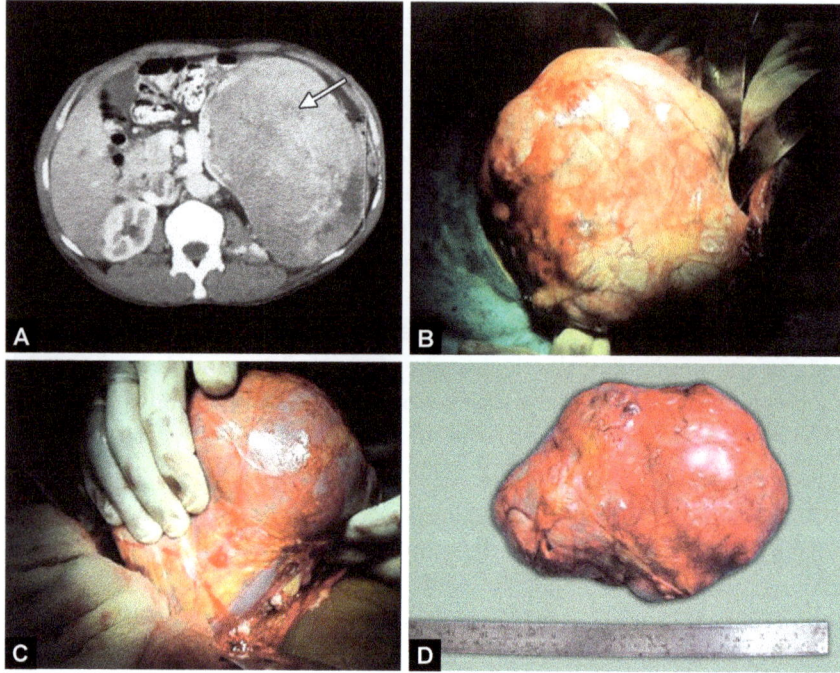

Figs. 3A to D: Radical nephrectomy for large left renal cell carcinoma (RCC): (A) Large RCC involving the left kidney (white arrow); (B) Intraoperative dissection and mobilization of the tumor bearing kidney; (C) Dissection of hilar structures prior to ligation and division; and (D) Tumor dimensions over 20 × 20 cm.

Nephron-sparing Surgery versus Radical Nephrectomy

Historically, partial nephrectomy has been reserved for bilateral tumors and tumors in solitary kidneys and radical nephrectomy was the standard treatment for all RCCs if the contralateral kidney was normal. However, radical nephrectomy has now been replaced by partial nephrectomy for all small renal masses (clinical T1a) even in the presence of a normal contralateral kidney, unless technical factors preclude it (Figs. 4A to D).

This change is based on the findings of several retrospective analyses of large databases which have suggested lower cardiac-specific mortality[35] as well as improved overall survival of partial nephrectomy as compared to radical nephrectomy in the long-term follow-up. The oncological safety (cancer specific survival and recurrence-free survival) of nephron sparing surgery has been demonstrated to be similar to radical nephrectomy and currently partial nephrectomy is the preferred treatment for most organ confined tumors, if technically feasible, since it preserves kidney function in a better way and delays development of metabolic as well as cardiovascular disorders in the long-term. In recent times, both radical and partial nephrectomies are being performed by laparoscopic approaches, thus

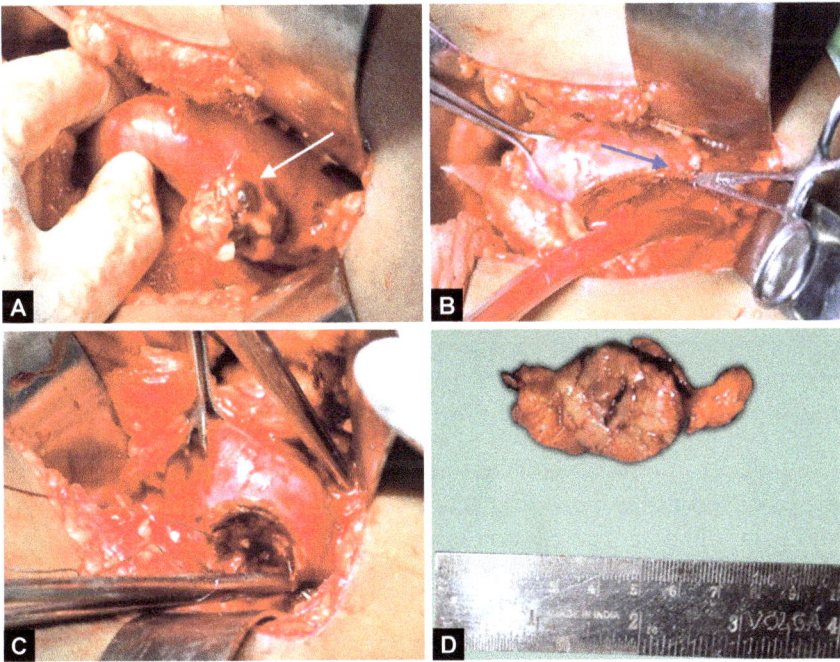

Figs. 4A to D: Partial nephrectomy: (A) An exophytic lesion over posterolateral aspect of kidney (white arrow); (B) Mass excised and bleeders being controlled (blue arrow); (C) Closure of the renal parenchymal defect; and (D) Approximately 4 cm renal mass after excision.

significantly reducing the perioperative morbidity without compromising the oncological outcomes. Both transperitoneal and retroperitoneoscopic approaches have been used with equal success and the choice is largely based on the surgeon preference and expertise. The introduction of robotic-assisted laparoscopic techniques has further reduced the morbidity and complications of radical and partial nephrectomies in the management of RCC.

Ablative Therapies

An upcoming advancement in the treatment of localized RCC (<4 cm) has been the use of thermal ablative therapies like cryoablation and radiofrequency ablation. These are suggested to provide equivalent outcomes to nephron sparing surgery in a minimally invasive manner.[36] For administering the thermal ablative therapies, the lesion can be accessed either percutaneously or by laparoscopic approach. Although the short-term outcomes in carefully selected patients are promising, the long-term data is lacking. The currently most suited patients for these modalities include elderly or surgically unfit patients with localized lesions, patients with multifocal tumors as in hereditary forms of renal cancer, patients who develop local recurrence following prior partial nephrectomy and patients with solitary tumor bearing kidney.

In a large study that compared partial nephrectomy (1,057 patients) to radiofrequency ablation (180 patients) and cryoablation (187 patients) for stage T1 tumors, the recurrence-free survival rates were similar. However, the metastasis-free survival was better with partial nephrectomy and cryoablation as compared to radiofrequency ablation although the follow up of patients in the thermal ablation groups was for a lesser period.[37] The potential complications of thermal ablative therapies include bleeding, paralytic ileus, inadvertent surrounding organ injury, infection, and renal injury.

TREATMENT OF LOCALLY ADVANCED RCC

Management of Locally Advanced Unresectable RCC

In surgically unresectable, locally advanced lesions, angioembolization of the renal vessels can provide effective palliation of symptoms like bleeding and pain. Although neoadjuvant targeted therapy to downstage the tumor has been tried but its use is largely investigational and is currently limited to clinical trials.

Management of RCC with Venous Tumor Thrombus

Development of tumor thrombus in the renal vein or IVC portrays an adverse prognosis. Aggressive surgical resection in form of radical nephrectomy and thrombectomy has been the preferred management option for patients with RCC and tumor thrombus extension.[38] All surgically fit patients without evidence of metastases and having RCC with venous tumor thrombus are candidates for radical surgery regardless of the level of venous involvement which can, however, have a bearing on the surgical approach required.[39] In patients having tumor thrombus extension into the right atrium, cardiopulmonary bypass techniques are utilized to ensure complete removal of the thrombus (Figs. 5A to D). Role of angioembolization prior to definitive surgical management has been debatable and few studies have reported increased blood loss, longer hospital stay and higher mortality with preoperative angioembolization.[40] Recently, many reports have appeared in the literature regarding use of laparoscopic and minimally invasive procedures in the setting of tumor thrombus leading to reduced morbidity and better perioperative outcomes.

Adjuvant Therapy

The role of adjuvant immunotherapy and targeted therapy in the setting of locally advanced RCC has been investigated by a number of randomized trials. However, no survival benefit has been attributable to adjuvant therapy in this setting. Likewise, use of tumor vaccines in locally advanced RCC

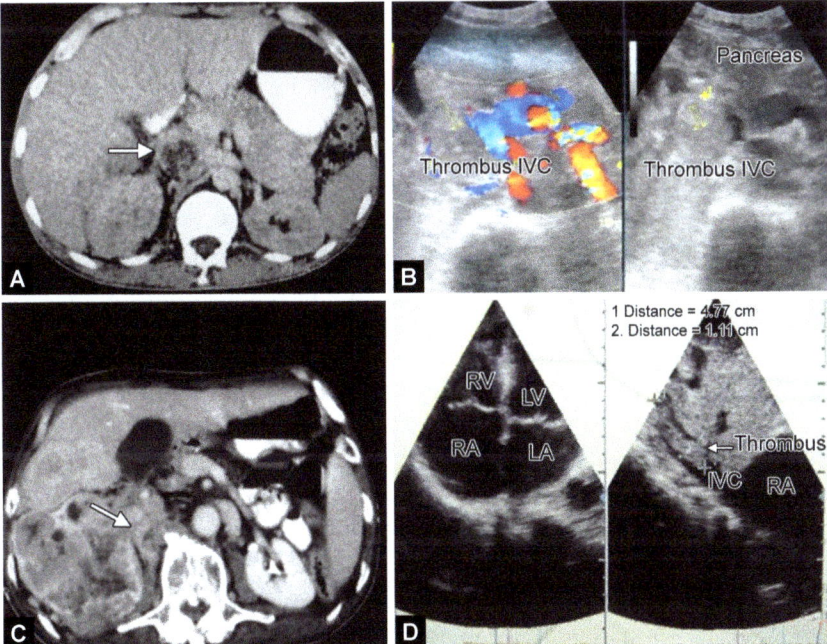

Figs. 5A to D: Renal cell carcinoma (RCC) with inferior vena cava (IVC) thrombus: (A) IVC thrombus seen as a filling defect in CT scan (white arrow); (B) Color Doppler showing the tumor thrombus; (C) Large right RCC with IVC tumor thrombus and enlarged hilar lymph nodes (white arrow); and (D) Two-dimensional echocardiography revealing tumor thrombus reaching up to the right atrium.

patients subjected to radical nephrectomy has failed to demonstrate any consistent benefit on the overall survival.[41]

Management of Clinically Positive Lymph Nodes (CN+)

Almost all guidelines agree about the necessity of performing a lymph node dissection in the presence of clinically enlarged regional lymph nodes. Nonetheless, the boundaries and the extent of lymphadenectomy remain a matter of controversy.

TREATMENT OF ADVANCED/METASTATIC RCC

Local Therapy

Cytoreductive Nephrectomy

Traditionally, debulking surgery in the form of cytoreductive nephrectomy has been widely practiced in those RCC patients with metastases who are surgically fit and have large primary lesions with limited metastatic disease.

The rationale underlying this policy is to improve the outcomes of adjuvant systemic therapy and provide local palliation.

In carefully selected fit patients with oligometastatic disease, radical nephrectomy with metastasectomy has been advised with a curative intent. This approach can provide a cure if all the metastases are surgically removed. A number of studies have reported higher overall survival in patients undergoing metastasectomy when compared to patients receiving systemic therapy alone or patients not undergoing any treatment.[42]

Cytoreductive nephrectomy is contraindicated in patients with high surgical risk, small primary tumors, sarcomatoid variants and high burden of metastatic disease. In these patients, angioembolization can be attempted to provide symptomatic relief from pain and/or bleeding.[43]

In patients with symptomatic bone metastases, local radiation, whether in the form of image guided radiotherapy (single dose or hypofractionated), conventional radiotherapy, or stereotactic body radiotherapy, provides not only better and longer lasting pain relief but also confers superior cancer specific survival and progression free survival.[44] Likewise, local excision and/or curettage and bone grafting with stabilization of involved bony sites has been shown to be superior to nonintervention group in terms of better symptom palliation and improved cancer specific survival.[45]

Similarly, various strategies for local palliation of brain metastases have been evaluated. These include whole brain radiotherapy (WBRT), stereotactic radiosurgery (SRS), a combination of SRS with WBRT, fractionated stereotactic radiotherapy (FSRT), and metastasectomy. The results of these studies are ambivalent and the small number of patients makes any meaningful interpretation difficult. In general, WBRT alone is believed to be inferior to other techniques and combined modalities.[46] Angioembolization of bone or spinal metastatic sites prior to resection has been shown to decrease intraoperative blood loss and by itself can provide symptomatic relief from painful metastases.[47]

SYSTEMIC THERAPY FOR ADVANCED/METASTATIC RENAL CELL CANCER

Chemotherapy

Unlike other malignancies, RCC has been resistant to conventional chemotherapy and the reported overall response in large meta-analyses has ranged around 5–6%.[48] A variety of chemotherapeutic agents have been tried alone and in various combinations without any significant benefit. These include 5-fluorouracil (5-FU), cisplatinum, gemcitabine, vinblastine, and bleomycin. A combination of 5-FU with immunotherapy (interferon-α) has been shown to have some therapeutic benefit in few studies but is not corroborated by other reports. A potential role of chemotherapy is in tumors with sarcomatoid components where a combination of gemcitabine and doxorubicin has been shown to have a modest therapeutic response.[49]

IMMUNOTHERAPY

Immunological factors have been postulated to be involved in the etiopathology and progression of RCC and immunotherapeutic agents have been used traditionally for metastatic RCC as a systemic therapy. However, the role of immunotherapy has been primarily in the clear cell RCC and less so for other histological subtypes. Interferons and interleukins have been the most widely used agents for systemic therapy of RCC.

Interferons

Interferons are cytokines with immunomodulatory properties besides a host of other functions in the body. A large number of studies have assessed the role of interferon-α in RCC immunotherapy and the overall response rate has ranged from 10% to 20%.[50] However, this efficacy has not been consistently demonstrated in all patients. The response has been better in patients with clear cell RCC having mainly pulmonary metastases and carrying favorable risk factors as per MSKCC criteria. Combination of interferon-α with bevacizumab has been shown to be superior to interferon-α alone in terms of progression-free survival.[51] Currently, the superiority of targeted therapy over interferon-α has resulted in decreased usage of the latter in management of metastatic RCC.

Interleukin-2

The interleukins have been used extensively in the treatment of metastatic RCC since mid-1908s. The reported response rate with interleukin-2 (IL-2) has been in the range of 10–25%.[52] Despite having a significantly higher toxicity as compared to interferon-α, IL-2 carries the potential to be completely curative in a small subset of patients. High-dose IL-2, which can produce a lasting response in certain patients, received FDA approval in 1992 for use in metastatic RCC. However, adverse effects like fluid retention, hypotension due to the vascular leak phenomenon, pulmonary complications, and multiorgan failure restrict its use and produce high morbidity and mortality.[53]

Newer Immunotherapy Strategies

Allogeneic hematopoietic stem cell transplantation, in which host immune components are replaced with hematopoietic stem cells from a compatible donor, is aimed at producing a sustained immune response against the tumor cells due to the "graft-versus-tumor effect". Initial response to this therapeutic approach has been promising in some trials and some patients have been reported to remission for up to 10 years.

Many phase III trials utilizing tumor vaccines in RCC are currently underway. These include tumor antigen 5T4 and monoclonal antibodies against PD-1 or its ligand (PD-1L).[54]

TARGETED THERAPIES

As newer insights have been obtained into the cellular pathways involved in the genesis of RCC, development of targeted therapeutic agents aimed at specific pathways has been the logical and rational sequelae. The development of vascular endothelial growth factor (VEGF) antagonists paved the way for such novel therapeutic interventions in management of RCC.

Von Hippel–Lindau (VHL) mutations with resultant HIF (hypoxia-inducible factor) accumulation lead to increased risk for developing bilateral, multifocal clear cell RCCs.[55] The accumulation of HIFs causes an upregulation of various growth factors, including VEGF, platelet-derived growth factor (PDGF), transforming growth factor-α, and erythropoietin, which play a vital part in the origin and evolution of clear cell RCC. The identification of this key pathway has provided the foundation for development of novel agents, which target specific components of this pathway in the treatment of metastatic clear cell RCC.

Vascular Endothelial Growth Factor Pathway Antagonists

Bevacizumab

Bevacizumab, a monoclonal antibody against VEGF-A, was the first VEGF antagonist used clinically. It has been tried as monotherapy and in combination with immunotherapeutic agents like interferon-α. Although the results of various trials are at inconsistent, there does appear to be a modest benefit in overall response rate when bevacizumab is used.[56] The exact role of bevacizumab in the sequencing of targeted therapeutic agents has been a matter of discussion.

Sorafenib

Receptor kinase inhibitors demonstrate activity against various receptors like VEGF and PDGF receptors. Sorafenib is an oral multi-kinase receptor inhibitor with significant inhibition of VEGF receptor-2, PDGF receptor-β, and raf-1. Despite being approved by the FDA in the management of metastatic RCC, sorafenib is not considered to be a first-line therapeutic agent in this setting owing to the availability of many other agents in the same class. Sorafenib is presently used in patients not responding to other targeted receptor inhibitors with modest success rates in small series of patients.

Sunitinib

The recommended and widely prescribed first-line therapeutic agent for metastatic RCC is sunitinib, another oral kinase inhibitor with significant action on VEGF receptor-2, PDGF receptor-β, c-Kit, and Flt3. The concurrent inhibition of both VGEF and PDGF receptors is believed to have a synergistic effect on the inhibition of angiogenesis.

Pazopanib

Pazopanib is a newer kinase receptor inhibitor, which is characterized by a selective activity against angiogenesis because of action on VEGFR without significantly inhibiting the other receptors like PDGFR. This is believed to have the same efficacy as sunitinib and sorafenib with lesser adverse effects and toxicity.

Axitinib

Axitinib is another newer oral selective inhibitor of VEGFs (VEGFR-1, -2, and -3). The currently recommended place of axitinib in therapy of advanced RCC is as a second-line agent in patients who have failed prior treatment with sunitinib.

Cabozantinib

Cabozantinib first received FDA approval for treatment of metastatic RCC as a second-line therapy, after failure of first-line angiogenesis inhibitors, in 2016. Subsequently, in December 2017, cabozantinib was granted approval by FDA for use as a first-line therapy for similar indications. Cabozantinib is also an oral tyrosine kinase inhibitor (TKI), with potent activity against VEGFR.

mTOR Inhibitors (Mammalian Target of Rapamycin)

The role of mTOR inhibitors as a treatment modality for different cancers has been the focus of extensive research in the last few years. This is based on the pivotal role played by mTOR in angiogenesis, protein synthesis, and cell metabolism including cell growth, development and survival. Elegantly conducted studies have already demonstrated that mTOR is set off in RCC due to a host of genetic alterations.[57] This activation of mTOR by genetic mutations is accompanied by an increase in HIF activity and leads to a genesis and growth of RCC.[58] The inhibitors of mTOR are believed to downregulate this increased HIF activity, largely in situations where mTOR pathway is abnormally activated. Thus, mTOR inhibitors are likely to be most efficacious in those RCCs in which the mTOR pathway is stimulated.

Temsirolimus

Temsirolimus is an inhibitor of mTOR. Current evidence, gathered from different trials, suggests that temsirolimus is most suited for poor risk RCC patients with nonclear cell histological subtypes. However, the role of temsirolimus in RCC refractory to conventional VGEF receptor antagonists is controversial with lack of definitive evidence from clinical trials.

Everolimus

Everolimus is an oral mTOR inhibitor, which is a serine-threonine kinase derivative of rapamycin. The role of everolimus has been evaluated in the setting of TKI refractory metastatic RCC.[59] Few trials have demonstrated the modest efficacy of everolimus in this subset of patients. The common adverse events include anemia, rashes, pneumonitis, hypophosphatemia, hyperglycemia, thrombocytopenia, and elevated liver function tests.

PROGNOSIS/5-YEAR SURVIVAL

The prognosis of RCC depends on a large number of factors which include stage, Fuhrman's grade, histological subtype, histological features such as sarcomatoid elements or microvascular invasion, performance status and a host of molecular factors like expression of hypoxia-inducible transcription factor, mutations in *VHL* gene, carbonic anhydrase expression, VEGF expression, loss of PTEN, p21 expression, etc. The overall reported 5-year survival rates for different stages are 90–95% for stage I, 70–85% for stage II, 40–60% for stage III, and less than 10% for stage IV tumors.[60]

CONCLUSION

There has been a significant increase in the incidence of RCC in recent decades, partly on account of incidental detection on non-related abdominal imaging and partly because of a real rise as reflected by the increase in incidence of advanced cancers. While surgical therapy still forms the cornerstone of therapy in RCC across all stages, the recent insights into pathophysiology and molecular pathways have opened up new avenues of therapy in the form of targeted therapy and mTOR inhibitors. Surgical therapy has seen major changes in the form of minimally invasive techniques, laparoscopic procedures and use of robotic assistance to minimize the treatment related morbidity without compromising the oncological safety. Another major change in management of RCC in recent times has been the growing influence of nephron sparing procedures in order to reduce the long-term morbidity associated with conventional surgical procedures. Despite the significant strides made over the last few decades, there is still a long way to go in understanding the etiopathology of RCC and develop newer treatment strategies in order to prolong the survival with minimal morbidity.

REFERENCES

1. Siegel RL, Miller KD, Jemal A. Cancer statistics, 2018. CA Cancer J Clin. 2018;68: 7-30.
2. Chow WH, Devesa SS, Warren JL, et al. Rising incidence of renal cell cancer in the United states. JAMA. 1999;281:1628-31.
3. Capitanio U, Montorsi F. Renal cancer. Lancet. 2016;387:894-906.
4. Vira MA, Novakovic KR, Pinto PA, et al. Genetic basis of kidney cancer: a model for developing molecular-targeted therapies. BJU Int. 2007;99:1223-9.
5. Ferlay J, Soerjomataram I, Ervik M, et al. GLOBOCAN 2012 v1.0, Cancer incidence and mortality worldwide: IARC Cancer Base No. 11. Lyon, France: International Agency for Research on Cancer; 2013.
6. Abraham G, Cherian T, Mahadevan P, et al. Detailed study of survival of patients with renal cell carcinoma in India. Indian J Cancer. 2016;53:572-4.
7. Pantuck AJ, Zisman A, Rauch MK, et al. Incidental renal tumors. Urology. 2000;56:190-6.
8. Wallen EM, Pruthi RS, Joyce GF, et al. Kidney cancer. J Urol. 2007;177:2006-19.
9. Lipworth L, Tarone RE, McLaughlin JK. The epidemiology of renal cell carcinoma. J Urol. 2006;176:2353-8.
10. Broecker B. Non-Wilms' renal tumors in children. Urol Clin North Am. 2000;27:463-9.
11. Sánchez-Ortiz RF, Rosser CJ, Madsen LT, et al. Young age is an independent prognostic factor for survival of sporadic renal cell carcinoma. J Urol. 2004b;171:2160-5.
12. Parker AS, Cerhan JR, Janney CA, et al. Smoking cessation and renal cell carcinoma. Ann Epidemiol. 2003b;13:245-51.
13. Calle EE, Kaaks R. Overweight, obesity and cancer: Epidemiological evidence and proposed mechanisms. Nat Rev Cancer. 2004;4:579-91.
14. Ljungberg B, Campbell SC, Choi HY, et al. The epidemiology of renal cell carcinoma. Eur Urol. 2011;60:615-21.
15. Linehan WM, Ricketts CJ. The metabolic basis of kidney cancer. Semin Cancer Biol. 2013;23:46-55.
16. Cho E, Curhan G, Hankinson SE, et al. Prospective evaluation of analgesic use and risk of renal cell cancer. Arch Intern Med. 2011;171:1487-93.
17. Cheng WS, Farrow GM, Zincke H. The incidence of multicentricity in renal cell carcinoma. J Urol. 1991;146:1221-3.
18. Fuhrman SA, Lasky LC, Limas C. Prognostic significance of morphologic parameters in renal cell carcinoma. Am J Surg Pathol. 1982;6:655-63.
19. Finley DS, Shuch B, Said JW, et al. The chromophobe tumor grading system is the preferred grading scheme for chromophobe renal cell carcinoma. J Urol. 2011;186:2168-74.

20. Jayson M, Sanders H. et al. Increased incidence of serendipitously discovered renal cell carcinoma. Urology. 1998;51:203-5.
21. Lee CT, Katz J, Fearn PA, et al. Mode of presentation of renal cell carcinoma provides prognostic information. Urol Oncol. 2002;7:135-40.
22. Kim HL, Dorey FJ, Figlin RA, et al. Paraneoplastic signs and symptoms of renal cell carcinoma: implications for prognosis. J Urol. 2003;170:1742.
23. Klatte T, Said JW, Belldegrun AS, et al. Differential diagnosis of hypercalcemia in renal malignancy. Urology. 2007;70:179.e7-8.
24. Giannakos G, Papanicolaou X, Trafalis D, et al. Stauffer's syndrome variant associated with renal cell carcinoma. Int J Urol. 2005;12:757-9.
25. Rosenkrantz AB, Hindman N, Fitzgerald EF, et al. MRI features of renal oncocytoma and chromophobe renal cell carcinoma. Am J Roentgenol. 2010; 195:W421.
26. Mueller-Lisse UG, Mueller-Lisse UL. Imaging of advanced renal cell carcinoma. World J Urol. 2010;28:253.
27. Park JW, Jo MK, Lee HM. Significance of 18F-fluorodeoxyglucose positron-emission tomography/computed tomography for the postoperative surveillance of advanced renal cell carcinoma. BJU Int. 2009;103:615.
28. Glazer A, Novick AC. Preoperative transesophageal echocardiography for assessment of vena caval tumor thrombi: a comparative study with vena cavography and magnetic resonance imaging. Urology. 1997;49:32-4.
29. Rini BI, McKiernan JM, Chang SS, et al. Kidney. In: Amin MB (Ed). AJCC Cancer Staging Manual, 8th edition. New York: Springer; 2017. pp. 739.
30. Lane BR, Abouassaly R, Gao T, et al. Active treatment of localized renal tumors may not impact overall survival in patients aged 75 years or older. Cancer. 2010;116:3119.
31. Robson CJ, Churchill BM, Anderson W. The results of radical nephrectomy for renal cell carcinoma. J Urol. 1969;101:297-301.
32. O'Malley RL, Godoy G, Kanofsky JA, et al. The necessity of adrenalectomy at the time of radical nephrectomy: a systematic review. J Urol. 2009;181:2009-17.
33. Phillips CK, Taneja SS. The role of lymphadenectomy in the surgical management of renal cell carcinoma. Urol Oncol. 2004;22:214-24.
34. Blute ML, Leibovich BC, Cheville JC, et al. A protocol for performing extended lymph node dissection using primary tumor pathological features for patients treated with radical nephrectomy for clear cell renal cell carcinoma. J Urol. 2004;172:465-9.
35. Huang WC, Elkin EB, Levey AS, et al. Partial nephrectomy versus radical nephrectomy in patients with small renal tumors: is there a difference in mortality and cardiovascular outcomes? J Urol. 2009;181:55-62.
36. Murphy DP, Gill IS. Energy-based renal tumor ablation: a review. Semin Urol Oncol. 2001;19:133-40.
37. Thompson RH, Atwell T, Schmit G, et al. Comparison of partial nephrectomy and percutaneous ablation for cT1 renal masses. Eur Urol. 2015;67:252.
38. Nesbitt JC, Soltero ER, Dinney CP, et al. Surgical management of renal cell carcinoma with inferior vena cava tumor thrombus. Ann Thorac Surg. 1997;63:1592.

39. Haferkamp A, Bastian PJ, Jakobi H, et al. Renal cell carcinoma with tumor thrombus extension into the vena cava: Prospective long-term follow-up. J Urol. 2007;177:1703.
40. Bissada NK, Yakout HH, Babanouri A, et al. Long-term experience with management of renal cell carcinoma involving the inferior vena cava. Urology. 2003;61:89.
41. Jocham D, Richter A, Hoffmann L, et al. Adjuvant autologous renal tumour cell vaccine and risk of tumour progression in patients with renal-cell carcinoma after radical nephrectomy: phase III, randomised controlled trial. Lancet. 2004;363:594.
42. Staehler MD, Kruse J, Haseke N, et al. Liver resection for metastatic disease prolongs survival in renal cell carcinoma: 12-year results from a retrospective comparative analysis. World J Urol. 2010;28:543.
43. Maxwell NJ, Saleem Amer N, Rogers E, et al. Renal artery embolisation in the palliative treatment of renal carcinoma. Br J Radiol. 2007;80:96.
44. Zelefsky MJ, Greco C, Motzer R, et al. Tumor control outcomes after hypofractionated and single-dose stereotactic image-guided intensity-modulated radiotherapy for extracranial metastases from renal cell carcinoma. Int J Radiat Oncol Biol Phys. 2012;82:1744.
45. Fuchs B, Trousdale RT, Rock MG, et al. Solitary bony metastasis from renal cell carcinoma: significance of surgical treatment. Clin Orthop Relat Res. 2005;(431):187-92.
46. Fokas E, Henzel M, Hamm K, et al. Radiotherapy for brain metastases from renal cell cancer: should whole-brain radiotherapy be added to stereotactic radiosurgery? Analysis of 88 patients. Strahlenther Onkol. 2010. 186: 210.
47. Forauer AR, Mavrogenis AF, Casadei R, et al. Selective palliative transcatheter embolization of bony metastases from renal cell carcinoma. Acta Oncol. 2007;46:1012.
48. Yagoda A, Abi-Rached B, Petrylak D. Chemotherapy for advanced renal-cell carcinoma: 1983-1993. Semin Oncol. 1995;22:42-60.
49. Haas NB, Lin X, Manola J, et al. A phase II trial of doxorubicin and gemcitabine in renal cell carcinoma with sarcomatoid features: ECOG 8802. Med Oncol. 2012;29:761.
50. Interferon-alpha and survival in metastatic renal carcinoma: early results of a randomised controlled trial. Medical Research Council Renal Cancer Collaborators. Lancet. 1999;353:14.
51. Escudier B, Pluzanska A, Koralewski P, et al. Bevacizumab plus interferon alfa-2a for treatment of metastatic renal cell carcinoma: A randomised, double-blind phase III trial. Lancet. 2007;370:2103.
52. McDermott DF, Regan MM, Clark JI, et al. Randomized phase III trial of high-dose interleukin-2 versus subcutaneous interleukin-2 and interferon in patients with metastatic renal cell carcinoma. J Clin Oncol. 2005;23:133.
53. Kammula US, White DE, Rosenberg SA. Trends in the safety of high dose bolus interleukin-2 administration in patients with metastatic cancer. Cancer. 1998;83:797-805.

54. Brahmer JR, Tykodi SS, Chow LQW, et al. Safety and activity of anti-PD-L1 antibody in patients with advanced cancer. N Engl J Med. 2012;366:2455.
55. Jaakkola P, Mole DR, Tian YM, et al. Targeting of HIF-α to the von Hippel-Lindau ubiquitylation complex by O_2-regulated prolyl hydroxylation. Science. 2001;292:468-72.
56. Escudier B, Bellmunt J, Négrier S et al. Phase III trial of bevacizumab plus interferon alfa-2a in patients with metastatic renal cell carcinoma (AVOREN): final analysis of overall survival. J Clin Oncol. 2010;28(13):2144-50.
57. Guertin DA, Sabatini DM. Defining the role of mTOR in cancer. Cancer Cell. 2007;12(1):9-22.
58. Hudson CC, Liu M, Chiang GG, et al. Regulation of hypoxia-inducible factor-1 alpha expression and function by the mammalian target of rapamycin. Mol Cell Biol. 2002;22:7004-14.
59. Calvo E, Escudier B, Motzer RJ, et al. Everolimus in metastatic renal cell carcinoma: Subgroup analysis of patients with 1 or 2 previous vascular endothelial growth factor receptor-tyrosine kinase inhibitor therapies enrolled in the phase III RECORD-1 study. Eur J Cancer. 2012;48:333.
60. Hollingsworth JM, Miller DC, Daignault S, et al. Five-year survival after surgical treatment for kidney cancer: A population-based competing risk analysis. Cancer. 2007;109:1763.

Chapter 11

Peritoneal Carcinomatosis

Shaifali Goel, Shivendra Singh

INTRODUCTION

Peritoneal carcinomatosis (PC) refers to the shedding, implantation and dissemination of a tumor, either localized or widespread to the peritoneum and serosal surfaces of the intraperitoneal viscera as well as the adjacent structures of the abdominal cavity. Usually this results from intracavitary dissemination of tumor that may arise from variety of primary sites such as gastrointestinal (GI), gynecologic, primary peritoneal or mesothelioma. The disease is often discovered at an advanced stage when ascites or intestinal obstruction develops. In 10-35% of patients with recurrent colorectal cancer (CRC) and in up to 50% of patients with recurrent gastric cancer (GC), peritoneal cavity is the most common site of recurrence. PC does not respond to systemic chemotherapy in the same fashion as liver and lung metastases. Life expectancy is limited and dependent on the pathology of the primary malignancy: between 3 and 6 months for gastric base PC, 11–21 months for colon/rectal PC and 14-24 months for ovarian PC. Systematic chemotherapy is the mainstay of treatment for peritoneal metastasis although with the recent available evidence it is now being considered as a metastatic disease eligible for a locoregional treatment in combination with systemic chemotherapy.

Surgery has been used as a palliative modality for PC for long. Extensive debulking for locally advanced ovarian cancers was described as early as 1930s by JV Meigs.[1] The concept of "debulking" was to reduce the tumor burden and eventually decrease the incidence of complications such as obstruction and perforation. He reported that in stage II and III ovarian cancers, residual tumor less than 1.6 cm was associated with better survival.[2] Another malignancy in which palliative surgery was used was pseudomyxoma peritonei (PMP) of appendiceal origin. Rationale behind debulking surgery in this group was that distant metastasis was rare and most important reason for morbidity and mortality was local disease causing bowel obstruction or perforation. In 1969, Alabama et al. showed improved survival with cytoreductive surgery

(CRS) and adjuvant chemotherapy in patients with PMP. He introduced the concept of intraperitoneal chemotherapy by administering alkylating agents.[3] After this there was a sudden increase in trials trying to establish the role of intraperitoneal (IP) chemotherapy in these cancers. Animal trials comparing intravenous (IV) and IP route of administration of cisplatin showed significantly higher intraperitoneal levels of drug compared to IV levels.[4] Multiple studies came up in 1970s and 1980s where IP chemotherapeutic drugs were administered at a concentration much higher than what could be safely administered IV. Most of the phase I and phase II trials showed efficacy of cytoreductive surgery (CRS) and IP chemotherapy in ovarian tumors. Concept of whole body hyperthermia in reducing the tumor burden levels was utilized in peritoneal malignancies and machines were developed to instill hyperthermic intraperitoneal chemotherapy (HIPEC). This gave way to use of intraperitoneal chemotherapy at higher temperatures with the hope that penetration into carcinoma cells would be better. Soon results of CRS and HIPEC showed that adequate cytoreduction is a must for complete benefit of HIPEC. The pioneering work of Dr Paul Sugarbaker in the field of CRS and HIPEC for malignancies gave a glimmer of hope for a select group of patients with peritoneal metastasis from malignancies.[5]

Although there is enough literature now to suggest that CRS and HIPEC is superior to systemic chemotherapy, it has not made its way into the routine management of stage IV disease as most of the treating surgeons and medical oncologists still consider this strategy to be experimental. Moreover, it is a very extensive surgery with relatively high morbidity. Management of peritoneal surface malignancies requires a dedicated multidisciplinary team comprising of a surgeon, medical oncologist, anesthesiologist, radiologist and intensivist.

DIAGNOSIS

Imaging

Preoperative diagnosis of PC is challenging. Imaging techniques computed tomography (CT) scan and magnetic resonance imaging (MRI)] are not only helpful in planning cytoreduction but also in preventing unwarranted laparotomy in patients with unresectable disease. The CT manifestations of peritoneal carcinomatosis include: (1) ascites; (2) soft-tissue permeation of fat, nodular to bulky cake-like tumors in the mesentery and greater omentum; (3) stellate pattern in the mesentery; (4) peritoneal implants along the perihepatic, subdiaphragmatic, anterior, or lateral margins of the peritoneal cavity and (5) bowel wall thickening with or without obstruction.[6] In a study by Koh et al. looking specifically at CRC-PC the authors found that CT significantly underestimated clinical peritoneal carcinomatosis index (PCI).

Sensitivity for CT detection of tumor nodules less than 0.5 cm and 1 cm was reported to be 11% and 25-50%, respectively. In fact sensitivity of small bowel involvement in each region ranged from 8% to 17% only.[7] Therefore, routine contrast CT is not very helpful in estimating the burden of PC. Fusion of PET and CT images allows accurate localization of increased metabolic activity, therefore differentiating normal physiological uptake (bowel and urinary tract) from disease processes. Imaging features of peritoneal malignancy on positron emission tomography (PET) shows avid 18F-FDG uptake within well-circumscribed nodules, to diffuse 18F-FDG uptake over peritoneal and serosal surfaces. Sensitivities and specificities of 78-97% and 55-90% have been reported in PET detection of peritoneal carcinomatosis of ovarian primary.[8-10] Previously occult nodal and extra-abdominal disease may also become detectable with PET/CT, potentially changing patient management (Table 1).

Magnetic resonance imaging, and particularly diffusion weighted images (DWI), has been demonstrated in prospective studies to have increased accuracy in detection of carcinomatosis within certain areas of the abdomen. The use of fat suppression, delayed post gadolinium-enhanced sequences and water-soluble enteric contrast agents has allowed detection sensitivities to surpass that of CT.[11] DWI has been shown to improve detection of peritoneal disease by showing restricted diffusion when combined with conventional contrast-enhanced MRI. Fuji et al. reported sensitivity and specificity of 90% and 95.5% in their study.[12] MRI however carries its own limitations due to the motion artifacts of peristalsis, cost, and the need for radiologists trained in their interpretation and interobserver variation.

Tumor Marker

Most tumor markers, including CEA, CA-125, CA 19-9, and CA 15-3, are not specific and are thus not helpful in determining the site of the primary tumor. They are generally not useful as diagnostic or prognostic tests. However, they are commonly elevated and may be useful in following the response to therapy. Also in ovarian cancer, CA-125 does not distinguish between localized or diffuse peritoneal disease.

Histological Diagnosis and Immunohistochemical Staining

Definite diagnosis can be made by performing ultrasonography (USG) or CT-guided biopsy from peritoneal deposits and subsequent histopathological examination. Tissue diagnosis is important not only for initiation of neoadjuvant therapy but also for prognostication. The diagnosis of PC from appendiceal mucinous neoplasm (AMN) depends largely on the presence of mucin on pathologic examination. Immunohistochemical (IHC) staining

Table 1: Noninvasive imaging for peritoneal carcinomatosis (PC) detection.

Imaging modality	Advantages	Disadvantages	Sensitivity and specificity as compared to surgical analysis[13]
Ultrasound	Inexpensive and effective for ascites. Often modality of choice for image-guided biopsy to achieve detection.	Limited PC nodule sensitivity, operator dependent.	Nonspecific
CT scan	Standard staging workup. Ease of access, fast image acquisition time, thin section scanning and multiplanar reformations	Limited small PC nodule (< 5 mm) sensitivity. Interobserver variability.	Sensitivity: 25–100%, with only 11–48% sensitivity for tumors less than 5 mm. Specificity: 78–100%
MRI	High PC sensitivity	Relatively expensive, peristalsis motion artifact, interobserver variability.	Sensitivity: 90% Specificity: 95% (diffusion weighted)
PET-CT	High PC sensitivity. Detection of extra-abdominal disease.	Relatively expensive, peristalsis motion artifact. False-negative results due to small tumor deposits, mucinous tumors (ovarian or colonic) or signet ring gastric cancers not taking up 18F-FDG. False-positive results due to nonmalignant and inflammatory lesions.	Sensitivity: 78–97% Specificity: 55–90%

(CT: computed tomography; MRI: magnetic resonance imaging; PET: positron emission tomography) is also successful in defining the tumor lineage of poorly differentiated neoplasms. AMN stain diffusely positive for CK20 (100%) and are often negative for CK7 (71%). For ovarian carcinoma, pathologists use a panel of IHC (CK7, WT-1, PAX8, CK20, and CDX-2) for confirmation of origin.[14]

Endoscopy

Upper GI endoscopy and colonoscopy are often indicated in preoperative workup of cases with mucinous peritoneal carcinomatosis with unknown primary in an attempt to identify the organ of origin. Colonoscopy should also be performed in patients with intra-abdominal metastases who have a cytokeratin (CK)20-positive/CK7-negative IHC staining pattern, a positive caudal-type homeobox transcription factor (CDX)-2 IHC stain, or a gene expression profile predictive of colorectal cancer.

Staging the Disease Burden: Peritoneal Carcinomatosis Index (Fig. 1)

It is a scoring system that quantifies the extent of carcinomatosis. It has been recognized as one of the most important prognostic indicators for the long-term outcomes of PC patients. The abdomen is divided into 13 regions: central region (0), right upper (1), epigastrium (2), left upper (3), left flank (4), left lower (5), pelvis (6), right lower (7), right flank (8), and the small bowel is divided into four regions: upper jejunum (9), lower jejunum (10), upper ileum (11), and lower ileum (12). Each one is assigned a lesion-size (LS) score of 0–3. LS-0 stands for no tumor seen, LS-1 indicates implants less than 0.25 cm, LS-2 indicates implants between 0.25 and 5 cm, and LS-3 indicates implants more than 5 cm or a confluence of disease. PCI score is a final numerical score of 0–39. A survival analysis according to the PCI of PC in colorectal cancer indicated that the 5-year overall survival (OS) rate was prominently higher in PC patients with a low PCI (<10) than in patients with a PCI ranging from 10 to 20 or a PCI of more than 20 (53%, 23%, and 12%, respectively. $p< 0.001$).[15] PCI is calculated on the basis of imaging as well as intraoperatively.

MANAGEMENT

Cytoreductive Surgery + Hyperthermic Intraperitoneal Chemotherapy

There are three routes by which a malignancy spreads: (1) hematogenous, (2) lymphatic and (3) transcoelomic. Transcoelomic route is responsible for PC. Usually PC can occur due to either exfoliation of cells through a tumor which has breached the serosa or during surgery. Thus, it should be

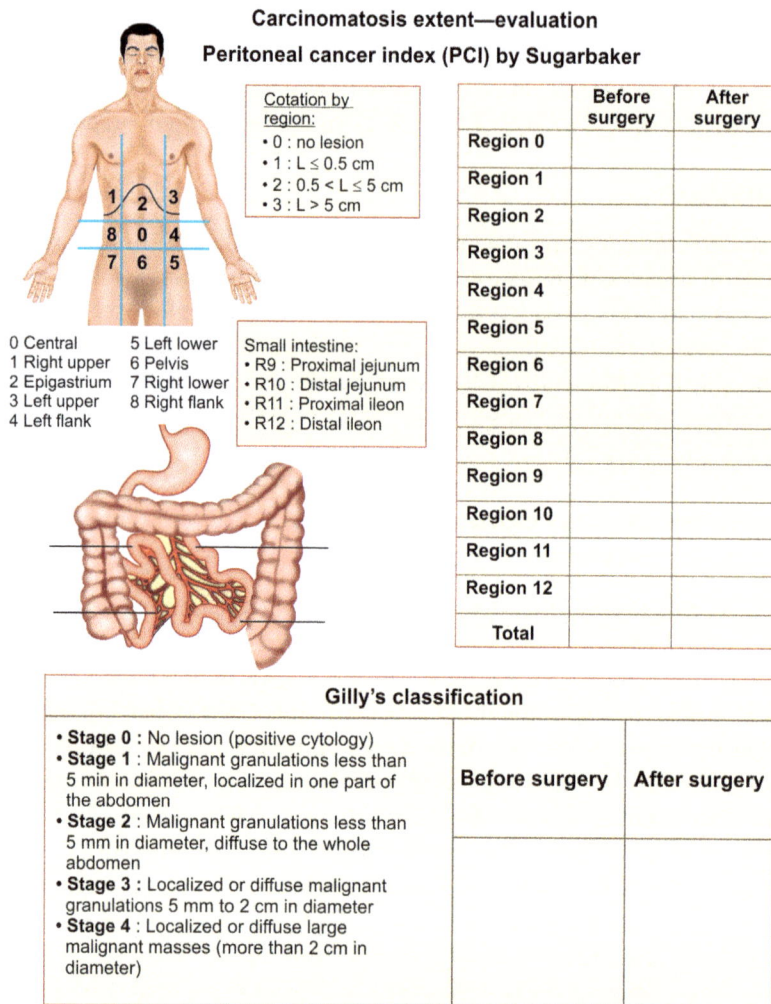

Fig. 1: Assessment of peritoneal carcinomatosis extent.

treated as local disease and not systemic disease. Unfortunately, systemic chemotherapy was considered by most as the treatment of choice for patients with peritoneal metastasis. Even with latest drugs, the survival is up to 16–20 months only. One of the main limiting factors governing dosimetry and thus efficacy of systemic chemotherapy is hematological toxicity. In other words, the actual dose given intravenously is not the dose one wants to give based on cytotoxicity studies, but rather the dose tolerated by the patient's hematological reserve.

In CRS with HIPEC, all the visible disease is removed (taking care of macroscopic disease) and chemotherapy is given at higher temperature intraperitoneally (taking care of microscopic disease). There are few drugs such as Mitomycin C which have a high intraperitoneal concentration and low plasma concentration when given intraperitoneally. Moreover, absorption into plasma is also slow thus giving more time for the anticancer drug to act on cancer nodules. This gives us an opportunity to give maximal dose of chemotherapy to the tumor cells without significant effect on hematological reserves. Another important characteristic which an intraperitoneal drug should possess is its ability to cross the cancer nodules and act on them. It has been found in various studies on rodent models that drugs like adriamycin have a very limited penetration in tumor nodules maximum being up to 1-2 mm. This finding has a very significant impact on the very premise on which concept of CRS and HIPEC is based. An adequate CRS (defined as CC-0 or CC-1) is a must for HIPEC to work. This implies that HIPEC would be effective only when residual tumor size is not more than 2 mm. Clinical studies have established the fact that completeness of cytoreduction is one the most significant factors affecting survival after HIPEC

Rationale Behind Hyperthermia

The rationale of HIPEC is the synergistic cytotoxic effect of heat (ideally 42–43°C) and the chemotherapeutic agent itself on tumor cells. Hyperthermia itself has got anticancer activity. Temperature above 41° causes selective cytotoxicity of malignant cells by various mechanisms like protein denaturation, impaired DNA repair and inhibition of oxidative metabolism. It causes vasodilation with improvement in tumor oxygenation improving the effects of chemotherapeutic agents. Heat also decreases interstitial pressure, allowing for optimal diffusion of chemotherapy and increases cytotoxicity, preferentially killing susceptible tumor cells. Various rat models have shown that adding hyperthermia to doxorubicin increased its concentration in peritoneum and doubled in the small bowel thus confirming that heat increases local tissue concentration.

Cytoreductive Surgery

Staging laparoscopy is done to assess the extent of small bowel disease and also the extent of hepatoduodenal ligament involvement if possible. However, limitations of laparoscopy in this subset of patients are that most of the patients have undergone prior surgery, sometimes even more than one prior surgery. Thus, there are intraoperative adhesions which might prevent complete visualization of small bowel. Recently BIG-RENAPE study concluded that laparoscopy may underestimate the extent of CRPM though it was found to be feasible in 88% of cases.[16] Moreover, disease in hepatoduodenal ligament is also difficult to visualize. Irrespective of these limitations, staging laparoscopy should be considered before contemplating CRS and HIPEC wherever possible.

Following evaluation, laparotomy is done from xiphoid process to pubis. The presence of macroscopic tumor deposits is recorded in 13 abdominal regions according to PCI chart (*see* Fig. 1). The procedure involves removal of peritoneum from all the five regions—right and left hemidiaphragm, right and left paracolic gutters and pelvic peritoneum (Figs. 2A to C). All the disease involving small bowel and its mesentery is also removed which may also involve resection and anastomosis of small bowel. In order to achieve complete cytoreduction, many times adjacent organs need to be resected like anterior resection for deposits on sigmoid and pouch of Douglas, distal gastrectomy, cholecystectomy, splenectomy, and colectomies. Other components of CRS are both greater and lesser omentectomies, Glissonian capsule removal (in case of involvement by mucinous tumors). The objective of cytoreduction is to leave no macroscopic tumor behind (CC-0; complete cytoreduction); but, if that could not be achieved, attempts are made to leave no residual tumor exceeding 2.5 mm in thickness (CC-1) as previously discussed. Main benefits for HIPEC are for CC-0 and CC-1. The limiting factor for complete cytoreduction in most of the cases is extensive small bowel involvement. Those with extensive small bowel involvement (with deposits on mesenteric side of small bowel) are difficult to treat as removing whole of the disease for a CC-0 or CC-1 would require multiple resection and anastomosis. Another factor which might prohibit complete cytoreduction is extensive involvement of hepatoduodenal ligament.

HIPEC

Various techniques of administering HIPEC have been proposed—open (coliseum technique), semiclosed and closed. In open technique, hyperthermic solution is administered in open abdomen and it is manually stirred with the aim to uniformly distribute the hyperthermic solution to all quadrants and whole of peritoneal surface. However, it runs the theoretical risk of exposure of chemotherapeutic drugs to the surgical team and operating room personnel. Till date, however no study has proved this risk in the care givers. Another side effect of open technique is the difficulty in maintaining the desired temperature of the hyperthermic solution. In semiclosed technique the abdomen is covered with a plastic sheet and a small opening is given in between through which the surgeon manually manipulates whole of solution. In closed technique, whole of the abdomen is closed and then HIPEC administered. It carries the benefit of earlier achievement of required temperature, safer for care givers but at the cost of nonuniform distribution of HIPEC solution in all quadrants. Till date, no trials have confirmed the benefit of one technique over the other. We prefer *closed technique* using

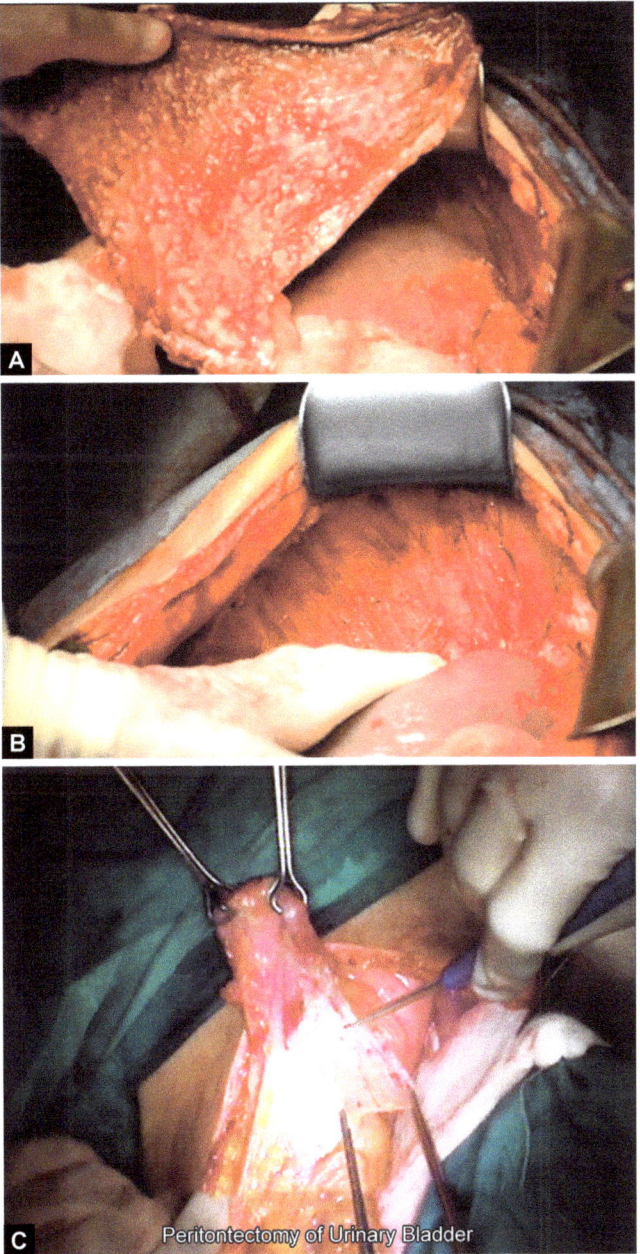

Figs. 2A to C: (A) Patient of pseudomyxoma peritonei with extensive diaphragmatic deposits, (B) Same patient after complete peritonectomy, and (C) Showing pelvic peritonectomy of the same patient.

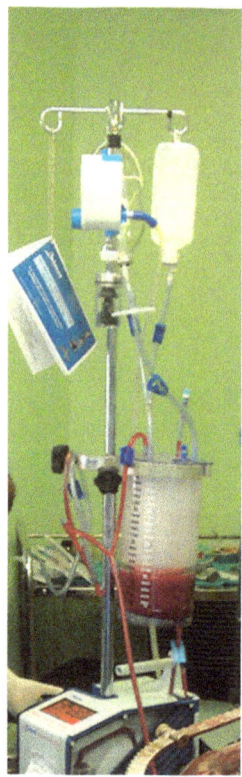

Fig 3: Belmont hyperthermia pump.

Belmont machine (Fig. 3). Perfusion is started with a minimum of 2 liters of isotonic dialysis fluid, with an inflow temperature of 43-44°C. As soon as the temperature in the abdomen is stable above 40°C in all the quadrants, chemotherapeutic agents are added to the perfusate and circulated for 90 min. Drug used for IP chemotherapy depends upon the primary disease. Even the duration of HIPEC depends on the type of drug used (30 minutes for Oxaliplatin, 90 minutes for Mitomycin C). Position of the patient is changed to allow for complete mixing of drug in whole of the abdomen. In open technique, whole of the drug is mixed manually so that it comes in contact with all the peritoneal surfaces. Patient is also given IV chemotherapy to increase the effect of IP chemotherapy (bidirectional chemotherapy). Before closing the abdomen the drains are inserted in all the five peritonectomy regions for the purpose of early postoperative chemotherapy.

Types of Intraperitoneal Chemotherapy Regimens

Neoadjuvant Intraperitoneal plus Intravenous Chemotherapy

This technique is used in patients in whom PC is diagnosed on staging laparoscopy. Patients are given both IP and IV chemotherapy with the aim to reduce or eradicate PC, checking the tumor biology and preventing the dissemination of disease to extra-abdominal spaces. Definitive surgery is done after 3-4 cycles of such therapies. Both radiological and clinical responses have been shown with this technique. However, it is not without complications. Firstly, there might be adhesions present due to prior surgical intervention and these might prevent the uniform distribution of drug. Moreover, extensive adhesive response from this technique might render future definitive CRS difficult and increase morbidity and mortality.

Intraoperative HIPEC plus Intravenous Chemotherapy

This is the most widely used technique. Here IP chemotherapy is given at the time of definitive surgery and is added after cytoreductive surgery.

Early Postoperative Intraperitoneal Chemotherapy

Early postoperative intraperitoneal chemotherapy (EPIC) is usually given immediately after definitive surgery. Drains are placed during primary surgery and chemotherapy is given through drainage catheters usually from postoperative day 1 to day 5. Drugs are given through one drain over 1 hour and all the drains are clamped for next 23 hours. Position of the patient is changed for effective mixing of drug in all the quadrants of the abdomen. Drug is allowed to flow out of the drains over next 1 hour. This process is repeated for next 4 days. Since adhesions have not formed, it allows for uniform distribution of drug throughout the peritoneal cavity and prevents the entrapment of cancer cells inside the fibrin deposits.

Adjuvant Intraperitoneal and Systemic Chemotherapy

Very few studies have been done on this approach. Usually used in the setting of incomplete cytoreduction in ovarian tumors, patients are given IP chemotherapy through port inserted at the time of first surgery. Additional systemic chemotherapy is also given. This type of technique can also be used a bridge between primary surgery and definitive or second look surgery later.

Indications for the Combined Treatment with CRS and HIPEC

- Peritoneal pseudomyxoma
- Peritoneal mesothelioma
- Primary colon and rectal cancer with peritoneal seeding of limited distribution and small volume
    - Perforated colon cancer
        - Colon cancer involving adjacent organs
        - Colon cancer disseminated to the ovaries

- Colon cancer with a positive peritoneal fluid cytology
 - Tumor rupture at a primary resection
- Recurrent colon and rectal cancer with carcinomatosis
 - Peritoneal seeding of limited distribution and small volume
 - Krukenberg tumor
 - Tumor rupture during resection of a recurrence
- Recurrent ovarian cancer with limited dissemination to the peritoneum
 - Prolonged disease free interval between initial treatment and recurrence
 - Limited or no options for chemotherapy via intravenous route
- Primary gastric cancer with limited peritoneal implants after a complete resection of both the primary and implant
- Peritoneal sarcomatosis
- Malignant ascites.

Contraindications to CRS and HIPEC

- Poor general status
- Presence of extraperitoneal metastases
- Diffuse widespread PC
- Presence of extensive liver metastases (relative)
- Evidence of ureteric or biliary obstruction
- More than one site of small bowel obstruction (relative)
- Extensive small bowel and mesenteric involvement
- Extensive disease in hepatoduodenal ligament area.

Complications of CRS and HIPEC

CRS ± HIPEC is a very extensive surgery involving extensive surgical resection and introduction of chemotherapeutic drug intraperitoneally. Both components add to the morbidity of the surgery. Overall morbidity and mortality of CRS and HIPEC is to the tune of 22-34% and 0.8-4.1%.[17] Various series have shown that mortality varies according to the primary disease.

Overall complications associated with CRS and HIPEC are hematological toxicity especially neutropenia, digestive fistulas, pneumonia, postoperative bleeding, septic infections like intra-abdominal abscess, wound infection and renal insufficiency. Respiratory complications ranged from 6% to 14%, GI complications including digestive fistulas ranged from 8% to 18.2%, renal 1-10% and hematological 6-20%. Various factors associated with higher morbidity and mortality are old age, hypoalbuminemia, poor performance status, high PCI score, high grade histology of tumors, associated bowel, diaphragmatic and pancreatic resections and surgeon experience. High PCI score has consistently been associated with higher morbidity. Reason behind this association may be due to extensive resection involved, associated bowel resection and poor general condition due to advanced disease. Surgeon experience has also been cited as an important factor determining the morbidity and mortality. One study showed that complications in first 70 cases were much higher compared to next 70 cases (30% vs 10%).[18] Learning curve, in this procedure, is not merely due to technical improvement but improved patient selection also plays an important role.[18]

Hematological toxicity is a common problem after HIPEC especially after use of mitomycin C. In our institution, neutropenia has been found in around 40% of the patients. Thus, we closely monitor leukocyte count especially after third postoperative day.

Pulmonary complications are one of the major concern post-CRS especially after subdiaphragmatic peritonectomy. It was hypothesized that after subdiaphragmatic peritoneal stripping, incidence of leakage of HIPEC fluid inside the pleural space increases. This increases the incidence of postoperative pneumonia, pleural effusion and respiratory distress. Although this theory has been quashed in a review by Sugarbaker,[19] only factor which was responsible for postoperative pulmonary complications was excessive blood transfusion. According to Müller and colleagues, the incidence of pulmonary complications can be decreased by restricting intraoperative fluids, intensified hyperglycemia management and reducing blood loss.[20] Oxaliplatin is associated with higher incidence of intra-abdominal bleeding and mild hepatotoxicity and cisplatin is associated with higher incidence of nephrotoxicity.

ROLE OF CYTOREDUCTIVE SURGERY AND HIPEC IN THE TREATMENT OF ABDOMINAL CARCINOMATOSIS FROM DIFFERENT PRIMARY MALIGNANCIES

Peritoneal Carcinomatosis from Colorectal Cancer

Peritoneal carcinomatosis is not an infrequent occurrence in patients with colorectal cancer (CRC, up to 8% at the time of primary surgery and up to 25% at the time of recurrent CRC).[21] Systemic chemotherapy alone is associated with a mean survival of 8–10 months. Complete CRS and HIPEC is associated with a significant increase in survival in patients of PC from CRC. Most commonly used drug for CRC is MMC. However, many European centers use oxaliplatin in HIPEC. Oxaliplatin has lower area under curve ratio, thus this drug being more easily absorbed systemically compared to MMC. Thus, dwell time of this drug is only 30 minutes compared to MMC whose dwell time is 90 minutes. 5-FU is used as bidirectional agent and as EPIC agent in CRC patients.

Verwaal J et al. conducted a randomized controlled trial (RCT) comparing systemic chemotherapy (5-FU and leucovorin) and palliative surgery versus CRS and HIPEC for PC from CRC. Median survival was 12.6 months with chemotherapy versus 22.3 months following CRS and HIPEC plus systemic chemotherapy. They concluded that CRS and HIPEC give better results in this group of patients compared to systemic chemotherapy alone.[22] Further follow-up over 8 years showed that 5-year DFS was 45% for patients with optimal cytoreduction compared to those who either received systemic chemotherapy alone or those who underwent incomplete cytoreduction. Major drawback of this study was the use of only 5-FU as a part of systemic chemotherapy protocol. Had oxaliplatin been used, results might have been different. But, same protocol was used as an adjunct to CRS and HIPEC.

Glehen published a multicenter study showing the results of CRS and HIPEC in PC from CRC. The study included 506 patients. Overall median survival was 19.2 months with patients having complete CRS having a median survival of 32.4 months.[23] Another multicenter study published by Elias et al. showed a median survival of 30.1 months following CRS and HIPEC with 5-year OS of 27% following. They concluded that CRS and HIPEC should be the gold standard treatment for limited PC from CRC.[24] Recently the early results of PRODIGE 7 trial were presented at ASCO meet in June 2018. The study included 265 patients who were randomized to CRS plus HIPEC with oxaliplatin or CRS alone, in association with systemic chemotherapy. The therapeutic management of PC from colorectal cancer by CRS showed satisfactory survival results. While the addition of HIPEC with oxaliplatin did not influence the OS while adding significantly to the morbidity, though a subclass of patients with intermediate PCI score, benefitted by addition of HIPEC to CRS.[25]

Peritoneal Carcinomatosis from Gastric Cancer

HIPEC has three roles in the management of peritoneal carcinomatosis from advanced gastric cancer—prophylactic HIPEC in advanced gastric cancer to prevent peritoneal carcinomatosis after curative surgery, HIPEC in established cases of peritoneal carcinomatosis and lastly, in palliative management of intractable ascites due to extensive peritoneal carcinomatosis. MMC and cisplatin are the most commonly used drugs for gastric cancer with PC. Cisplatin is also used for ovarian malignancies. It has low AUC. It is nephrotoxic and ototoxic. Metal binding agents such as sodium thiosulfate and amifostine are used to prevent tubular damage. Other drugs used are taxanes.

Various studies have been published after Fujimoto first published their experience of HIPEC in established cases of gastric cancer and peritoneal carcinomatosis in which they showed 2-year survival of upto 45% after HIPEC compared to 0% after surgery alone.[26,27] Such dismal results were improved for first time by Yonemura et al. who reported 5-year survival of 11%.[28]

Glehen et al. reported data from West showing overall median survival of 10.3 months with 5-year survival reaching upto 16%.[29] Largest series till date has been from France. It was a multi-institutional study involving 159 patients. Patients had a median PCI score of 9.4. It also showed overall median survival of 9.2 months with 5-year survival of 13% while patients having complete cytoreduction had a median survival of 15 months with 5-year survival of 23%.[30] First RCT came from Yang et al. who showed a significantly higher median survival of 11 months for CRS and HIPEC group compared to 6.5 months for CRS alone group.[31] Median PCI score was 15 in this study. However, selection criteria in most of the studies have varied considerably. Also the drugs used have also varied although most have used the combination of cisplatin and mitomycin.

PSEUDOMYXOMA PERITONEI

Pseudomyxoma peritonei (PMP), a syndrome firstly described by Rokitansky in 1842, is an enigmatic, often fatal intra-abdominal disease characterized by gelatinous ascites and multifocal peritoneal epithelial implants secreting copious globules of extracellular mucin. This condition is almost always due to a perforated epithelial appendix cancer. Histopathologically, they can be divided into three categories—disseminated peritoneal adenomucinosis (DPAM), PMCA with intermediate (well differentiated) features and peritoneal mucinous carcinomatosis (PMCA).[32] DPAM is associated with better prognosis compared to PMCA. Overall disease has very good prognosis because of absence of extra-abdominal metastasis and lower propensity to involve small bowel. Complete cytoreduction is associated with very good results. Sugarbaker and Chua et al. reviewed 2,300 patients of pseudomyxoma peritonei of appendiceal origin from 16 centers with a mean PCI of 20 and found that following CRS + HIPEC, median survival rate was astonishingly, 16.3 years. The overall 3, 5, 10, and 15-year survival rates were 80%, 74%, 63%, and 59%, respectively. CC0/1 was achieved in 83%, mortality was 2% and major morbidity was 24%.[33]

PERITONEAL MESOTHELIOMA

Malignant peritoneal mesothelioma is a very aggressive disease with uniformly fatal outcome. It is an uncommon tumor arising from the serosal layer of pleura, peritoneum, pericardium and tunica vaginalis testi. It is associated with ascites and intra-abdominal mesenteric or small bowel nodules. It has three variants—epithelioid, sarcomatoid and mixed. Epithelioid variant is associated with superior outcome. CRS and HIPEC with or without EPIC and systemic chemotherapy is the treatment of choice for peritoneal malignant mesothelioma. Patients with PCI score less than 20 are considered to be ideal candidates. Prognosis dips progressively as the extent of small bowel involvement increases. CC-0 and CC-1, epithelioid variants and presence of ascites in the absence of small bowel involvement are associated with improved survival. With morbidity and mortality of 30–40% and 2–4%, respectively, a median survival of 30–92 months has been achieved following adequate CRS and HIPEC.[34] Yan et al.[35] in a multi-institutional study examined 407 patients affected by peritoneal mesothelioma treated with CRS and HIPEC in 7 different surgical centers. Eighty nine percent of the cases were epithelial mesothelioma while 11% were sarcomatoid or biphasic. CC0-CC1 rates was achieved in 46% of cases, lymph nodes metastases were find in 6% and distant metastases in 3% of the patients. After a mean follow-up of 30 months, the median survival was 53 months independent prognostic factor are the histological type of the mesothelioma, level of cytoreduction achieved, lymph node metastases, and the possibility to perform HIPEC.

PERITONEAL CARCINOMATOSIS FROM OVARIAN CANCER

Epithelial cancers of ovarian, fallopian tubal and peritoneal origin exhibit similar clinical characteristics and behavior and are referred to as epithelial ovarian cancer (EOC). It is the most common cause of death among women with gynecologic malignancies. Majority of cases are stage III (disease that has spread throughout the peritoneal cavity or that involves lymph nodes) or stage IV (disease spread to more distant sites) disease at diagnosis.

Primary surgical cytoreduction followed by systemic chemotherapy is the preferred initial management for women with stage III or IV EOC. For women with optimally reduced disease (<1 cm of residual disease), there are two options: intravenous (IV) chemotherapy alone or a combination of IV and intraperitoneal (IP) chemotherapy (IV/IP therapy). Women with suboptimally reduced disease (≥1 cm of residual disease) are not candidates for IP therapy due to limited penetration into larger tumors; different studies demonstrated that a progressively more aggressive surgical effort is associated with improvements in disease-free and overall survival rates. The OS ranges between 46 months and 106 months for patients with complete CRS (no residual disease) and between 12 months and 39 months for incomplete CRS (residual disease of more than 1 cm).[36-43] Up to now, the majority of available series report cases treated with the standard systemic platinum-taxanes chemotherapy and CRS. Three phase III randomized trials and two meta-analyses have demonstrated the favorable impact of platinum-based primary intraperitoneal chemotherapy following an attempt at maximal surgical cytoreduction in advanced EOC in terms of both progression-free and OS.[44-49] The drugs used are paclitaxel and cisplatin.

CONCLUSION

Peritoneal carcinomatosis is a challenging situation for oncologists and surgeons, for which multimodality treatment is the only way forward. Substantial differences exist in treating the different form of PC from different diseases among different centers and countries. Cytoreductive surgery + HIPEC is a promising therapeutic technique to improve long-term survival and may even cure selected patients with peritoneal carcinomatosis secondary to tumors arising from the ovaries, appendix, colorectal or GI tract. The key to successful HIPEC is proper patient selection and adequate CRS with limited blood loss. A dedicated multidisciplinary team approach yields the best long-term results in this difficult group of patients.

REFERENCES

1. Neuwirth MG, Alexander HR, Karakousis GC. Then and now: cytoreductive surgery with hyperthermic intraperitoneal chemotherapy (HIPEC), a historical perspective. J Gastrointest Oncol. 2016;7(1):18-28.
2. Griffiths CT. Surgical resection of tumor bulk in the primary treatment of ovarian carcinoma. Natl Cancer Inst Monogr. 1975;42:101-4.
3. Long RT, Spratt JS Jr, Dowling E. Pseudomyxoma peritonei: New concepts in management with a report of seventeen patients. Am J Surg. 1969;117:162-9.
4. Pretorius RG, Petrilli ES, Kean CK, et al. Comparison of the IV and IP routes of administration of cisplatin in dogs. Cancer Treat Rep. 1981;65:1055-62.
5. Sugarbaker PH. Peritonectomy procedures. Ann Surg. 1995; 221:29-42.
6. Jeffrey RB Jr. CT demonstration of peritoneal implants. AJR. 1980;135:323-6.
7. Koh JL, Yan TD, Glenn D, Morris DL. Evaluation of preoperative computed tomography in estimating peritoneal cancer index in colorectal peritoneal carcinomatosis. Ann Surg Oncol. 2008;16:327-33.
8. Turlakow A, Yeung HW, Salmon AS, et al. Peritoneal carcinomatosis: role of (18) F-FDG PET. J Nucl Med. 2003;44:1407-12.
9. Kitajima K, Murakami K, Yamasaki E, et al. Diagnostic accuracy of integrated FDG-PET/contrast-enhanced CT in staging ovarian cancer: comparison with enhanced CT. Eur J Nucl Med Mol Imaging. 2008;35:191-220.
10. Dirisamer A, Schima W, Heinisch M, et al. Detection of histologically proven peritoneal carcinomatosis with fused 18F-FDGPET/MDCT. Eur J Radiol. 2009;69:536-41.
11. Low RN, Barone RM, Lacey C, et al. Peritoneal tumor: MR imaging with dilute oral barium and intravenous gadolinium-containing contrast agents compared with unenhanced MR imaging and CT. Radiology. 1997;204: 513-20.
12. Fujii S, Matsusue E, Kanasaki Y, et al. Detection of peritoneal dissemination in gynecological malignancy: evaluation by diffusion-weighted MR imaging. Eur Radiol. 2008;18:18-23.

13. Baratti D, Kusamura S, Deraco M. The Fifth International Workshop on Peritoneal Surface Malignancy (Milan, Italy, December 4-6, 2006): methodology of disease-specific consensus. J Surg Oncol. 2008;98:258-62.
14. Greco FA, Lennington WJ, Spigel DR, et al. Poorly differentiated neoplasms of unknown primary site: diagnostic usefulness of a molecular cancer classifier assay. Mol Diagn Ther. 2015;19:91.
15. Goéré D, Malka D, Tzanis D, et al. "Is there a possibility of a cure in patients with colorectal peritoneal carcinomatosis amenable to complete cytoreductive surgery and intraperitoneal chemotherapy?" Ann Surg. 2013;257(6)1065-71.
16. Passot G, Dumont F, Goéré D, et al. Multicentre study of laparoscopic or open assessment of the peritoneal cancer index (BIG-RENAPE). Br J Surg. 2018;105(6):663-7.
17. Newton AD, Bartlett EK, Karakousis GC. Cytoreductive surgery and hyperthermic intraperitoneal chemotherapy: a review of factors contributing to morbidity and mortality. J Gastrointest Oncol. 2016;7(1):99-111.
18. Yan TD, Links M, Fransi S, et al. Learning curve for cytoreductive surgery and perioperative intraperitoneal chemotherapy for peritoneal surface malignancy—a journey to becoming a nationally funded peritonectomy center. Ann Surg Oncol. 2007;14:2270-8.
19. Preti V, Chang D, Sugarbaker PH. Pulmonary Complications following Cytoreductive Surgery and Perioperative Chemotherapy in 147 Consecutive Patients. Gastroenterol Res Pract. 2012;2012:635314.
20. Müller H, Hahn M, Weller L, et al. Strategies to reduce perioperative morbidity in cytoreductive surgery. Hepato-Gastroenterology. 2008;55(86-87):1523-9.
21. American Cancer Society. Cancer Facts & Figures. 2012. [online] Available from http://www.cancer.org. [Accessed December, 2018].
22. Verwaal VJ, van Ruth S, de Bree E, et al. Randomized trial of cytoreduction and hyperthermic intraperitoneal chemotherapy versus systemic chemotherapy and palliative surgery in patients with peritoneal carcinomatosis of colorectal cancer. J Clin Oncol. 2003;21(20):3737-43.
23. Glehen O, Kwiatkowski F, Sugarbaker PH, et al. Cytoreductive surgery combined with perioperative intraperitoneal chemotherapy for the management of peritoneal carcinomatosis from colorectal cancer: a multi-institutional study. J Clin Oncol. 2004;22(16):3284-92.
24. Elias D, Gilly F, Boutitie F, et al. Peritoneal colorectal carcinomatosis treated with surgery and perioperative intraperitoneal chemotherapy: retrospective analysis of 523 patients from a multicentric French study. J Clin Oncol. 2010;28(1):63-8.
25. ASCO. Abstract. [online] Available from https://meetinglibrary.asco.org/record/158740/abstract. [Accessed December, 2018].
26. Fujimoto S, Shrestha RD, Kokubun M, et al. Intraperitoneal hyperthermic perfusion combined with surgery effective for gastric cancer patients with peritoneal seeding. Ann Surg. 1988;208(1):36-41.
27. Fujimoto S, Shrestha RD, Kokubun M, et al. Positive results of combined therapy of surgery and intraperitoneal hyperthermic perfusion for far-advanced gastric cancer. Ann Surg. 1990;212(5):592-6.

28. Yonemura Y, Fujimura T, Nishimura G, et al. Effects of intraoperative chemohyperthermia in patients with gastric cancer with peritoneal dissemination. Surgery. 1996;119(4):437-44.
29. Glehen O, Schreiber V, Cotte E, et al. Cytoreductive surgery and intraperitoneal chemohyperthermia for peritoneal carcinomatosis arising from gastric cancer. Arch Surg Chic Ill 1960. 2004;139(1):20-6.
30. Glehen O, Gilly FN, Arvieux C, et al. Peritoneal carcinomatosis from gastric cancer: a multi-institutional study of 159 patients treated by cytoreductive surgery combined with perioperative intraperitoneal chemotherapy. Ann Surg Oncol. 2010;17(9):2370-7.
31. Yang X-J, Huang C-Q, Suo T, et al. Cytoreductive surgery and hyperthermic intraperitoneal chemotherapy improves survival of patients with peritoneal carcinomatosis from gastric cancer: final results of a phase III randomized clinical trial. Ann Surg Oncol. 2011 Jun;18(6):1575–81.
32. Ronnett BM, Zahn CM, Kurman RJ, et al. Disseminated peritoneal adenomucinosis and peritoneal mucinous carcinomatosis. A clinicopathologic analysis of 109 cases with emphasis on distinguishing pathologic features, site of origin, prognosis, and relationship to "pseudomyxoma peritonei". Am J Surg Pathol. 1995;19:1390-408.
33. Chua TC, Moran BJ, Sugarbaker PH, et al. Early- and long-term outcome data of patients with pseudomyxoma peritonei from appendiceal origin treated by a strategy of cytoreductive surgery and hyperthermic intraperitoneal chemotherapy. J Clin Oncol. 2012;30(20):2449-56.
34. Alexander HR Jr, Burke AP. Diagnosis and management of patients with malignant peritoneal mesothelioma. J Gastrointest Oncol. 2016;7(1):79-86.
35. Yan TD, Deraco M, Baratti D, et al. Cytoreductive surgery and hyperthermic intraperitoneal chemotherapy for malignant peritoneal mesothelioma: multi-institutional experience. J Clin Oncol. 2009;27(36):6237-42.
36. Armstrong DK, Bundy B, Wenzel L, et al. Intraperitoneal cisplatin and paclitaxel in ovarian cancer. N Engl J Med. 2006;354: 34-43.
37. Ozols RF, Bundy BN, Greer BE, et al. Phase III trial of carboplatin and paclitaxel compared with cisplatin and paclitaxel in patients with optimally resected stage III ovarian cancer: a Gynecologic Oncology Group study. J Clin Oncol. 2003;21:3194-200.
38. Bereder J, Glehen O, Habre J, et al. Cytoreductive surgery combined with perioperative intraperitoneal chemotherapy for the management of peritoneal carcinomatosis from ovarian cancer: a multi-institutional study of 246 patients. J Clin Oncol. 2009;27:5542.
39. Song YJ, Lim MC, Kang S, et al. Extended cytoreduction of tumor at the porta hepatis by an interdisciplinary team approach in patients with epithelial ovarian cancer. Gynecol Oncol. 2011;121:253-7.
40. Wimberger P, Lehmann N, Kimmig R, et al. Prognostic factors for complete debulking in advanced ovarian cancer and its impact on survival. An exploratory analysis of a prospectively randomized phase III study of the ArbeitsgemeinschaftGynaekologischeOnkologie Ovarian Cancer Study Group (AGO-OVAR). Gynecol Oncol. 2007;106:69-74.

41. Salani R, Zahurak ML, Santillan A, et al. Survival impact of multiple bowel resections in patients undergoing primary cytoreductive surgery for advanced ovarian cancer: a case-control study. Gynecol Oncol. 2007;107:495-9.
42. Bookman MA, Brady MF, McGuire WP, et al. Evaluation of new platinum based treatment regimens in advanced-stage ovarian cancer: a Phase III Trial of the Gynecologic Cancer Intergroup. J Clin Oncol. 2009;27:1419-25.
43. Jaaback K, Johnson N. Intraperitoneal chemotherapy for the initial management of primary epithelial ovarian cancer. Cochrane Database Syst Rev. 2006;CD005340.
44. Hess LM, Benham-Hutchins M, Herzog TJ, et al. A meta-analysis of the efficacy of intraperitoneal cisplatin for the front-line treatment of ovarian cancer. Int J Gynecol Cancer. 2007;17:561.
45. Tewari D, Java JJ, Salani R, et al. Long-term survival advantage and prognostic factors associated with intraperitoneal chemotherapy treatment in advanced ovarian cancer: A gynecologic oncology group study. J Clin Oncol. 2015;33: 1460-6.
46. Wright AA, Cronin A, Milne DE, et al. Use and effectiveness of intraperitoneal chemotherapy for treatment of ovarian cancer. J Clin Oncol. 2015;33:2841-7.
47. Armstrong DK, Bundy B, Wenzel L, et al. Intraperitoneal cisplatin and paclitaxel in ovarian cancer. N Engl J Med. 2006;354:34.
48. Neuwirth MG, Alexander HR, Karakousis GC. Then and now: cytoreductive surgery with hyperthermic intraperitoneal chemotherapy (HIPEC), a historical perspective. J Gastrointest Oncol. 2016;7(1):18-28.
49. Griffiths CT. Surgical resection of tumor bulk in the primary treatment of ovarian carcinoma. Natl Cancer Inst Monogr. 1975;42:101-4.

12
Chapter

Drug Resistance in Cancer

Sujith Kumar M, Jaya Ghosh

INTRODUCTION

Cancer is one of the most significant noncommunicable diseases of current times in terms of both mortality and morbidity. The overall incidence of cancer is on an increasing trend and the global cancer burden in 2018 is 18 million cases.[1] The advancements in chemotherapy, targeted therapy and recently immunotherapy along with other modalities such as surgery and radiation therapy have reduced cancer mortality and morbidity. However, tumor resistance to chemotherapy and molecularly targeted therapies limits their effectiveness.

As with antibiotics, the issue of resistance to chemotherapy has been described since a longtime.[2] This resistance could be present inherently in a tumor or acquired after exposure to the drug.[3] The different hallmarks of anticancer drug resistance have been well described.[4] Multidrug resistance (MDR) occurs, when these mechanisms act individually or synergistically making the cell resistant to a variety of structurally and mechanistically unrelated drugs in addition to the drug initially administered.[5] Resistance thus occurs as a result of changes within the cancer cell itself or in its microenvironment in the struggle for survival against the onslaught of chemotherapy.[4,6,7] In this chapter, the various mechanisms of drug resistance in oncology are summarized along with a brief section on the ways to overcome the problem and the way forward. Figure 1 depicts the various mechanisms of drug resistance.

PRINCIPLES OF DRUG RESISTANCE

The pharmacokinetic properties of chemotherapy or targeted therapy drugs including absorption, distribution, metabolism, and excretion determine fundamentally the cellular availability of drugs to cause its effects.[5] The action of drug inside the cells (pharmacodynamics) is in-turn influenced by

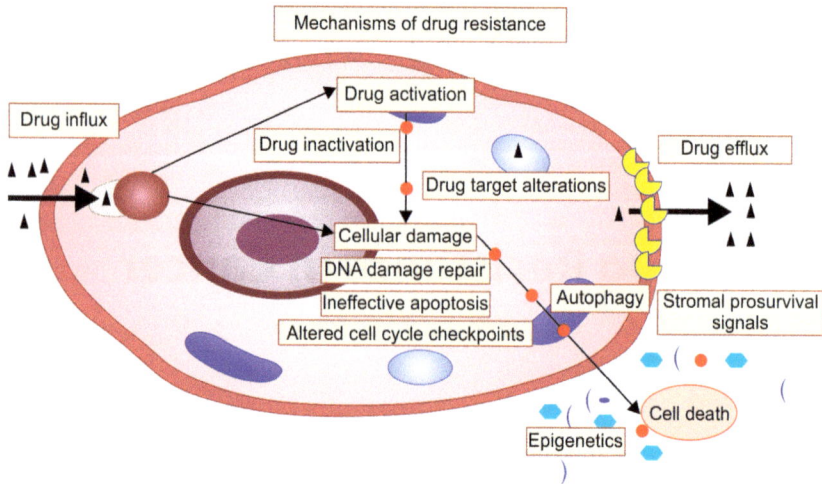

Fig. 1: Mechanisms of drug resistance in oncology.

the internal milieu comprised by the drug targets and the enzymatic system in the cell apart from presence of intrinsic mechanisms, which may reduce the availability of the drug inside.[8] Reduced drug influx or excessive efflux; drug inactivation; alterations in drug target; and dysfunctional apoptosis, intracellular, or external prosurvival signals can negatively influence the anticancer effects of drug.[8] Positive selection of a drug-resistant tumor subpopulation in a heterogeneous tumor due to selective anticancer action can also lead on to drug resistance.[9] The different mechanisms of drug resistance are briefly described below.

DIFFERENT MECHANISMS OF DRUG RESISTANCE

Reduced Drug Influx

Passive diffusion via the lipid membrane (e.g. doxorubicin and vinblastine) or facilitated transport with help of transporters (e.g. nucleoside analog) are two main ways of drug uptake.[5] Only a few drugs enter by endocytosis (pinocytosis).[5] These processes can either be specific or nonspecific.[5] Any decrease in the endocytosis or receptor-mediated drug uptake can result in drug resistance.[5] Decreased expression of reduced folate carrier and polymorphisms in its gene significantly hamper a patient's response to methotrexate[5] similarly decreased endocytosis and receptor-mediated transporters reduce cisplatin uptake.[5]

Increased Drug Efflux and Multidrug Resistance

Drug efflux has been extensively studied as a major mechanism of drug resistance. Adenosine triphosphate (ATP)-binding cassette (ABC) transporters are transmembrane proteins with two distinct domains—a highly conserved nucleotide binding domain and a more variable transmembrane domain exists not only in cancer cells but also various types of human cells such as epithelium of liver, intestine, and blood brain barrier.[3,4] There are 49 known members of the ABC family in humans of which three transporters: (1) P glycoprotein (Pgp), (2) MDR (Multidrug resistance)-associated protein 1 (MRP1), and (3) breast cancer resistance protein (BCRP) are important in drug resistance.[5,8]

The *MDR1* (multidrug resistance) gene, which produces P glycoprotein (Pgp), was the first one of the efflux pumps to be described.[5,8] Drug binding to Pgp results in activation of one of the ATP-binding domains and the subsequent hydrolysis of ATP causes conformational change in Pgp and leads to expulsion of the drug from the cancer cell.[5] Thus, the ATP-binding domain acts like an engine driving the Pgp to pump out drugs.[4,5,8] The binding of Pgp to the drug is not specific and thus there is cross-resistance against multiple unrelated drugs that are structurally and/or functionally different resulting in MDR.[4,5] MDR can be intrinsic or acquired resulting from an upregulation of the efflux pumps.[5,8] Tumors such as colon cancer, renal cancer, liver cancer as well as some in some lymphoma, leukemia, and myeloma upregulate MDR1.[5,8,10] Related transporters MRP1 or BCRP are involved in drug resistance in tissues such as lung and breast cancers.[5,8] Chemotherapy drugs such as anthracyclines, vinca alkaloids, epipodophyllotoxins, actinomycin D, taxanes, and antimetabolites are substrates for MDR.[5,8] Some molecularly targeted agents, gefitinib, erlotinib, and sunitinib are also substrates for MDR.[4,8] Thus, the ABC family of efflux pumps plays an important role in resistance of both important chemotherapy and some molecularly targeted agents.

Cisplatin is a one of the drugs, which is not a substrate for MDR efflux pump.[3] It is transported by copper influx and efflux transporters and a gain of function of the efflux transporters would result in resistance.[3] This noncross resistance to Pgp transporters makes platinum compound in the management of many cancers.

Drug Inactivation

Drug metabolism in the cell can lead on to its activation or deactivation. This involves phase I or oxidative metabolism and phase II reactions involving conjugation steps.[11] The cytochrome P450 enzymes (CYP), such as CYP3A, CYP2D6, CYP2C family of microsomal enzymes metabolize most chemotherapeutic drugs and are genetically highly polymorphic.[11] The variable expression of these enzymes among genetically different population has impact on the response outcomes to drug including efficacy and toxicity.[11]

They are also implicated in intrinsic and acquired drug resistance for drugs like cyclophosphamide.[11]

Phase II enzymes are involved in conjugation reactions using enzymes such as glutathione S-transferase (GST), uridine 5′-diphospho glucuronosyltransferases (UGT), and sulfotransferases, which transform the reactive species into hydrophilic nontoxic metabolite conjugates, which undergo drug efflux.[11] Inactivation of enzymes converting prodrugs to active compounds also leads to resistance. For example, methylation and thus silencing of gene encoding for thymidine phosphorylase, which convert capecitabine into active compound 5-fluorouracil (5-FU) leads to its resistance.[8] Thus decreased drug activation or increased inactivation due to defect in the enzymatic system can lead on to drug resistance.

Deoxyribonucleic Acid Damage Repair

Different chemotherapy drugs act on deoxyribonucleic acid (DNA) as their target leading on to structural alterations such as crosslinking as in case of alkylating agents or platinum compounds causing defective replication, which lead on to cell death.[8] There are several repair pathways such as mismatch repair (MMR), nucleotide excision repair (NER), base excision repair (BER), the homologous recombination (HR), and the nonhomologous end joining (NHEJ) pathway.[8] Thus, increased repair of the DNA damage caused by chemotherapy through any of these pathways leads to resistance.[8]

Mismatch repair acts as a sensor of DNA damage, which then activates the apoptotic pathway resulting in cell death.[12,13] Drugs acting via causing DNA damage thus need the MMR to recognize the damage and cause tumor cell kill by apoptosis.[13] Hence, MMR deficiency caused by either germline mutation in MLH1, MSH2, MSH6, and PMS2 or methylation of MLH1 results in resistance to alkylating agents such as busulfan and methylating agents like procarbazine and temozolomide, and also low level resistance to topoisomerase II inhibitors like doxorubicin and etoposide.[12,13] It is interesting to note that cisplatin and carboplatin DNA adducts are recognized by MMR but oxaliplatin is not.[12,13] Hence, MMR deficiency causes resistance to cisplatin and carboplatin but not to oxaliplatin.[12,13] It also causes resistance to 5-FU.[12] Thus in colorectal cancers adjuvant 5-FU based chemotherapy is not recommended in stage II, if they are MMR deficient.[12] Thus knowledge of MMR deficiency helps to personalize the choice of chemotherapy drugs used.

Nucleotide excision repair pathway especially the excision repair cross-complementing 1 (ERCC1) is involved in repairing DNA adducts caused by cisplatin.[8,14] Thus, high expression of ERCC1 is a predictor of platinum resistance and poor response to platinum-based therapy in non-small cell lung, gastric, and ovarian cancer.[8,14]

The BRCA is an important component of the HR repair pathway.[15] Polyadenosine diphosphate (ADP)-ribose polymerase (PARP) is needed for BER.[15] Thus, if one arm of the repair pathway is already deficient like in those with BRCA mutation and the other arm is inhibited by PARP inhibitors then it results in cell death by "synthetic lethality", as the cell is unable to repair double-stranded breaks.[15] PARP inhibitors have thus provided a major breakthrough in the treatment of patients with BRCA mutation especially in ovarian cancers.[16] However, resistance to PARP has been reported due to in frame deletions, which restore its DNA repair function.[8,17] Thus, though PARP inhibitors are a major break through the cancer cells have already found means to circumvent them and cause resistance.

Ineffective Apoptosis and Autophagy

Dysfunctional apoptosis can reduce the efficiency with which drug-induced DNA damage results in cell death.[8] Both apoptotic and non-apoptotic mechanisms such as autophagy are involved in the regulation of the final step in cancer drug effect that is cell death. Chemotherapy-induced resistance occurs primarily via the mitochondrial pathway and regulated by the BCL2 family of genes, which are predominantly antiapoptotic. BCL2 inhibitors such as venetoclax have shown excellent response in relapsed or refractory chronic lymphocytic leukemia.[18]

TUMOR MICROENVIRONMENT: THE PROTECTIVE NICHE FOR SURVIVAL

The homeless tumor cell away from its microenvironment is more likely to be die (undergo apoptosis) after exposure to chemotherapy than those securely at home adherent to their extracellular matrix.[19] Once home, they are also more likely to proliferate.[19] This cell adhesion-mediated drug resistance (CAM-DR) was demonstrated in myeloma cell, where increase in β_1 integrin resulting in cell adhesion was shown to reduce DNA damage and apoptosis caused by chemotherapy.[19] Other stromal cells such as cancer-associated fibroblasts may also provide prosurvival signals resulting in resistance.[7] The new disorganized leaky tumor vasculature with high interstitial pressures impairs drug delivery also contributing to resistance.[7] The tumor stroma thus provides a protective niche to the cancer cells against chemotherapy.

Some cancer cells are transformed and become more hardy and resistant capable of travelling to distant sites and producing metastasis. This transformation is brought about by epithelial to mesenchymal transition (EMT).[20] This transition also leads to drug resistance.[20] Cytotoxic insult further stimulates the prosurvival signals for EMT from the extracellular stroma.[20] Thus, EMT contributes toward drug resistance. Cytotoxic chemotherapy while killing some cancer cells also recruits immune suppressive macrophages, which in-turn promotes cancer cell survival.[7] This paradoxical effect reduces the effect of chemotherapy. The immune cells in the tumor microenvironment are an important determinant of both inherent and acquired drug resistance.[7]

TUMOR HETEROGENEITY, CANCER STEM CELLS AND CLONAL EVOLUTION: THE PROBLEM OF CHANGING TARGETS

Tumors have a mixed clonal population of chemosensitive relative fitter cells, which constitute the major bulk, and the chemoresistant cells, which spend most of their energy in maintaining resistance mechanism, and hence are less fit and fewer in numbers.[9] With the onslaught of chemotherapy, the tumor shrinks mainly by killing of the chemosensitive cells.[9] This releases the competitive pressure allowing the resistant clones to proliferate.[9] Also cytotoxic stress induces some of the epithelial cells to transform into cancer stem cell via EMT leading to expansion and diversification of resistant clones.[21] This transition and clonal evolution may be brought about by genetic or epigenetic events.[22] Thus chemotherapy by killing chemosensitive clones paradoxically increases the chemoresistant clones.

Targeted therapy, which was hailed as magic bullets,[23] too have met with resistance. Unlike chronic myeloid leukemia which is more like the palm tree with a single trunk (driver mutation), most solid tumors are complex like the baobab or chestnut trees with multiple trunks and branches (driver and subclonal mutations).[24] Thus, it is easy to fell down the palm tree by striking at the trunk while in most solid tumors cutting one trunk leads to the growth of other trunks and thus resistance.[24,25] Hence, though long-term remission is achieved with imatinib 83% survival at 10 years.[26] In case of anti-epidermal growth factor receptor (EGFR), tyrosine kinase inhibitors (TKIs) such as gefitinib and erlotinib there are initial good response rates (60–70%) but within a year, nearly 50% develop resistance. *EGFR-T790M* gatekeeper mutations are detected in more than 60% cases and mandates change of therapy to osimertinib.[27] Thus, clonal evolution leads to only modest benefit with many targeted therapy.[24,25]

Immunotherapy a major breakthrough in science has also met with resistance. When the brakes on immune system [programmed cell death receptor- ligand-1 (PDL 1) or cytotoxic T-lymphocyte–associated antigen 4 (CTLA 4) inhibitors] are released, there is an increased immune attack on the tumor cells.[28] In an attempt to escape this, there is decreased antigen production, presentation, or altered expression by the tumor so that it is not recognized by the immune cells thus leading to resistance.[28] Hence although the responses are durable only about one-fourth of patients respond to immunotherapy.[28]

CHEMOTHERAPY SENSITIVITY AND RESISTANCE ASSAYS: CAN THE CHOICE BE PERSONALIZED?

Antibiotic sensitivity assays have long been used to guide effective therapy. So, it was intuitive to design assays to test chemotherapy sensitivity and resistance with the hope that it would help to personalize treatment. These assays culture tumor cells *in vitro* with different chemotherapy drugs and the sensitivity assessed by tests of tumor cell viability.[29] Though these tests are able to predict drug resistance, there is insufficient evidence in clinical trials that assay directed therapy improves survival compared to empiric therapy.[29,30] Thus, the American Society of Clinical Oncology (ASCO) guidelines do not recommend using these tests outside of clinical trials.[30] In the realm of targeted therapy, however, testing for resistance has been of clinical relevance. Imatinib resistance mutation analysis helps in choosing second-line TKIs based on the mutation detected.[31] Thus though evaluating for resistance or sensitivity by testing for specific mutation has helped in the choice of targeted therapy, there is a long way to go before choosing the right chemotherapy using drug sensitivity assay becomes a reality.

OVERCOMING RESISTANCE: CHALLENGING PRESENT DOGMAS

Traditionally, chemotherapy drugs with synergistic efficacy and differing toxicities have been combined to overcome resistance.[4] Combining targeted therapy and immunotherapy with chemotherapy have helped to achieve a multipronged approach to attack cancer cells.[32] Targeted therapy with antiangiogenic agent and chemotherapy has shown some improvement in ovarian cancer.[33] Combination of immunotherapy with chemotherapy has been proven successful in different cancers like lung.[34] The concept of "synthetic lethality" where deficiency of one target or pathway is ineffective in killing the cancer cell but knocking down another target or pathway results in cell death has been used successfully.[15,32] This strategy has effectively been used in ovarian with the use of PARP in ovarian cancers with BRCA deficiency.[16]

Apart from the above mechanisms, it is proposed also that drug ineffectiveness also is resulted from tumor-host interactions and clear understanding of the same is needed to combat the problem.[35] A paradigm change in the way we combat cancer is probably needed. Traditionally, chemotherapy used at maximally tolerated dose results is killing of chemosensitive cells and shrinkage of primary tumor but paradoxically gives the less fit chemoresistant cells a survival advantage resulting in their escape and metastasis.[9] Hence, researchers are now exploiting Darwin's evolutionary model and planning newer adaptive dose protocols whereby chemotherapy kills some but not all sensitive cells, thus allowing competitive inhibition of resistant cells, thereby achieving stability.[36,37] Repurposing drugs and using metronomic doses of conventional chemotherapy have helped, are treatment of chemoresistant cancers such as angiosarcoma.[38] Thus, using different dosing and scheduling of the same chemotherapy drug may help to overcome resistance.

LOOKING INTO FUTURE, REACHING THE MOON: IS THE WAY THROUGH THE WAR ZONE?

The "War on Cancer" was declared in 1971, however, now close to half a century later though a few battles have been won the war continues.[32] A renewed effort in pursuit of the elusive cure for cancer, the "moonshot" was declared in 2016 by accelerating research and sharing data.[39] However, introspection is needed on the strategy to be used to achieve this aim. Metronomic and adoptive dosing and activating the immune system may be some of the approaches. Another interesting concept is the potential possibility of reverting cancer to normal cells.[40,41] This has been demonstrated *in vitro* and drugs such as sertraline and thioridazine have the potential to restore wild type p53 function and thereby restore its function.[41,42] Tumor reversion is a rare event and understanding its mechanism to achieve stable reversions which is clinically relevant remains a challenge.[40] Thus, newer ways to reach the moon needs to be sought.

CONCLUSION

Progress has been made in understanding and overcoming various mechanisms of resistance. Looking at the battlefield as a whole, adopting different strategies, discovering new armamentarium, and working together combining several different forces would help to win more wars. However, the possibility of a true victory probably lies in winning over our enemies and transforming foes to friends. Thus, working together, changing our strategy, and expanding our vision would be the way forward.

REFERENCES

1. Bray F, Ferlay J, Soerjomataram I, et al. Global cancer statistics 2018: GLOBOCAN estimates of incidence and mortality worldwide for 36 cancers in 185 countries. CA Cancer J Clin. 2018;68(6):394-424.
2. Welch AD. The problem of drug resistance in cancer chemotherapy. Cancer Res. 1959;19(4):359-71.

3. Gottesman MM, Lavi O, Hall MD, et al. Toward a better understanding of the complexity of cancer drug resistance. Annu Rev Pharmacol Toxicol. 2016;56:85-102.
4. Cree IA, Charlton P. Molecular chess? Hallmarks of anti-cancer drug resistance. BMC Cancer. 2017;17(1):10.
5. Gottesman MM. Mechanisms of cancer drug resistance. Annu Rev Med. 2002;53(1):615-27.
6. Tredan O, Galmarini CM, Patel K, et al. Drug resistance and the solid tumor microenvironment. J Natl Cancer Inst. 2007;99(19):1441-54.
7. Junttila MR, de Sauvage FJ. Influence of tumour micro-environment heterogeneity on therapeutic response. Nature. 2013;501(7467):346-54.
8. Holohan C, Van Schaeybroeck S, Longley DB, et al. Cancer drug resistance: an evolving paradigm. Nat Rev Cancer. 2013;13(10):714-26.
9. McGranahan N, Swanton C. Clonal Heterogeneity and Tumor Evolution: Past, Present, and the Future. Cell. 2017;168(4):613-28.
10. Nass J, Efferth T. Drug targets and resistance mechanisms in multiple myeloma. Cancer Drug Resist. 2018;1:87-117.
11. Gillet JP, Gottesman MM. Mechanisms of multidrug resistance in cancer. Methods Mol Biol. 2010;596:47-76.
12. Sinicrope FA, Sargent DJ. Molecular pathways: microsatellite instability in colorectal cancer: prognostic, predictive, and therapeutic implications. Clin Cancer Res. 2012;18(6):1506-12.
13. Fink D, Aebi S, Howell SB. The role of DNA mismatch repair in drug resistance. Clin Cancer Res. 1998;4(1):1-6.
14. Kirschner K, Melton DW. Multiple roles of the ERCC1-XPF endonuclease in DNA repair and resistance to anticancer drugs. Anticancer Res. 2010;30(9):3223-32.
15. Iglehart JD, Silver DP. Synthetic lethality: a new direction in cancer-drug development. N Engl J Med. 2009;361(2):189-91.
16. Mirza MR, Monk BJ, Herrstedt J, et al. Niraparib maintenance therapy in platinum-sensitive, recurrent ovarian cancer. N Engl J Med. 2016;375(22):2154-64.
17. Patch AM, Christie EL, Etemadmoghadam D, et al. Whole-genome characterization of chemoresistant ovarian cancer. Nature. 2015;521(7553):489-94.
18. Jones J, Choi MY, Mato AR, et al. Venetoclax (VEN) monotherapy for patients with chronic lymphocytic leukemia (CLL) who relapsed after or were refractory to ibrutinib or idelalisib. Blood. 2016;128(22):637.
19. Hazlehurst LA, Landowski TH, Dalton WS. Role of the tumor microenvironment in mediating *de novo* resistance to drugs and physiological mediators of cell death. Oncogene. 2003;22(47):7396-402.
20. Nurwidya F, Takahashi F, Murakami A, et al. Epithelial mesenchymal transition in drug resistance and metastasis of lung cancer. Cancer Res Treat. 2012;44(3):151-6.
21. Agliano A, Calvo A, Box C. The challenge of targeting cancer stem cells to halt metastasis. Semin Cancer Biol. 2017;44:25-42.
22. Salgia R, Kulkarni P. The Genetic/Non-genetic Duality of Drug 'Resistance' in Cancer. Trends Cancer. 2018;4(2):110-8.

23. Strebhardt K, Ullrich A. Paul Ehrlich's magic bullet concept: 100 years of progress. Nat Rev Cancer. 2008;8(6):473-80.
24. Yap TA, Gerlinger M, Futreal PA, et al. Intratumor Heterogeneity: Seeing the Wood for the Trees. Sci Transl Med. 2012;4(127):127ps10.
25. Turner NC, Reis-Filho JS. Genetic heterogeneity and cancer drug resistance. Lancet Oncol. 2012;13(4):e178-85.
26. Hochhaus A, Larson RA, Guilhot F, et al. Long-term outcomes of imatinib treatment for chronic myeloid leukemia. N Engl J Med. 2017;376(10):917-27.
27. Mok TS, Wu YL, Ahn MJ, et al. Osimertinib or Platinum–Pemetrexed in EGFR T790M-Positive Lung Cancer. N Engl J Med. 2017;376(7):629-40.
28. Sharma P, Hu-Lieskovan S, Wargo JA, et al. Primary, Adaptive, and Acquired Resistance to Cancer Immunotherapy. Cell. 2017;168(4):707-23.
29. Schrag D, Garewal HS, Burstein HJ, et al. American Society of Clinical Oncology Technology Assessment: chemotherapy sensitivity and resistance assays. J Clin Oncol. 2004;22(17):3631-8.
30. Burstein HJ, Mangu PB, Somerfield MR, et al. American Society of Clinical Oncology clinical practice guideline update on the use of chemotherapy sensitivity and resistance assays. J Clin Oncol. 2011;29(24):3328-30.
31. Bixby D, Talpaz M. Seeking the causes and solutions to imatinib-resistance in chronic myeloid leukemia. Leukemia. 2010;25(1):7-22.
32. Hanahan D. Rethinking the war on cancer. Lancet. 2014;383(9916):558-63.
33. Oza AM, Cook AD, Pfisterer J, et al. Standard chemotherapy with or without bevacizumab for women with newly diagnosed ovarian cancer (ICON7): overall survival results of a phase 3 randomised trial. Lancet Oncol. 2015;16(8):928-36.
34. Garon EB, Rizvi NA, Hui R, et al. Pembrolizumab for the treatment of non–small-cell lung cancer. N Engl J Med. 2015;372(21):2018-28.
35. Alfarouk KO, Stock CM, Taylor S, et al. Resistance to cancer chemotherapy: failure in drug response from ADME to P-gp. Cancer Cell Int. 2015;15:71.
36. Gatenby RA, Silva AS, Gillies RJ, et al. Adaptive therapy. Cancer Res. 2009;69(11):4894-903.
37. Enriquez-Navas PM, Kam Y, Das T, et al. Exploiting evolutionary principles to prolong tumor control in preclinical models of breast cancer. Sci Transl Med. 2016;8(327):327ra24.
38. Pasquier E, André N, Street J, et al. Effective management of advanced angiosarcoma by the synergistic combination of propranolol and vinblastine-based metronomic chemotherapy: A bench-to-bedside Study. EBioMedicine. 2016;6:87-95.
39. Barlas S. The White House Launches a Cancer Moonshot: Despite Funding Questions, the Progress Appears Promising. PT. 2016;41(5):290-5.
40. Powers S, Pollack RE. Inducing stable reversion to achieve cancer control. Nat Rev Cancer. 2016;16(4):266-70.
41. Amson R, Karp JE, Telerman A. Lessons from tumor reversion for cancer treatment. Curr Opin Oncol. 2013;25(1):59-65.
42. Tuynder M, Fiucci G, Prieur S, et al. Translationally controlled tumor protein is a target of tumor reversion. Proc Natl Acad Sci USA. 2004;101(43):15364-9.

Chapter 13

Vascular Malformations

Satyendra K Tiwary, Ajay K Khanna

INTRODUCTION

Vascular malformations are always a challenge for correct clinical diagnosis and proper therapeutic approach. Even with increasing awareness of rare diseases along with availability of diagnostic tools, it remains an uphill task to diagnose, classify and intervene properly in vascular anomalies which are an important group of congenital disorders mostly associated with complex clinical presentation in medicine. Vascular anomalies may be either vascular tumors or vascular malformations. Proliferation of endothelial cells is basic aberration in vascular tumors while angiogenetic and mesenchymal components are affected in vascular malformations.[1,2] Basic difference between vascular tumor and vascular malformation underlies in natural course with possibility of regression with increasing age in vascular tumor while vascular malformations never decrease in size without intervention.

Considering the components involved, vascular malformations may be classified into venous, arterial, capillary, lymphatic or combined. Most frequently observed are venous malformations (VMs) in almost 70 % of vascular malformations.[3] Lymphatic malformations (LMs) are in about 12% cases and arteriovenous malformations (AVM) in 8%. Capillary malformations (CMs) are in only 4% while different syndromes with multiple vascular components in 6%. Classification system with clarity is required for precise diagnosis and proper therapeutic decisions. Landmark work with publication in 1982 by Mulliken and Glowacki about vascular anomalies was based on clinical features and biological behavior and an elaborate classification was prepared which was followed for about 30 years in understanding vasculogenesis and angiogenesis.[4]

Two broad categories have been identified with proliferative or vascular neoplasms and vascular malformations which were last updated (Table 1) in

Table 1: The International Society for the Study of Vascular Anomalies (ISSVA) classification of vascular anomalies.

Vascular tumors	Vascular malformations		
	Simple	Complex	Flow
• Hemangioma	• Capillary (CM)	• Lymphaticovenous (LVM)	
• Pyogenic granuloma	• Venous (VM)	• Capillary lymphaticovenous	Slow
• Hemangiopericytoma	• Lymphatic (LM)		
• Hemangioendothelioma	• Arterial	Capillary arteriovenous	
• Tufted angioma	• Arteriovenous (AVM)		Fast

2014.[5] Vascular anomalies require dedicated interdisciplinary management which should include all medical disciplines involved for achieving optimum and adequate results.

CLASSIFICATION OF VASCULAR MALFORMATIONS

Vascular malformations, based on angiogenetic and vasculogenetic dysplastic disorder, are always present at birth and never regress spontaneously. They may be quiescent for a long time, before mechanical or hormonal influence stimulates them to grow. Diagnosis should include complete morphology, lesion extension, dominant vessel type, flow velocity, and potential complications regarding dermal, orthopedic, neurological, muscular, and specific organ manifestations. Vascular malformations are classified as *simple malformations, combined malformations, vascular malformations of major named vessels* and *vascular malformations associated with other anomalies*.[5] Simple malformations are the most common with mostly containing only one type of vasculature either vein, capillaries or lymphatics.

Venous Malformations

Venous malformations (VMs) are the most frequent vascular malformations (70%). At clinical presentation, multiple common diagnostic features are detected easily. It can be superficial or deep and may be localized, multicentric or diffuse (Box 1). VMs are soft compressible masses with skin changes, mostly in the form of color change with bluish skin discoloration without any signs of bruit, pulsation, tenderness or local redness. Sometimes tiny dark blue spots over the skin are visible which indicate phleboliths due to recurrent thrombophlebitis (Fig. 1). Cutaneous and musculoskeletal locations (Fig. 2) of vascular malformations lead to cutaneous, subcutaneous, epifascial, subfascial, muscular or osseous type.[6]

Box 1: Classification of venous malformations (VMs).

- Common VM (*TIE2* somatic)
- Familial VM cutaneomucosal (*TIE2*)
- Blue rubber bleb nevus syndrome
- Glomuvenous malformation (glomulin)
- Cerebral cavernous malformation (CCM)
- Others

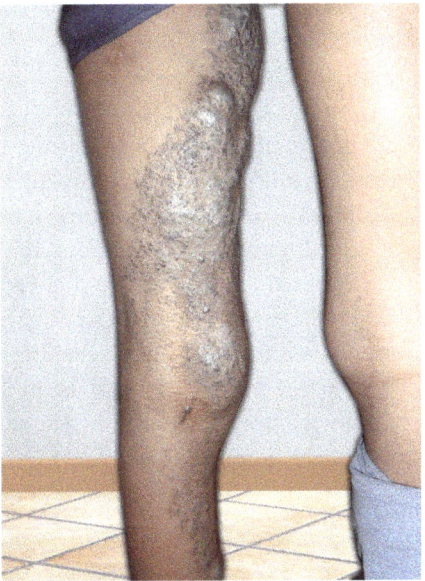

Fig. 1: Extensive involvement of right lower limb by vascular malformations.

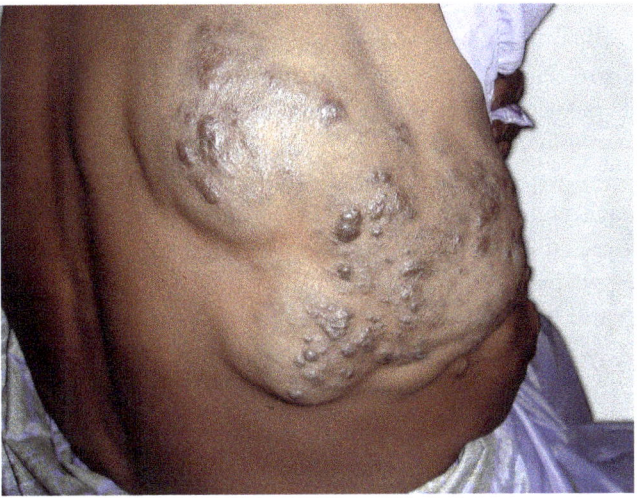

Fig. 2: Extensive involvement of trunk in vascular malformations.

X-ray sometimes reveals, phleboliths surrounding the venous malformation indicative of progressive calcification due to recurrent thrombophlebitis. Key tool in investigating venous malformations is ultrasound. The flow pattern of VMs on Doppler ultrasound is slow flow or no flow in case of thrombosis. Classical character in USG is hypoechogenic clusters of compressible, dysplastic veins in every tissue layer. Puig classification differentiates VM into four types as[7,8]
1. Type I VM without venous drainage
2. Type II VM draining into normal veins
3. Type III VM draining into dysplastic veins
4. Type IV VM draining into dilated veins.

Venous malformations sometimes may extend into adjoining structures with bony involvement and role of MRI becomes pivotal for assessment initially as well as during follow-up even after treatment. Intense hyperintense signal in T2 is characteristic of venous malformations, but isointense imaging to muscular tissue in pre-contrast T1-weighted sequences and hyperintensity in post-contrast T1-weighted sequences is always observed due to contrast pooling in malformations.[9] CT is rarely used but very important investigative tool to map bony involvement in VMs as well as mobility and stability. Percutaneous phlebography is rarely used and it may outline lesion during sclerotherapy treatment.[10]

Lymphatic Malformations

Head and neck region is mostly affected by lymphatic malformations (LMs) in around 70% of all LMs and may present with troublesome features such as swallowing and breathing discomfort due to hemorrhage in lesion causing pressure over adjoining structures. Clinically, lymphatic malformations may manifest with quite troublesome local swelling, skin discoloration (red/purple/brown), pain and infection. About 25% of LMs are observed in the chest wall and extremities and 5% inside the organs.[11] Classifications of LMs are based on consistency and size, extension and location of the cysts. They are classified as macrocystic, microcystic, mixed cystic decided by size, and localized or generalized (extension) or cutaneous, subcutaneous, fatty, intramuscular (Location or level)[5] (Box 2). Capillary malformations are associated usually with LMs but sometimes multiple and combined malformations may be the feature. Serological marker, podoplanin D2-40 is positive in lymphatic malformations due to abundance of lymphatic endothelium in lesions.[11]

Ultrasound is the first investigative tool detecting mostly thin-fluid pattern without flow enclosed in a cavity surrounded by thin wall of the cyst. No echo or poor echoes are frequent finding with ultrasound. Altered echogenicity either hyper or hypo may be detected in case of hemorrhage or inflammation

> **Box 2:** Classification of lymphatic malformations (LMs).
>
> - *Common (cystic) LM*:
>   - Macrocystic LM
>   - Microcystic LM
>   - Mixed cystic LM
> - Generalized lymphatic anomaly
> - LM in Gorham-Stout disease
> - Channel-type LM
> - *Primary lymphedema*:
>   - Nonne-Milroy syndrome (*FLT4/VEGFR3*)
>   - Primary hereditary lymphedema (*VEGFC, GfC2*/connexin 47)
>   - Lymphedema-distichiasis (*FOXC2*)
>   - Hypertrichosis-lymphedema-telangiectasia (*SOX18*)
>   - Primary lymphedema with myelodysplasia (*GATA2*)
>   - Primary generalized lymphatic anomaly (*CCBE1*)
>   - Microcephaly ± chorioretinopathy, lymphedema, or mental retardation syndrome (*KIF11*)
>   - Lymphedema-choanal atresia (*PTPN14*)

leading to increased density of contents inside cavity and may be one sign in bacterial infection.[8] MRI is used as the preferred imaging modality in most cases during workup plan for intervention as best assessment of lymphatic malformations is done by T2-weighted and T-1 weighted MRI. Macrocystic, microcystic or mixed LMs are better defined with pattern of enhancement of administered contrast. CT is always second choice as intervention requires detailed information which is not possible with CT as compared to MRI.

Arteriovenous Malformations

Absent intervening capillary bed between arteries and veins leads to high flow malformations termed as arteriovenous malformations (AVMs) notorious for rapid progression, arterialization of veins and recurrence. Effective and optimum treatment is always a challenge due to high flow in lesions (Fig. 3). AVMs usually present clinically with pulsatile swelling with palpable thrill detected on examination. It is associated with pain sometimes but heaviness of the affected part is more common. Complications are likely to be observed in neglected cases with longer duration or rapidly progressive disease with bleeding, ulceration or inflammation. The classification for AVMs by Schobinger is an important tool in evaluation as well in treatment protocol decided by risk assessment and timing to intervene (Table 2).[12-14]

First line investigation is duplex ultrasonography which is more useful for superficial lesions and characteristic pattern of feeding arteries and draining veins with intervening nidus are detected. Site, size, number, contents, nidus, feeding arteries, draining veins, mapping of adjoining affected structures are essential before final intervention in AVMs. Magnetic resonance angiography (MRA) with dynamic contrast enhancement may best outline feeder arteries,

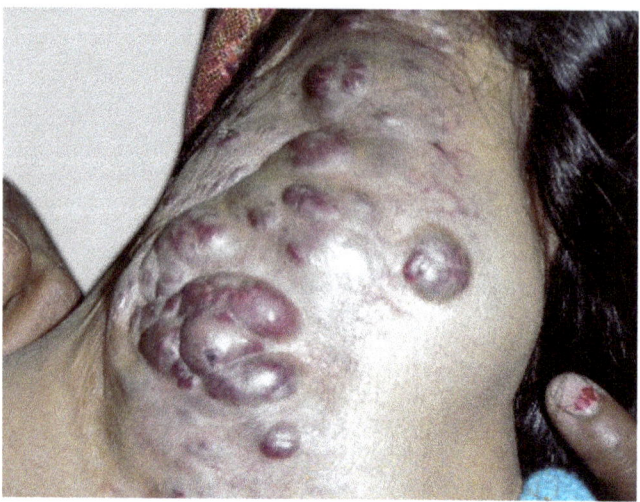

Fig. 3: Rapid progression of arteriovenous malformation.

Table 2: Schobinger clinical staging system for arteriovenous malformations.[51]

Stage	Description	Findings
I	Quiescence	Cutaneous blush or warmth
II	Expansion	Bruit or thrill, increasing size, pulsation, no pain
III	Local destruction	Pain, bleeding, infection, skin necrosis or ulceration
IV	Decompensation	High-output cardiac failure

draining veins, size and site of nidus.[15] Alternative to MRA is now 4D-CT-angiography which is being used in clinical practice more and more for assessment of triad of feeding arteries, nidus and draining veins by analysis of perfusion and flow dynamics. Identification of nidus is essential before planning embolotherapy followed by required excision of AVM. MRA and CT angiography are still far behind gold-standard catheter angiography which is best diagnostic tool in treatment of arteriovenous malformations. Utility of catheter-directed angiography is beyond comparison to any other mode of investigations as multiple routes of access available through artery, vein, skin or nidus for angiography as well as therapeutic embolization in a single intervention.[16,17]

Capillary Malformations

Capillary malformations (CMs) are congenital and cosmetic concern is core component in clinical evaluation and assessment. Cutaneous or mucosal lesions conventionally known as birth marks or port-wine stains (PWS) are pink in color.[18] Initially flat in appearance but may be elevated in appearance later on with red to purple discoloration. Sturge-Weber syndrome (SWS) comprises CMs in face and intracranial components affecting meninges along with trigeminal nerve distribution involvement. Intracranial component in SWS gives rise to neurological manifestations in the form of hemiparesis, weakness, epilepsy, glaucoma and mental retardation. MRI is the investigation of choice at birth, if any features observed at birth or later on.

Combined Vascular Malformations

In contrast to simple malformations where only one type of vessel was affected, combined malformations always composed of two or more than two types of vessels. CMs are mostly one component with venous, lymphatic or arteriovenous other components, Complexity of this group is always associated with multiple combinations of slow-flow and fast-flow vascular anomalies (Box 3).

Vascular Malformations of Major Vessels

Sometimes major named arteries, veins or lymphatics are affected which are major vascular channels. Embryonic vessels may persist and are included in this section. Other type is arteriovenous fistulas (AVFs) of congenital origin.

Vascular Malformations with Other Anomalies

Sometimes in addition to vascular components osseous, muscular, fascial or visceral involvement in malformations are present and they are termed syndrome (Box 4). Clinical presentation in such combined malformations is according to components or parts affected and may present with skin changes, swelling usually multiple due to overgrowth of bone, muscle or fascia and deformity due to aplasia or hyperplasia resulting in disturbed gait.[18] Klippel-Trenaunay syndrome (KTS) is combined vascular malformation involving capillaries, veins and lymphatics with limb hypertrophy. Absent or hypoplastic deep veins, recurrent thrombophlebitis, dilated superficial veins, lower limb ulcer, disturbed gait and bleeding are presenting features.[18] Timely multidisciplinary intervention, surveillance and proper follow-up to correct

---

Box 3: Combined vascular malformations.

- CM + VM (CVM)
- LM + VM (LVM)
- CM + LM + VM (CLVM)
- CM + AVM + VM (CAVM)
- CM + LM + AVM + VM (CLAVM)

(CM: capillary malformation; VM: venous malformation; LM: lymphatic malformation; CVM: combined vascular malformation; AVM: arteriovenous malformation; LVM: lymphaticovenous malformation; CLVM: capillary lymphaticovenous malformation; CAVM: capillary arteriovenous malformation; CLAVM: capillary lymphatic-arteriovenous malformation)

> **Box 4:** Vascular malformations associated with other anomalies.
> - Klippel-Trenaunay syndrome
> - Parkes Weber syndrome (*RASA1*)
> - Servelle-Martorell syndrome
> - Sturge-Weber syndrome (*GNAQ*)
> - Limb CM + congenital nonprogressive limb hypertrophy
> - Maffucci syndrome (VM ± spindle cell hemangioma + enchondroma)
> - Macrocephaly-CM (*PIK3CA*)
> - Macrocephaly-CM (*STAMBP*)
> - CLOVES (LM + VM + CM ± AVM + lipomatous overgrowth) (*PIK3CA*)
> - *Proteus* syndrome (CM, VM, and/or LM + asymmetric somatic overgrowth) (*AKT1*)
> - Bannayan-Rilay-Ruvalcaba syndrome (AVM + VM + macrocephaly, lipomatous overgrowth) (*PTEN*)

(CM: capillary malformation; VM: venous malformation; LM: lymphatic malformation; AVM: arteriovenous malformation)

the components involved earliest with required intervention are important in this group of disorders.[19]

Another interesting malformation affecting lymphatics and bones is Gorham Stout syndrome (GTS). Microcystic lymphatic malformation is present in area of destroyed bone. It is also called as vanishing bone syndrome.[20] Complex vascular malformations usually combined or associated with anomalies are mostly due to mutations in somatic cell line but in syndromes where hyperplasia or enlargement of the parts affected is the clinical finding, mutations in germ cell lines is observed which can be therapeutically targeted selectively for treatment as well as diagnosis.[21]

DIAGNOSIS

Adequate history with correct clinical examination leading to proper diagnosis is mandatory. Multidisciplinary approach with team of surgeons, vascular surgeons, plastic surgeons, orthopedic surgeons, dermatologists, radiologists, and interventional radiologists are the key factors for acceptable outcome of complex disorder. Important points in clinical examination are color change of skin or mucosa, obvious swelling either localized or diffuse, gait and movement disorders, bruit, deformity in the bones, wounds or bleeding. In detailed history each and every vascular event should be noted as thrombophlebitis, coagulopathy, immobilization, superficial vein thrombosis, deep vein thrombosis, trauma, bleeding, drug history, family history, pregnancy and congenital heart diseases. In initial hematological investigations, complete blood count is done in every patient with hemoglobin and platelet count included. In large, extensive or complex malformations D-dimer is always assayed as chances and risk of coagulopathy is in more than one-third patients. Once D-dimer elevated, fibrinogen is estimated and total coagulation profile is recommended to detect any cause of coagulopathy. Routine tests should include renal function tests, thyroid profile, liver function tests, full blood count, complete coagulation profile, fibrinogen, and D-dimer.

Diagnostic tool in vascular malformations include ultrasound with color Doppler, which provide basic information about lesion regarding size, site, number, location, depth, flow velocity and structure affected. Slow flow and fast flow malformations are two basic groups decided by color Doppler for further intervention. CT (Fig. 4) and MRI are the next line of investigations but MRI always better and preferred as it is always superior in all malformations except bony involvement where CT is better and recommended. Ultrasound and MRI are two integral and key investigations with color Doppler examination always included in each and every patient of vascular malformation. MRI (Fig. 5) being most informative and elaborative in defining the size and extent of malformation with mapping of adjoining structures affected is recommended before intervention for adequate and proper therapeutic intervention. Finally, percutaneous, trans-arterial or transvenous angiography in the form of digital subtraction angiography is best mode to map-out malformations before any intervention is planned either endovascular, surgical, radiological or medical.

Every VMs should be assessed by its symptoms, likely complications with treatment and without treatment and available treatment options with all merits and demerits. Intervention is recommended only when benefits of intervention always outweighs risks. Multidisciplinary team decides mode of therapy in every case after complete clinical examination, complications of disease and treatment and color Doppler ultrasound. Two categories of

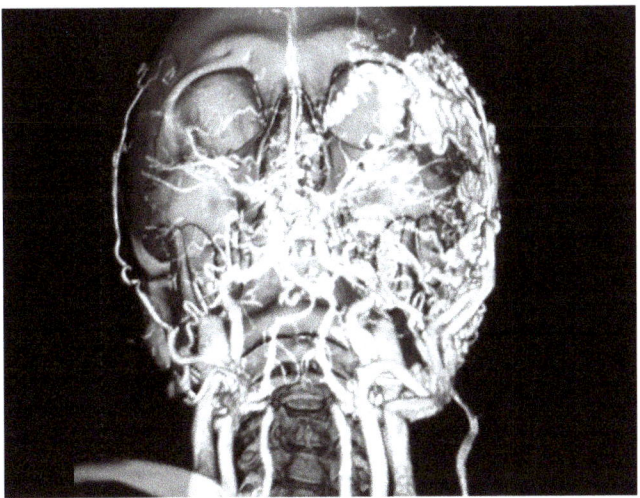

Fig. 4: CT angiogram with reconstruction image of face showing feeding vessels in arteriovenous malformations.

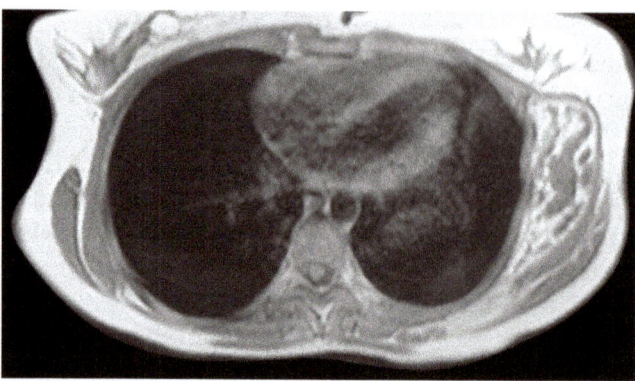

Fig. 5: Extensive chest wall involvement in vascular malformations with marked hyperintensity signal in T2-weighted MRI.

slow-flow and fast-flow malformations require different therapeutic approaches. Informed consent includes details about disease, complications, treatment options, risk and benefits of each mode of treatment and possibility of further treatment as 100% cure is seldom achieved in vascular malformations.

TREATMENT

Therapeutic workup in vascular malformations is determined by morphology, hemodynamics and structures involved. Broad division of vascular malformations with color Doppler study into slow-flow and fast-flow is first basic step deciding the mode of intervention required for treatment.[4,5,22] As randomized control trials are not available in literature with sufficient evidence, vascular malformations are still a big challenge to manage. Despite all odds and complexity, single point of consensus is treatment should be in multidisciplinary settings and multimodal intervention is central point in treatment plan. Vascular surgeon and interventional radiologist are two key players always to define, decide and do the work in vascular malformations. Surgical, medical and radiological issues are always incorporated which necessitates knowledge of surgical intervention, reconstruction, sclerotherapy or angioembolization. Conservative approach with wait and watch policy combined with anticoagulation, compression stockings, antibiotic, wound care are also important where complications are more likely with active or aggressive intervention.[22]

Therapy of Venous Malformations

The most common vascular malformations are VM in 70% cases with solitary lesion in almost 90% cases. Venous malformations with multifocal locations usually have some associated anomaly in the form of syndromes like Klippel-Trenaunay syndrome, blue rubber bleb nevus syndrome.[23,24] Absolute indications of treatment in VMs are pain, bleeding, ulceration, thrombosis, unacceptable cosmesis, functional disability, vital structures threatened due to close associations.

Sclerotherapy is the treatment of choice[23] but best results are with surgical excision where complete resection is possible without significant functional or structural disturbance. Localized intravascular coagulopathy is very frequent in large and complex VMs diagnosed by elevated D-dimer and reduced fibrinogen.[25,26] Phleboliths, as palpable nodules are pathognomonic feature which are detected easily on X ray and even confirmed on ultrasound. But, ultrasound always and MRI in most cases are needed for proper evaluation, assessment, treatment plan and follow-up.[27]

Medical Management

Management of VMs medically is always an option to delay the progress of natural course of the disease and integral part of treatment in any complications such as wound, thrombosis, pain, deformity. Compression stockings, limb elevation, exercise and physiotherapy are definite players to reduce pain, swelling and deformity with delaying the progress of the disease.[28] Pain killers are required always in thrombophlebitis or thrombosis. Low-molecular-weight heparin (LMWH) is the key drug to prevent thrombosis as well as to treat thrombosis and prophylactic use is well established in high-risk patients undergoing interventions.[25,26] Effective medical treatment of VMs is still not well established due to inferior results but some studies have shown that mechanistic target of rapamycin (mTOR) inhibitors in the form of sirolimus have effects on regression of VMs.[29-33] Role of sirolimus is still in infancy and still a long path to get it established as medical management of choice in VMs only after randomized-controlled trials and long-term results are available.

Sclerotherapy

Sclerotherapy is the treatment of choice in VMs.[34] It is combined on one hand with medical treatment to alleviate bleeding, discomfort, swelling, pain, indicated in conjunction with conservative management in symptomatic VMs to reduce pain, disfigurement, hemorrhage, deformity, risk to adjoining vital structures, thrombosis and thromboembolism. It is always a central role of sclerotherapy to be combined with medical management on one hand and other definitive approach-like laser or surgical excision on the other complete the spectrum of treatment but proper communication between patient and intervening specialists with documentation is essential considering limitations of any mode of intervention, weak evidence and limited study.[35]

The principle of sclerotherapy is to disrupt the endothelial layer leading to inflammation, thrombosis, and fibrosis, obliteration of lumen and collapse of walls leading to reduced size or disappearance of VMs.[36] A number of sclerosants work by different modes and are available in the form of ethyl alcohol, ethanol gel, polidocanol, sodium tetradecyl sulfate, and bleomycin. Superior sclerosing agent in terms of effectiveness is still not established as systematic reviews are inadequate.[36-40] Deciding factors of selection of sclerosant should be fewer side effects of agent to be used. Foam is always better than liquid as it occupies more surface area better displaces luminal blood, contact time is more and occlusion rate is higher.

Phlebography of VMs should be obtained before intervention in Type I lesions, VMs having no venous drainage, Type II normal-sized, Type III enlarged venous drainage, respectively, and Type IV lesions are composed of basically ectatic dysplastic vein. Phlebographic patterns with large draining veins Type III likely to have more complications in sclerotherapy.[7] Under ultrasonic guidance, the sclerosant should be injected slowly in the malformation Occlusion of outflow always practiced with thumb, tourniquet or pneumatic cuff to lessen the hazard of spillage into the deep veins. Single or multiple interventions may be done by USG guidance for best results but care should be taken during injection to avoid extravasation.[41] Pain felt by the patient, resistance during injection are alarming signs to stop the injection.

Endovenous Intervention

Two modes of endovenous approaches are endovenous laser ablation (EVLA) or endovenous radiofrequency ablation (RFA) which are useful for large venous channels of embryonic origin in syndromes or associated anomalies such as KTS.[42,43]

Surgical Excision

Localized, simple and single VM is surgically excised (Fig. 6) with best results and always an integral component in management and combined with endovascular intervention as required.

Laser Excision

Superficial VMs are excised completely, safely and effectively with long wavelength laser such as neodymium-doped:yttrium aluminum garnet (Nd:YAG) laser.[23]

Follow-up

Compression stockings after intervention are very helpful in control of symptoms and regression of the malformation. Elevation of the limb above

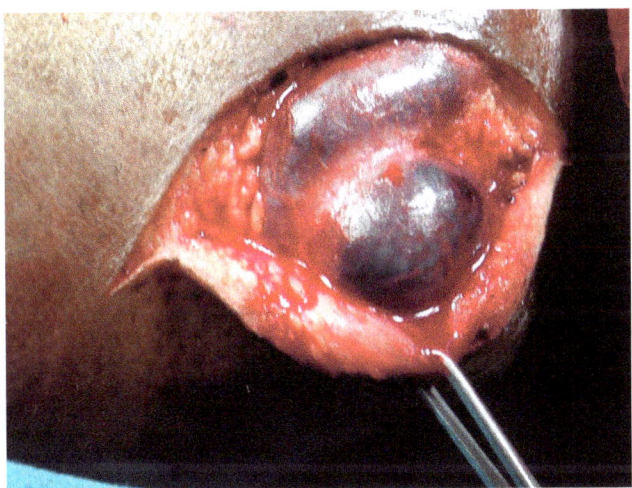

Fig. 6: Exposure of venous malformation of elbow region during surgical excision.

the level of the heart, cold ice packs, and analgesics are advised. Prophylactic anticoagulation with LMWH is recommended to prevent and to exclude DVT. Ultrasound should be performed after 24 hours.[34]

Therapy of Lymphatic Malformations

Lymphatic malformations (LMs) are slow flow vascular anomalies and are the second most common type of peripheral vascular malformation besides venous malformations. Lymphatic system is affected with cystic spaces containing lymphatic fluid and dilated lymphatics and is classified microcystic, macrocystic (>1 cm), and mixed.[34] As compared to VMs which were 90% solitary. LMs are most commonly associated with syndromes like Klippel-Trenaunay-Weber syndrome, CLOVES syndrome or *Proteus* syndrome.[23] The most common location is in the head and neck area of the body followed by the axilla and pelvis respectively.[44] Diagnosis of LMs is established by history and clinical examination. Extension of the proper mapping of the LMs is done by USG color Doppler study and MRI. In MRI, septae and walls are enhanced in contrast study to differentiate microcystic and macrocystic lesions making contrast-enhanced MRI with T1 and T2 images as an integral part of investigation before intervention.

Expectant Therapy

Small and asymptomatic LMs can be managed even with monitoring and just waiting without any immediate treatment. Analgesic, antibiotic and compression therapy are used to relieve pain, treat infection and reduce swelling. Sirolimus is a mTOR inhibitor and studies had shown some promising results in extensive LMs.[45,46]

Sclerotherapy

Major mode and preferred form of treatment is sclerotherapy and intervention is indicated in complicated LMs such as recurrent bleeding, recurrent inflammation, cosmetic disfigurement and threatened vital neighboring structures.[44] Microcystic and mixed LMs are treated by sclerotherapy.[44] Sclerosants used commonly in LMs are picibanil (OK-432), bleomycin, and doxycycline. Picibanil is a lyophilized mixture and acts by extensive fibrosis and preferred in macrocystic lesions.[43-45] Bleomycin is the preferred sclerosant in patients with macrocystic LMs. It should be used in very small doses to avoid toxicity, e.g. pulmonary fibrosis.[46-47] Doxycycline is used in treatment of macrocystic and mixed lymphatic malformations.[48-50] Cysts are punctured with a needle under ultrasound guidance. Aspirating the contents before instillation of contrast or sclerosant confirms the diagnosis and before injection whole cavity fluid should be aspirated out and finally sclerosant instilled.[50]

Laser Therapy

Lasers are being used in LMs with effectiveness of CO_2 laser, Nd:YAG laser, erbium laser and pulsed dye laser in small, cutaneous or mucosal lesions.

Surgery

Lymphatic malformations are usually non-operable and when surgical option is exercised, incomplete excision has poor satisfactory result.

Follow-up

Postoperative pain control with analgesic and compression stockings are recommended in all patients undergoing intervention. Effects of sclerotherapy are achieved completely only after 4–6 weeks.

Therapy of Capillary Malformations

Capillary malformations are congenital and manifest right from the birth.[23] It includes two principal groups: port-wine stain and Sturge-Weber syndrome. Treatment of choice is laser therapy in CMs. Pulsed dye laser therapy (PDLT) is most common mode of intervention in CMs. Cryogen spray cooling combined with PDLT reduces adverse effects and improves outcome. Other effective lasers are Nd: YAG, potassium titanyl phosphate lasers. Alternative and second-line therapy is photodynamic therapy (PDT) with chemical photosensitizer administered intravenously. Surgical option should be very limited, focused, patient-oriented with proper timing and include excision, direct suturing, split-skin grafting, skin flaps, tissue expansion and reconstructions.[23]

Therapy of Fast-Flow Vascular Malformations

Therapy of Arteriovenous Malformation and Arteriovenous Fistula

Arteries and veins are connected pathologically rather than physiologically and intervening capillary bed is absent in fast-flow vascular malformations leading to formation of abnormal shunts between arteries and veins. Nidus is a network of vessels where arterial blood is shunted into venous blood in arteriovenous malformations. In a single arterialized vein, blood is shunted in AVF.[34] Features may be expansile masses, raised temperature, or bruit. Arterializations of veins, bleeding or ischemia, ulcerations are likely complications in late stages.[51] Considering the aggressive nature of AVM and AVF, recurrence after therapy is always a possibility.

Arteriovenous malformations are diagnosed primarily by color Doppler ultrasound and MRI.[52] Analysis of flow patterns and fluid dynamics is useful to establish the diagnosis of fast-flow malformations. Once bone involvement is associated with AVM or AVF, Computed tomography (CT) can be performed. Arteriography is gold standard and always performed before intervention.

Medical Therapy

Compression stockings can improve symptoms and quality of life. Chronic pain should be managed preferably by a specialist. mTOR inhibitors for the treatment of aggressive AVMs is disappointing.

Embolotherapy

Schobinger classification is main guideline for intervention. Embolization is the gold standard therapy as it offers treatment with least morbidity and better results but is prone to recurrence. In some cases, preoperative embolization is exercised even when complete surgical resection of the nidus is achievable. Occlusion of the nidus or fistula completely by embolotherapy should be aim in treatment. Ethanols, N-butyl cyanoacrylate (NBCA), ethylene-vinyl-alcohol-copolymer (EVOH) are commonly used for embolothearpy. Role of coils sometimes and vascular plugs in selected cases is used to control hemodynamics for adequate treatment. A combination of the embolic agents can be ideal sometimes for the endovascular treatment of complex and fast-flow malformations.[53]

Embolization technique: Diagnostic angiography is the first part to determine the flow dynamics, physiology and morphology. Most types of AVMs can initially be embolized via a transarterial approach is the initial and preferred approach. If there is dominant venous drainage (type II), the nidus can be embolized by retrograde transvenous embolization technique. Direct puncture of the nidus is suitable in type II and IIIb lesions. Non-feeding parenchymal arteries should never be embolized.[34]

Surgery

Surgery combined with embolotherapy gives best outcome in terms of complete cure and postoperative outcome. Usual time duration after embolotherpy is 24–48 hours and a margin of 5–10 mm is preferred for complete excision of the lesion. Sometimes feeder vessels are ligated before excision to control the bleeding and better outcome, but if duration is increased between ligation and excision, poor results are likely. Key step is control of nidus in AVM for and that should be either complete occlusion by embolotherapy or complete excision by surgery.

CONCLUSION

Vascular malformations are congenital conditions of complex clinical characteristics, it is evaluated clinically as well as with color Doppler for correct classification and complete diagnosis. Conservative approach, compression garments, care of wounds are better recommended in low flow type (VM, CM, LM or combined) malformations with sclerotherapy, laser, and excision either alone or combined for definitive treatment. Percutaneous sclerotherapy is the treatment of choice for venous and lymphatic malformations. Gold standard treatment for CMs is lasers in the form of pulsed dye laser therapy and photodynamic therapy. High flow malformations either AVF or AVM are always managed aggressively with complete occlusion of nidus by catheter directed or direct puncture embolotherapy followed by surgical excision. Complications are an integral part of the disease and treatment both, so it must be evaluated in terms of outcome and complications before deciding the mode of intervention in multimodal approach which is always better in vascular malformations. The radiologist and vascular surgeon are two key players in multidisciplinary team needed for management of vascular malformations.

REFERENCES

1. Nosher JL, Murillo PG, Liszewski M, et al. Vascular anomalies: a pictorial review of Nomenclature, Diagnosis and Treatment. World J Radiol. 2014;28:677-92.
2. Ricci KW. Advances in the Medical Management of Vascular Anomalies. Semin Intervent Radiol. 2017;34:239-49.
3. Adams DM, Brandão LR, Peterman CM, et al. Vascular anomaly cases for the pediatric hematologist oncologists: An interdisciplinary review. 2017:65(3); e26716.
4. Mulliken JB, Glowacki J. Hemangiomas and vascular malformations in infants and children: a classification based on endothelial characterisitics. Plast Reconstr Surg. 1982;69:412-22.

5. Wassef M, Blei F, Adams D, et al. Vascular anomalies classification: Recommendations from the international society for the study of vascular Anomalies. Pediatrics. 2015;136:e203-14.
6. Lee BB, Baumgartner I, Berlien P, et al. Diagnosis and Treatment of Venous Malformations Consensus Document of the International Union of Phlebology (IUP): updated 2013. Int Angiol. 2015;34:97-149.
7. Puig S, Aref H, Chigot V, et al. Classification of venous malformations in children and implications for sclerotherapy. Pediatr Radiol. 2003;33:99-103.
8. Sadick M, Müller-Wille R, Wildgruber M, et al. Vascular anomalies (Part I): Classification and Diagnostics of vascular anomalies. Rofo. 2018;190:825-35.
9. Hammer S, Uller W, Manger F, et al. Time-resolved magnetic resonance angiography (MRA) at 3.0 Tesla for evaluation of hemodynamic characteristics of vascular malformations: Description of distinct subgroups. Eur Radiol. 2017;27:296-305.
10. Vahlensieck M, Beltz L. The value of plain X-ray diagnosis and phlebography in the thoracic outlet syndrome. Aktuelle Radiol. 1991;1:244-48.
11. Smith MC, Zimmermann B, Burke DK, et al. Efficacy and Safety of OK-432 Immunotherapy of Lymphatic Malformations. Laryngoscope. 2009;119:107-15.
12. Clemens RK, Pfammatter T, Meier TO, et al. Vascular malformations revisited. Vasa. 2015;44:5-22.
13. Weitz NA, Lauren CT, Behr GG, et al. Clinical spectrum of capillary malformation-arteriovenous malformation syndrome presenting to a pediatric dermatology practice: a retrospective study. Pediatr Dermatol. 2015;32:76-84.
14. Gilbert P, Dubois J, Giroux MF, et al. New treatment approaches to arteriovenous malformations. Semin Intervent Radiol. 2017;34:258-71.
15. Wohlgemuth WA, Müller-Wille R, Teusch VI, et al. The Retrograde Transvenous Push-through Method: a Novel Treatment of Peripheral Arteriovenous Malformations with Dominant Venous Outflow. Cardiovasc Intervent Radiol. 2015;38:623-31.
16. MacDonald ME, Dolati P, Mitha AP, et al. Flow and pressure measurements in aneurysms and arteriovenous malformations with phase contrast MR imaging. Magn Reson Imaging. 2016;34:1322-8.
17. Gnannt R, Clemens RK, Pfammatter T. Transvenous embolization of an acquired arteriovenous malformation of the arm. J Vasc Interv Radiol. 2015;26:1585-7.
18. Greene AK, Liu AS, Mulliken JB, et al. Vascular anomalies in 5621 patients: Guidelines for referral. J Pediatr Surg. 2011;46:1784-9.
19. Sadick M, Dally FJ, Schönberg SO, et al. Strategies in interventional radiology: Formation of an interdisciplinary center of vascular anomalies—chances and challenges for effective and efficient patient management. Rofo. 2017;189:957-66.
20. Nikolaou VS, Chytas D, Korres D, et al. Vanishing bone disease (Gorham-Stout syndrome): a review of a rare entity. World J Orthop. 2014;18:694-8.
21. Nguyen HL, Boon LM, Vikkula M. Vascular anomalies caused by abnormal signaling within endothelial cells: Targets for novel therapies. Semin Intervent Radiol. 2017;34:233-8.

22. Horbach SER, Utami AM, Meijer-Jorna LB, et al. Discrepancy between the clinical and histopathologic diagnosis of soft tissue vascular malformations. J Am Acad Dermatol. 2017;77:920-9.
23. Zhang B, Lin Ma. Updated classification and therapy of vascular malformations in pediatric patients. Pediatr Invest. 2018;2:119-23.
24. Nozaki T, Nosaka S, Miyazaki O, et al. Syndromes associated with vascular tumors and malformations: a pictorial review. Radiographics. 2013;33:175-95.
25. Mazoyer E, Enjolras O, Bisdorff A, et al. Coagulation disorders in patients with venous malformation of the limbs and trunk: a case series of 118 patients. Arch Dermatol. 2008;144:861-7.
26. Zhuo KY, Russell S, Wargon O, et al. Localised intravascular coagulation complicating venous malformations in children: Associations and therapeutic options. J Paediatr Child Health. 2017;53:737-41
27. Sierre S, Teplisky D, Lipsich J. Vascular malformations: an update on imaging and management. Arch Argent Pediatr. 2016;114:167-76 .
28. Legiehn GM, Heran MK. A step-by-step practical approach to imaging diagnosis and interventional radiologic therapy in vascular malformations. Semin Intervent Radiol. 2010;27:209-31.
29. Kim D, Benjamin L, Wysong A, et al. Treatment of complex periorbital venolymphatic malformation in a neonate with a combination therapy of sirolimus and prednisolone. Dermatol Ther. 2015;28:218-21.
30. Triana P, Dore M, Cerezo VN, et al. Sirolimus in the treatment of vascular anomalies. Eur J Pediatr Surg. 2017;27:86-90.
31. Yesil S, Tanyildiz HG, Bozkurt C, et al. Single-center experience with sirolimus therapy for vascular malformations. Pediatr Hematol Oncol. 2016;33:219-25.
32. Goldenberg DC, Carvas M, Adams D, et al. Successful treatment of a complex vascular malformation with sirolimus and surgical resection. J Pediatr Hematol Oncol. 2017;39:e191-5.
33. Salloum R, Fox CE, Alvarez-Allende CR, et al. Response of blue rubber bleb nevus syndrome to sirolimus treatment. Pediatr Blood Cancer. 2016;63:1911-4.
34. Müller-Wille R, Wildgruber M, Sadick M, et al. Vascular Anomalies (Part II): Interventional therapy of peripheral venous malformations. Rofo. 2018;190:927-37.
35. van der Vleuten CJ, Kater A, Wijnen MH, et al. Effectiveness of sclerotherapy, surgery, and laser therapy in patients with venous malformations: a systematic review. Cardiovasc Intervent Radiol. 2014;37:977-89.
36. Green D. Mechanism of action of sclerotherapy. Semin Dermatol. 1993;12:88-97.
37. Horbach SE, Lokhorst MM, Saeed P, et al. Sclerotherapy for low-flow vascular malformations of the head and neck: A systematic review of sclerosing agents. J Plast Reconstr Aesthet Surg. 2016;69:295-304.
38. Qiu Y, Chen H, Lin X, et al. Outcomes and complications of sclerotherapy for venous malformations. Vasc Endovascular Surg. 2013;47:454-61.
39. Ali S, Mitchell SE. Outcomes of venous malformation sclerotherapy: A review of study methodology and long-term results. Semin Intervent Radiol. 2017;34:288-93.

40. Steiner F, FitzJohn T, Tan ST. Ethanol sclerotherapy for venous malformation. ANZ J Surg.2016;86:790-95.
41. Lackner H, Karastaneva A, Schwinger W, et al. Sirolimus for the treatment of children with various complicated vascular anomalies. Eur J Pediatr. 2015;174:1579-84.
42. Thomas DM, Wieck MM, Grant CN, et al. Doxycycline sclerotherapy is superior in the treatment of pediatric lymphatic malformations. J Vasc Interv Radiol. 2016; 27:1846-56.
43. Rebuffini E, Zuccarino L, Grecchi E, et al. Picibanil (OK-432) in the treatment of head and neck lymphangiomas in children. Dent Res J (Isfahan). 2012;9:S192-6.
44. Motz KM, Nickley KB, Bedwell JR, et al. OK432 versus doxycycline for treatment of macrocystic lymphatic malformations. Ann Otol Rhinol Laryngol. 2014;123:81-8.
45. Ravindranathan H, Gillis J, Lord DJ. Intensive care experience with sclerotherapy for cervicofacial lymphatic malformations. Pediatr Crit Care Med. 2008;9:304-9.
46. Yura J, Hashimoto T, Tsuruga N. et al. Bleomycin treatment for cystic hygroma in children. Nihon Geka Hokan. 1977;46:607-14.
47. Yang Y, Sun M, Ma Q, et al. Bleomycin A5 sclerotherapy for cervicofacial lymphatic malformations. J Vasc Surg. 2011;53:150-5.
48. Cheng J. Doxycycline sclerotherapy in children with head and neck lymphatic malformations. J Pediatr Surg. 2015;50:2143-6.
49. Shergill A, John P, Amaral JG. Doxycycline sclerotherapy in children with lymphatic malformations: outcomes, complications and clinical efficacy. Pediatr Radiol. 2012;42:1080-8.
50. Burrows PE, Mitri RK, Alomari A, et al. Percutaneous sclerotherapy of lymphatic malformations with doxycycline. Lymphat Res Biol. 2008;6:209-16.
51. Dunham GM, Ingraham CR, Maki JH, et al. Finding the nidus: Detection and workup of non-central nervous system arteriovenous malformations. Radiographics. 2016;36:891-903.
52. Grigg C, Anderson D, Earnshaw J. Diagnosis and treatment of hereditary hemorrhagic telangiectasia. Ochsner J. 2017;17:157-61.
53. Cho SK, Do YS, Shin SW, et al. Arteriovenous malformations of the body and extremities: analysis of therapeutic outcomes and approaches according to a modified angiographic classification. J Endovasc Ther. 2006;13:527-38.

14
Chapter

Triple-negative Breast Cancer

Seema Khanna, RN Meena, Rahul Khanna

INTRODUCTION

Breast cancer is the most common cancer and the leading cause of cancer-related deaths among women all over the world. It is believed to be a heterogeneous group of diseases characterized by different morphologies, biological behaviors, forms of presentation, and clinical evolution.[1] Triple-negative breast cancer (TNBC) was first described as a unique subset of breast cancer patients in 2005. It is characterized by the absence of estrogen and progesterone receptors (ER and PR) and a lack of amplification of the human epidermal growth factor receptor 2 (HER2) gene.[2] The usual biological behavior of TNBC patients is thought to be much more aggressive with a higher incidence of visceral and central nervous system metastases as compared to non-TNBC patients.

MOLECULAR CLASSIFICATION OF BREAST CANCER

Traditionally surgeons and pathologists have relied on the "histological grade" of breast cancer to determine its biological aggressiveness and to accordingly modify the therapeutic options. The Nottingham modification of the Bloom Richardson system is still used in histopathology reports and influences the choice of adjuvant therapy considerably. It takes into account: (i) Tubule formation, (ii) Nuclear pleomorphism, and (iii) Mitotic count.[3] The score can range from 3 (best histology) to 9 (worst histology). The score is considered in the context of the TNM staging system to guide treatment planning and to predict prognosis.

With the advent of microarray-based technology and addition of immunohistochemistry technique to routine histological evaluation, a breast cancer classification system based on tumor biology rather than morphology was developed. Perou and Sorlie first described the "molecular

Table 1: Major molecular subtypes of breast cancer.

Molecular subtype	Gene expression pattern	Response to treatment	Prognosis
Luminal A	• ER/PR positive • HER2/neu negative	• Response to endocrine therapy • Variable response to chemotherapy	Good
Luminal B	• ER/PR positive • HER2/neu variable • Ki67 positive	• Response to endocrine therapy less than luminal A • Response to chemotherapy better than luminal A	Not as good as luminal A
HER2/neu	• ER/PR weak expression • HER2/neu over expression • High proliferation index	• Response to trastuzumab • Response to anthracycline	Unfavorable
Basal like	• ER/PR weak expression • HER2/neu weak expression • High expression of basal cytokeratins	• No response to endocrine therapy or trastuzumab • Sensitive to platinum-based chemotherapy and PARP inhibitors	Unfavorable

classification" of breast cancer based on differences in gene expression.[4] On the basis of immunohistochemical expression of ER, PR and HER2/neu status, breast cancer was categorized into: luminal type A, luminal type B, HER2/neu enriched and the basal variety (Table 1). The distinction between luminal type A and type B was stronger expression of hormone receptors in type A and higher proliferation index as evidenced by Ki67 expression in type B variety. The HER2/neu enriched variety has an over expression of HER2/neu (3+ or above) and the basal variety is characterized by expression of basal epithelial and cytokeratin genes. A "normal-like" group was described, which represents samples with low tumor content and a higher normal tissue component.[5]

Taking cognizance of the importance of the biological characteristics, the European Institute of Oncology (EIO) has suggested the tumor, node, metastasis (TNM) EIO system of staging breast cancer. Besides the anatomical details, this staging system includes the biological properties such as ER, PR, and HER2 expresssion.[6]

DEFINITION OF TRIPLE-NEGATIVE BREAST CANCER

As the name suggests, TNBCs lack expression of ER, PR, and HER-2/neu. It accounts for 15–20% of all breast cancer in Europe and America.[7] The prevalence of TNBC among African-American women is almost twice as high. Our own study on Indian breast cancer patients visiting surgical OPD in Banaras Hindu University found an incidence of 32.6% of TNBC among the 196 consecutive breast cancer patients evaluated.[8] Other centers from India have reported prevalence of TNBC to vary from 26% to 46%. Large studies recruiting several thousand patients have reported the prevalence rates of 12.5% from USA, 16.37% from UK, and 12.1% from China (Table 2). The reason for this wide variation has not been entirely explained although it is most likely to be due to genetic and social differences rather than geographical or environmental factors. Another reason could be the methodology employed by different laboratories and the cutoff values used to determine ER and PR positivity as well as HER2 expression. Tumors with HER2, 2+ score on IHC require fluorescent in situ hybridization (FISH) for accurate categorization and presence or absence of FISH facilities could have a bearing on the interpretation of results and the reported prevalence rate from that center.[8-15]

Is Triple-negative Breast Cancer Synonymous with Basal-like Breast Cancer?

Many physicians perceive TNBC to be identical to the basal-like breast cancer described in Perou's molecular classification. There is a great overlap between the two entities with about 75% of TNBC tumors showing basal-like gene expression and vice versa, yet they are not entirely similar. Basal-like breast cancers arise from the myoepithelial cells of the breast while TNBC are generally ductal carcinomas. Basal-like breast cancer expresses basal membrane cytokeratin 5/6 and HER1 (EGFR) receptor. Although most basal-like varieties can be ER, PR or even HER2 positive. Conversely 19% of the TNBC tumors do not express basal-like markers.[10] Expression of CK 5/6 which is representative of basal or myoepithelial cells is regarded as the

Table 2: Prevalence of triple-negative breast cancer (TNBC) among breast cancer patients in different countries.

Author	Year	Country	Number of cases	Prevalence of TNBC
Bauer et al.[9]	2007	USA	92,358	12.5%
Rakha et al.[10]	2007	UK	1,726	16.3%
Li et al.[11]	2013	China	21,749	12.18%
Zubeda et al.[12]	2013	India	619	46%
Sharma et al.[13]	2015	India	972	31.9%
Akhtar et al.[14]	2015	India	85	43.5%
Lakshmaiah et al.[15]	2016	India	322	26%
Khanna et al.[8]	2017	India	196	32.6%

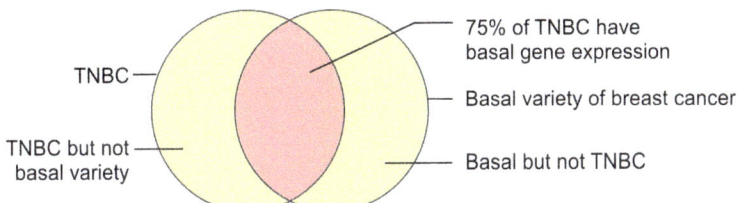

Fig. 1: Relationship between triple-negative breast cancer (TNBC) and basal variety of breast cancer.

most useful marker for identification of basal-like breast cancer. Therefore in spite of the great deal of overlap, TNBC and basal-like breast cancer may vary is about 25% of patients and should not be considered to be synonymous (Fig. 1).

NATURAL HISTORY OF TRIPLE-NEGATIVE BREAST CANCER

Triple-negative breast cancers are histologically high-grade invasive ductal carcinoma of no special type.[16] They are more rapidly growing and occur in younger woman compared to non-TNBC tumors. As mammographic screening is usually done in women over the age of 40 years, they are less likely to be diagnosed on a screening protocol. The rapid growth means that their probability of being detected as interval cancers between two episodes of screening is considerable. They are more likely to metastasize to viscera, especially to lungs and brain and less likely to metastasize to bones compared to non-TNBC tumors.[17] Also they are more likely to recur locally after therapy compared to their hormone positive counterparts.[18]

Survival among TNBC patients during the first 5 years is poorer compared to non-TNBC patients. However, distant relapse after 5 years is much less common and after 10 years, relapse among ER positive patients is more frequent than ER negative patients.[19] Although TNBC lesions are biologically aggressive, a fair percentage are still potentially curable.

TRIPLE-NEGATIVE BREAST CANCER IMAGING STUDIES

Because of their rapid growth, TNBC may be missed at routine mammographic screening and are likely to present as interval cancers. Further, there is a relative lack of typical microcalcifications which is the sine qua non for the mammographic diagnosis of breast cancer. Ultrasonogram of the breast is also less reliable because TNBC lesions appear as well circumscribed masses which is more typical for benign rather than malignant lesions. Thus, both mammogram and ultrasonogram are quite likely to miss a TNBC lesion.

Magnetic resonance imaging of TNBC lesions shows specific features such as rim enhancement and very high intratumoral signal intensity on T2-weighted images which are fairly suggestive as these features are not prominent among ER/PR positive and HER2 negative cancers.[20] On FDC-PET scan, TNBC lesions show a higher FDG uptake due to enhanced glycolysis. Patients with TNBC should have a careful evaluation of their internal mammary, supraclavicular and infraclavicular nodes in addition to the axillary lymph nodes by an ultrasound examination.

PROGNOSIS OF TRIPLE-NEGATIVE BREAST CANCER

Triple-negative breast cancer has a much poorer prognosis compared to non-TNBC patients. This is on account of their biological aggressive behavior, rapid growth, and greater propensity for local recurrence and visceral metastasis. Further contributing to their dismal prognosis is their nonresponsiveness to endocrine therapy and targeted therapy against HER2. Some TNBC tumors show good to excellent sensitivity to chemotherapy and have a better prognosis and may even be potentially curable. HER2-positive breast cancers were also associated with a poor prognosis, but now with availability of trastuzumab which targets HER2/neu, their prognosis has significantly improved. Trastuzumab monoclonal antibody therapy is expensive (Rs. 50,000/month) and for HER2-positive patients unable to afford it, prognosis will be as poor if not worse than TNBC patients.

TREATMENT IN TRIPLE-NEGATIVE BREAST CANCER

Patients with TNBC do not respond to endocrine therapy or trastuzumab and this is responsible to a great extent for the poor prognosis besides the aggressive biological behavior per se. The sheet anchor of treatment is surgery with adjuvant chemotherapy and some newly emerging options of targeted therapy.

SURGERY IN TRIPLE-NEGATIVE BREAST CANCER

Recommended surgical options for TNBC stage for stage are similar to those for non-TNBC patients. Considering the aggressive nature and the greater propensity for locoregional recurrence, most surgeons would recommend a modified radical mastectomy rather than breast conserving procedure. For the same rationale axillary clearance would be advised over a sentinel node biopsy protocol even in N0 patients. However, a retrospective study of patients with TNBC treated with mastectomy compared with breast conserving surgery (BCS) concluded that BCS should be considered as an option in selected TNBC patients.[21] This was because recurrence after BCS was found to be equivalent in TNBC and non-TNBC patients.

CHEMOTHERAPY IN TRIPLE-NEGATIVE BREAST CANCER

Generally, TNBC lesions are more sensitive to chemotherapy than non-TNBC. Response to chemotherapy is probably the most important prognostic criteria in TNBC patients. TNBC patients on neoadjuvant chemotherapy who have a complete pathological response have an excellent outcome while the outcome for those who demonstrate a partial response is relatively poor.[19] Analysis of several trials suggests than a combination of taxanes and anthracycline-containing regimen will show a better response than the usual cyclophosphamide, adriamycin 5-fluorouracil regimen in TNBC.[22] Rouzier et al. used a taxane and anthracycline combination in the neoadjuvant setting and found a 45% complete pathological remission in basaloid tumors compared to only 6% for luminal tumors.[23] The fact that TNBC is associated with a higher incidence of *BRCA1* dysfunction is the basis for use of cisplatin and carboplatin in the patients. Neoadjuvant use of cisplatin results in a high rate of complete pathological response in patients who have *BRCA1* mutation and also in TNBC patients.[24]

Based on current evidence combination therapy with anthracyclines and taxanes may be recommended as first-line and even neoadjuvant regimen of choice for TNBC patients. However, TNBC patients who do not achieve a complete pathological response would have a poor outcome compared to non-TNBC patients stage for stage. To reduce the cumulative cardiotoxicity of adriamycin, liposomal or pegylated variety may be incorporate in the regimen.

Ixabepilone is a microtubule stabilizer. It has been shown to be effective in cancers which are insensitive to paclitaxel.[25] Ixabepilone in combination with capecitabine has demonstrated effectiveness in the treatment of TNBC patients and a longer time to progression among patients who have failed to respond to anthracycline plus taxane combination.[26] The role of platinums is being reconsidered considering the high percentage of *BRCA1* gene dysfunction in TNBC patients. Ongoing trials in the adjuvant, neoadjuvant, and metastatic setting are examining the role of various combinations such as carboplatin versus docetaxel, epirubicin and cyclophosphamide, gemcitabine and cisplatinum, gemcitabine and oxaliplatin with variable results.[27]

TARGETED THERAPY IN TRIPLE-NEGATIVE BREAST CANCER

Clearly TNBC patients are not going to respond to conventional therapies targeting ER, PR, and HER2/neu. However, there are other potential targets such as angiogenesis [vascular endothelial growth factor (VEGF)], tyrosine kinase, mammalian target of rapamycin (mTOR) and poly (ADP-ribose) polymerase (PARP) which have been the subject of considerable interest over the last decade.

Angiogenesis Inhibitors

Bevacizumab is a monoclonal antibody which targets VEGF. It is recommended as first-line therapy as combination of bevacizumab with paclitxel has shown a response rate of 36.9% versus 21.2% with paclitaxel monotherapy.[28] The RIBBON-1 study has used bevacizumab in combination with different drugs such as capecitabine, nab-pactitaxel, docetaxel or anthracyclines.[29]

Tyrosine Kinase Inhibitors

Tyrosine kinases are a family of enzymes which catalyze phosphorylation of tyrosine and are important mediators of signal transduction process leading to cell proliferation, differentiation, migration, metabolism, and programmed cell death. Tyrosine kinase inhibitors such as sunitinib and sorafenib have shown same antitumor activity in TNBC patients. Sunitinib whose targets include VEGF and platelet-derived growth factor (PDGF) was not found to be effective enough to be recommended as monotherapy in treatment of breast cancer.

Sorafenib a potent multikinase inhibitor with antiangiogenic and antiproliferative activity is used primarily for advanced renal cell carcinoma and unresectable hepatocellular carcinoma. It has shown modest activity against breast cancer and has been used in combination with capecitabine and paclitaxel.[30] The dose limiting toxicity with sorafenib is hand-foot syndrome.

Poly (ADP-ribose) Polymerase Inhibitors

Poly (ADP-ribose) polymerase is a family of proteins involved in a number of cellular processes such as DNA repair, genomic stability, and programmed cell death.[31] The main role of PARP (found in the cell nucleus) is the detect and initiate an immediate cellular response to metabolic, chemical or radiation-induced single strand DNA breast (SSB) by signaling the enzymatic machinery involved in the SSB repair.

Poly (ADP-ribose) polymerase inhibitors (such as iniparib, olaparib, and veliparib) interfere with the DNA damage repair mechanism and induce synthetic lethality. The best results of PARP inhibitors have been obtained in combination with cisplatin or carboplatin as well as with topotecan and temozolamide and response rates in BRCA-related tumors of up to 73%.[32] However, results from various other trials have produced conflicting results and PARP inhibitors are still under investigations (Table 3).

Table 3: Potential therapeutic targets, agents under trial and outcome in triple-negative breast cancer (TNBC) patients.

Potential target	Agent used	Outcome
Angiogenesis (VEGF)	Bevacizumab	Promising results in combination with paclitaxel
Tyrosine kinase	• Sunitinib • Sorafenib	Modest results
PARP	• Iniparib • Olaparib • Veliparib	Conflicting results
mTOR	• Rapamycin • Everolimus	Promising results in combination with taxanes/anthracycline and bevacizumab
Immune system (PD-L1)	• Atezolizumab • Pembrolizumab	Promising results in combination with paclitaxel

Mammalian Target of Rapamycin Inhibitors

Mammalian target of rapamycin is a member of the phosphatidylinositol 3-kinase-related kinase family of protein kinases. It regulates cell growth, cell proliferation, cell motility, cell survival, protein synthesis, autophagy, and transcription.[33] Rapamycin was the first mTOR inhibitor discovered in 1975 in a soil sample from Easter Island of South Pacific. Studies on the rapamycin analog everolimus have yielded promising results in TNBC. When everolimus was combined with T-FEC (paclitaxel, 5FU, epirubicin and cyclophosphamide) the 12 weeks response rate improved from 30% to 48%.[34]

IMMUNOTHERAPY

Atezolizumab is a fully humanized, engineered monoclonal antibody of IgG1 isotype against the protein programmed cell death ligand 1 (PD-L1). It is an immunotherapy drug used to boost the power of the immune system to find and kill cancer cells by blocking PD-L1, a protein which may help cancer cells escape detection by the immune system. In early TNBC patients, the neoadjuvant I-SPY2 trial demonstrated a 40% improvement in pathological complete response when pembrolizumab was added to paclitaxel.[35]

RADIOTHERAPY IN TRIPLE-NEGATIVE BREAST CANCER

As per the limited available literature the role of radiotherapy in TNBC, the indications and efficacy of postmastectomy radiotherapy is similar as per non-TNBC patients. If a BCS is chosen, postoperative radiotherapy is mandatory. Studies have confirmed the beneficial impact of postmastectomy radiotherapy on the local recurrence rate and the disease-free surgical in high risk TNBC (stage T3-T4 and/or N2-N3).[36] In low-risk TNBC patients presence of lymphovascular invasion on histopathology could be an indication for postmastectomy radiotherapy.

CONCEPT OF BRCAness

Tumors that share molecular features of *BRCA* mutant tumors are said to possess "BRCAness". These tumors may share similar biologic behaviors and response to treatment.[37] Only 5–10% of breast cancer patients in women are attributed to *BRCA1* and *BRCA2* mutations. Conversely women with harmful mutations in either *BRCA1* or *BRCA2* have a five times higher risk of developing breast cancer and a 10 to 30-fold higher risk for developing ovarian cancer.[38] Among TNBC patients the prevalence of BRCA mutation has been reported to be 30.8%.[39] The prevalence of genetic mutation is higher in younger women (43.8% at less than 40 years of age versus 16.6% at over 70 years of age). It can also vary according to ethnicity and race. Loss or inactivation of *BRCA* gene results in inefficient repair mechanism.

The *BRCA* status is considered a predictive factor for response to chemotherapy and PARP inhibitors. Tumors lacking functional *BRCA* gene are more sensitive to platinum (DNA crosslinking agents) and anthracycline (DNA damaging agents) based chemotherapy.[40] The Olympiad trial recruited 302 metastatic breast cancer patients who had *BRCA* mutations. It was found that response rate to olaparib (PARP inhibitor) was 59.9% compared to 28.8% in patients receiving single-agent chemotherapy (capecitabine, eribulin or vinorelbine).[41] In January 2018, the US Food and Drug Administration approved the use of olaparib in BRCA-mutated metastatic breast cancer.

QUADRUPLE-NEGATIVE BREAST CANCER

The subgroup of TNBC patients who lack an androgen receptor (AR) as well have been termed as quadruple-negative breast cancer (QNBC).[42] The presence of AR in TNBC is associated with a luminal subtype on gene microarray while most of AR negative TNBC (also called QNBC) exhibit a basal-like molecular subtype while TNBC has the potential of a therapeutic target in the AR, QNBC has been shown to express unique proteins which may be available for the development of a therapeutic target. One such protein is the fatty acid activating enzyme, long chain fatty acyl-COA synthetase 4 (ACSL4).

CONCLUSION

The incidence of TNBC in the Indian subcontinent is 2–3 times higher than that reported from Europe and America. It may be diagnosed preoperatively, if a core needle biopsy specimen is subjected to IHC studies for ER, PR, and HER2 status. Patients being treated on basis of their FNAC report are going to be diagnosed when their postoperative specimen histopathology and IHC reports become available. TNBC patients requiring neoadjuvant therapy should preferentially receive a taxane-anthracycline combination upfront rather than cyclophosphamide-5Fu-adriamycin regimen. Recommendations of surgical treatment in TNBC and non-TNBC patients are similar although most surgeons are likely to opt for a modified radical mastectomy rather than a BCS. Similarly node-negative TNBC patients are likely to receive an axillary clearance rather than a sentinel node biopsy. Thus decision is based on the rational that TNBC is a more aggressive lesion with a higher chance of locoregional recurrence. Postoperative endocrine therapy and trastuzumab is not an option for TNBC patients. However, there are other potential therapeutic targets such as angiogenesis, PARP, mTOR, tyrosine kinase, and immunotherapy which over various clinical trials have demonstrated modest to encouraging results.

REFERENCES

1. Chacón RD, Costanzo MV. Triple-negative breast cancer. Breast Cancer Res. 2010;12 (Suppl 2):S3.
2. Brenton JD, Carey LA, Ahmed AA, et al. Molecular classification and molecular forecasting of breast cancer: ready for clinical application. J Clin Oncol. 2005;23(29):7350-60.
3. Meyer JS, Alvarez C, Milikowski C, et al. Breast carcinoma malignancy grading by Bloom-Richardson system vs proliferation index: reproducibility of grade and advantages of proliferation index. Mod Pathol. 2005;18(8):1067-78.
4. Perou CM, Sørlie T, Eisen MB, et al. Molecular portraits of human breast tumours. Nature. 2000;406(6797):747-52.
5. Eliyatkın N, Yalçın E, Zengel B, et al. Molecular Classification of Breast Carcinoma: From Traditional, Old-Fashioned Way to A New Age, and A New Way. J Breast Health. 2015;11(2):59-66.
6. Veronesi U, Viale G, Rotmensz N, et al. Rethinking TNM: breast cancer TNM classification for treatment decision-making and research. Breast. 2006;15(1):3-8.
7. Hurvitz S, Mead M. Triple-negative breast cancer: advancements in characterization and treatment approach. Curr Opin Obstet Gynecol. 2016;28(1):59-69.
8. Khanna R, Meena RN, Bansal A, et al. Triple Negative Breast Cancer: Experience from a North Indian Tertiary Care Center. Indian J Surg. 2018;80:474-8.
9. Bauer KR, Brown M, Cress RD, et al. Descriptive analysis of estrogen receptor (ER)-negative, progesterone receptor (PR)-negative, and HER2-negative invasive breast cancer, the so-called triple-negative phenotype: a population-based study from the California cancer Registry. Cancer. 2007;109(9):1721-8.
10. Rakha EA, Tan DS, Foulkes WD, et al. Are triple-negative tumours and basal-like breast cancer synonymous? Breast Cancer Res. 2007;9(6):404.

11. Li CY, Zhang S, Zhang XB, et al. Clinicopathological and prognostic characteristics of triple-negative breast cancer (TNBC) in Chinese patients: A retrospective study. Asian Pac J Cancer Prev. 2013;14(6):3779-84.
12. Zubeda S, Kaipa PR, Shaik NA, et al. Her-2/neu status: a neglected marker of prognostication and management of breast cancer patients in India. Asian Pac J Cancer Prev. 2013;14(4):2231-5.
13. Sharma M, Sharma JD, Sarma A, et al. Triple negative breast cancer in people of North East India: critical insights gained at a regional cancer centre. Asian Pac J Cancer Prev. 2014;15(11):4507-11.
14. Akhtar M, Dasgupta S, Rangwala M. Triple negative breast cancer: an Indian perspective. Breast Cancer (Dove Med Press). 2015;7:239-43.
15. Lakshmaiah KC, Das U, Suresh TM, et al. A study of triple negative breast cancer at a tertiary cancer care center in southern India. Ann Med Health Sci Res. 2014;4(6):933-7.
16. Foulkes WD, Smith IE, Reis-Filho JS. Triple-negative breast cancer. N Engl J Med. 2010;363(20):1938-48.
17. Dent R, Hanna WM, Trudeau M, et al. Pattern of metastatic spread in triple-negative breast cancer. Breast Cancer Res Treat. 2009;115(2):423-8.
18. Voduc KD, Cheang MC, Tyldesley S, et al. Breast cancer subtypes and the risk of local and regional relapse. J Clin Oncol. 2010;28(10):1684-91.
19. Liedtke C, Mazouni C, Hess KR, et al. Response to neoadjuvant therapy and long-term survival in patients with triple-negative breast cancer. J Clin Oncol. 2008;26(8):1275-81.
20. Uematsu T, Kasami M, Yuen S. Triple-negative breast cancer: correlation between MR imaging and pathologic findings. Radiology. 2009;250(3):638-47.
21. Freedman GM, Anderson PR, Li T, et al. Locoregional recurrence of triple-negative breast cancer after breast-conserving surgery and radiation. Cancer. 2009;115(5):946-51.
22. Ellis P, Barrett-Lee P, Johnson L, et al. Sequential docetaxel as adjuvant chemotherapy for early breast cancer (TACT): an open-label, phase III, randomised controlled trial. Lancet. 2009;373(9676):1681-92.
23. Rouzier R, Perou CM, Symmans WF, et al. Breast cancer molecular subtypes respond differently to preoperative chemotherapy. Clin Cancer Res. 2005;11(16):5678-85.
24. Silver DP, Richardson AL, Eklund AC, et al. Efficacy of neoadjuvant Cisplatin in triple-negative breast cancer. J Clin Oncol. 2010;28(7):1145-53.
25. Goodin S. Ixabepilone: a novel microtubule-stabilizing agent for the treatment of metastatic breast cancer. Am J Health Syst Pharm. 2008;65(21):2017-26.
26. Thomas ES, Gomez HL, Li RK, et al. Ixabepilone plus capecitabine for metastatic breast cancer progressing after anthracycline and taxane treatment. J Clin Oncol. 2007;25(33):5210-7.
27. Tan AR, Swain SM. Therapeutic strategies for triple-negative breast cancer. Cancer J. 2008;14(6):343-51.
28. Miller K, Wang M, Gralow J, et al. Paclitaxel plus bevacizumab versus paclitaxel alone for metastatic breast cancer. N Engl J Med. 2007;357(26):2666-76.

29. Robert NJ, Dieras V, Glaspy J, et al. RIBBON-1: Randomized, double-blind, placebo-controlled, phase III trial of chemotherapy with or without bevacizumab (B) for first-line treatment of HER2-negative locally recurrent or metastatic breast cancer (MBC). J Clin Oncol. 2009;27(15 Suppl):1005.
30. Gradishar WJ, Kaklamani V, Sahoo TP, et al. A double-blind, randomised, placebo-controlled, phase 2b study evaluating sorafenib in combination with paclitaxel as a first-line therapy in patients with HER2-negative advanced breast cancer. Eur J Cancer. 2013;49(2):312-22.
31. Herceg Z, Wang ZQ. Functions of poly(ADP-ribose) polymerase (PARP) in DNA repair, genomic integrity and cell death. Mutat Res. 2001;477(1-2):97-110.
32. Pahuja S, Beumer JH, Appleman LJ, et al. A phase I study of veliparib (ABT-888) in combination with weekly carboplatin and paclitaxel in advanced solid malignancies and enriched for triple-negative breast cancer (TNBC). J Clin Oncol. 2015;33:(15 Suppl):1015.
33. Lipton JO, Sahin M. The neurology of mTOR. Neuron. 2014;84(2):275-91.
34. Gonzalez-Angulo AM, Akcakanat A, Liu S, et al. Open-label randomized clinical trial of standard neoadjuvant chemotherapy with paclitaxel followed by FEC versus the combination of paclitaxel and everolimus followed by FEC in women with triple receptor-negative breast cancer. Ann Oncol. 2014;25(6):1122-7.
35. Nanda R, Liu MC, Yau C, et al. Pembrolizumab plus standard neoadjuvant therapy for high-risk breast cancer (BC): Results from I-SPY 2. J Clin Oncol. 2017;35(15 Suppl):506.
36. Chen X, Yu X, Chen J, et al. Radiotherapy can improve the disease-free survival rate in triple-negative breast cancer patients with T1-T2 disease and one to three positive lymph nodes after mastectomy. Oncologist. 2013;18(2):141-7.
37. Lord CJ, Ashworth A. BRCAness revisited. Nat Rev Cancer. 2016;16(2):110-20.
38. National Cancer Institute (2009). *BRCA1* and *BRCA2*: Cancer rist and genetic testing. [online]. Available from *https://pdfs.semanticscholar.org/b2a5/5fd78d46 d1344b5e37e102b012835362e38b.pdf* [Accessed December, 2018].
39. Greenup R, Buchanan A, Lorizio W, et al. Prevalence of *BRCA* mutations among women with triple-negative breast cancer (TNBC) in a genetic counseling cohort. Ann Surg Oncol. 2013;20(10):3254-8.
40. Wang C, Zhang J, Wang Y, et al. Prevalence of BRCA1 mutations and responses to neoadjuvant chemotherapy among BRCA1 carriers and non-carriers with triple-negative breast cancer. Ann Oncol. 2015;26(3):523-8.
41. Chen ZJ, Shi Y, Sun Y, et al. Fresh versus frozen embryos for infertility in the polycystic ovary syndrome. N Engl J Med. 2016;375(6):523-33.
42. Hon JD, Singh B, Sahin A, et al. Breast cancer molecular subtypes: from TNBC to QNBC. Am J Cancer Res. 2016;6(9):1864-72.

15
Chapter

Hormone Therapy for Breast Cancer

Ramya VC, Gaurav Agarwal

A lady with growth neoplastic
Thought castration was just a bit drastic
She preferred that her ill could be cured with a pill
Today it's no longer fantastic.

Elwood Jensen and Craig Jordan*

INTRODUCTION

The outcomes of breast cancer, the most common cancer in women, have improved considerably over the last few decades. This is attributable largely to multimodality treatment protocols. Systemic treatment including chemotherapy, hormonal therapy, and molecular targeted therapy has contributed in improving survival of breast cancer patients of all stages. Extensive basic research has provided insights into pathophysiological pathways linking estrogens and breast oncogenesis, and the effect hormonal manipulations can have on the breast cancer initiation and progression. High quality and large clinical trials have established the efficacy of hormone therapy (HT) in hormone receptor positive (HR+) breast cancers. A large proportion of breast cancers are HR+. HT, given mainly as antiestrogenic therapy, is the mainstay of adjuvant systemic treatment in HR+, early stage breast cancer patients and one of the important components of multimodality adjuvant systemic therapy in locally advanced as well as metastatic breast cancers (MBCs). Treatment of breast cancer by manipulation of hormonal *milieu* by various modalities has been in use for many decades and has undergone interesting changes overtime. This chapter intends to provide the reader an account of basic physiology of hormonal manipulation, their effects and their current evidence based clinical applications.

---

*As told by Elwood Jensen to JJ Moore in an interview

EVOLUTION OF HORMONAL THERAPY IN BREAST CANCER

Discovery of the effect of ovarian hormones on breast cancer is serendipitous like most medical discoveries. The effect of ovarian hormones on carcinoma breast was first observed by Thomas William Nunn.[1] Beatson was first to provide a scientific report of benefits of oophorectomy in breast cancer patients in 1896.[1] Estrogen receptor (ER) was first described by Elwood Jensen and colleagues in 1958,[2] while the progesterone receptor (PR) was isolated by the laboratories of Pierre Chambon, Edwin Milgrom, and Bert O'Malley in 1980s.[3] Though the drug tamoxifen (the first antiestrogen drug used in treatment of breast cancer), a selective ER modulator was developed to be used as a contraceptive, the early recognition of its use in mice in prevention of breast tumors resulted in its usage for treatment of postmenopausal patients with metastatic breast cancer in 1973. Tamoxifen came into routine clinical use from early 1970's for metastatic breast cancer followed in late 1970's as an adjuvant therapy in early stage breast cancer. The concept of HT and usage of antiestrogenic therapy in breast cancer went through many changes until 1988 when the meta-analysis by the Early Breast Cancer Trialists' Collaborative Group (EBCTCG) suggested that ovarian ablation achieved either with a surgical oophorectomy or by radiation increased disease-free and overall survival in breast cancer patients.

Hormone receptors are widely expressed in many normal tissues and few tumors. About 60–75% of breast cancers retain their steroid HR expression (ER, PR)—whereas rest of them loose expression as they dedifferentiate.[4] The natural history of HR+ and HR negative (HR–) tumors differs significantly, with the HR+ patients having better survival than HR– disease as established by numerous studies including major trials such as National Surgical Adjuvant Breast and Bowel Project (NSABP)-06.[4] Apart from the intrinsic biological differences between them, the chance to administer endocrine therapy targeting these receptors has made outcomes better for HR+ tumors.

The steroid hormone 17β-estradiol (E2) derived from the ovary in premenopausal women, and as the conversion product of adrenal steroid androstenedione by aromatase in peripheral tissues (especially adipose tissue) in postmenopausal women, is the most potent estrogen and main ligand for these receptors. Physiologically, E2 is essential in growth, proliferation, differentiation, and maintenance of cells in various tissues, including the breast parenchymal and ductal cells. Because HT is such an effective intervention, proven over long period of time in large trials to improve outcomes of breast cancer, it remains an issue of great research interest. As a result, newer and more effective, yet safer HT modalities continue to be discovered and integrated in multimodal breast cancer treatment protocols.

ESTROGEN EXPOSURE AS A RISK-FACTOR FOR BREAST CANCER

A systematic review of epidemiological studies suggests that increased cumulative exposure to unopposed estrogen (without progesterone exposure) in situations like nulliparity, delayed child-bearing (first child-birth after age of 35 years), early menarche, late menopause; or estrogen synthesis in adipose tissue and greater bioavailability as in case of postmenopausal obesity are significantly associated with increased risk of breast cancer. These result in higher risk of HR+ breast cancer, however their role in causation or risk of HR– cancers is less clear. The etiological role of exogenous estrogen use [oral contraceptive pills (OCPs) and hormone replacement therapy (HRT)] is not proven.[5] However, there is some evidence that in women with genetic predisposition to breast cancer, OCPs may increase the risk though not necessarily result in HR+ tumors.[6] Life-style factors like alcohol consumption and smoking are also associated with higher risk of breast cancer.

PHYSIOLOGICAL BASIS OF ANTIESTROGEN THERAPY IN BREAST CANCER

The estrogen-mediated intracellular signaling is complex. The age-old simplistic model of intranuclear ER-mediated DNA expression has been discarded. The ER has been classified under the superfamily of nuclear HR (NHR). It is mainly located but not restricted to, in the nucleus of the cells. It is highly mobile within the nuclear matrix and is in close physical association with the target DNA. The extranuclear locations include plasma membrane and mitochondria. Apart from the E2 itself, the estrogen response elements (EREs), intracellular and transmembrane proteins, coregulators, post-translational modifications, and epigenetic mechanisms contribute to the execution of varied ER functions.

Two subtypes of ER identified so far, ERα and ERβ differ in N-terminus structure.[7] They have differential expression and functions in various locations within the cell and in various tissues. ERα is present predominantly in epithelial cells of normal breast tissue whereas the ERβ is present in epithelial as well as stromal elements. ERα is essential for normal growth and development of breast tissue.[8] ERα expression is increased and ERβ expression is decreased in breast tumor tissue.[9] ERα has been found to be the prime receptor subtype based on knock-out studies in mice, in many tissues including the breast, uterus, cervix, vagina, and other organs. Different

pathways of estrogen-dependent response signaling pathways have been proposed,[10] namely:
- *Estrogen receptor-mediated nuclear signaling*: ERE-dependent (transcription factors mediated) and ERE-independent [peptide growth factor mediated *viz* epidermal growth factor (EGF), insulin-like growth factor 1 (IGF-1), etc.]
- Estrogen receptor-mediated membrane signaling
- Estrogen receptor-mediated mitochondrial events. Estrogens are potent stimuli for cell proliferation.

ASSESSMENT OF BREAST CANCERS FOR HORMONE RECEPTOR POSITIVITY

Establishing the presence of ER is of great predictive and prognostic significance, and indicates HT responsiveness. The assessment of breast cancers for presence or expression of ER and PR is essentially done by immuno-histochemical staining (IHC) for these in paraffin-embedded sections of the tumor tissue. There has been considerable debate in past about the cut-off based on intensity of staining and percentage of cancer cells staining for ER and/or PR for it to be reported as ER and/or PR positive. This has now been set to rest, and the current American Society of Clinical Oncology or College of American Pathologists (ASCO or CAP) guidelines suggest that even if immunoreactivity of tumor cell nuclei is more than or equal to 1%, it should be reported as positive[11] when performed on sufficiently large-sized cores of tissue that are assessed soon after the biopsy was performed. This cut-off of ER+ status even at such low proportion of cells staining for it is based on the observation that HT is effective even in patients with such low levels of ER positivity. The laboratories performing the test should be internally and externally validated and accredited. Though the HR assessment can be performed by reverse transcriptase-polymerase chain reaction (RT-PCR) also, IHC is found to be comparable to RT-PCR, and is now the standard and recommended method of HR assessment in breast cancer.[12] Breast tumors show heterogeneity in expression of ER within different areas of tumors as well as circulating tumor cells showing positivity and negativity for ER staining.[13] There are various scoring systems devised to account for the heterogenous immunostaining of ER. The commonly used "Allred" scoring system uses percentage and intensity of staining of ER to give the final score.

Progesterone Receptors in Breast Cancer

While the main focus of endocrine therapy in breast cancer is via ER manipulation, the role of progestins has been contentious with no consistent and encouraging results. Data suggests that PR positivity can be of protective or good prognostic effect in breast cancer.[14] Though progestins like medroxy-progesterone acetate, hydroxy-progesterone caproate, and megestrol acetate which act by anti-androgenic and anti-estrogenic effects have been investigated in breast cancer, the role of therapy directed via PR is not well established. So, anti-progestins as treatment modality of breast cancer are not in routine use as of now. There is some recent evidence that PR expression in ER expressing tumors has prognostic importance suggesting that loss of PR expression worsens the outcomes in ER+, human epidermal growth factor receptor 2 (HER 2) neu negative cancers.[14]

MODALITIES OF HORMONAL THERAPY FOR BREAST CANCER

Surgery (bilateral salpingo-oophorectomy), radiation (to the ovaries), and medical therapies have been evaluated as hormone treatment for HR+ breast cancers. Surgery is safe and is the modality that can have an early, permanent, and complete ovarian function suppression in pre-menopausal women. Though radiotherapy-based ovarian function ablation was in vogue in the past, it has fallen out of favor in the current times, owing to the relatively unpredictable and variable efficacy, and concerns about its safety. Various drug categories used in hormonal manipulation of HR+ breast cancers include (Table 1):

- Selective ER modulators (SERM)
- Selective ER degraders (SERD)—also known as anti-estrogens
- Aromatase inhibitors (AIs)
- Gonadotropin releasing hormone (GnRH) analogs—mainly luteinizing hormone releasing hormone, (LHRH) analogs, and
- Progestins.

The initial efforts in developing anti-estrogens were intended for contraception and subsequently found to have anti-cancer effects. SERMs are non-steroidal, synthetic molecules (>70 described so far) that can bind to ER in a competitive manner and block the cell cycle in G1 phase.[15] The most common and most effective SERM in use is tamoxifen, efficacy of which in breast cancer treatment has been established by multiple extensive trials. SERMs have differential actions in tissues based on differences in the downstream pathways that are stimulated via ER. They have anti-estrogenic effect in breast and stimulatory effect in uterus, cardio-vascular system, blood lipids and bones. Therefore, the SERMs help in improvement in bone mineral density through anti-resorptive action, decreasing risk of contralateral breast cancer, maintaining cardiac health, and maintaining a favorable cholesterol profile, but these increase the risk of endometrial carcinoma,

Table 1: Summary of commonly used class of hormone therapeutic agents, their mode of actions, and clinical usage.

Category of drug	Drugs	Mechanism of action	Specific indications	Side-effects	Recommended therapy monitoring
Selective estrogen receptor modulators (SERMs)	Tamoxifen Raloxifene Toremifene	Estrogen antagonists in breast tissue, partial agonists in bone, CVS, and uterus	Tamoxifen—First-line HT in premenopausal women with ER+ tumors, DCIS, IDC, as adjuvant therapy. HR+ MBC; Chemoprevention in high-risk women Raloxifene: Osteoporosis and chemoprevention	Hot flushes, thrombo-embolic events, and endometrial carcinoma	Monitor endometrial thickness (by pelvic or transvaginal USG)
Selective ER degraders (SERDs)	Fulvestrant	Irreversible down-regulation of ER	First or second line therapy in HR+ MBC, as monotherapy or in combination with CDK 5/6 inhibitors	Nausea, hot flushes, osteoporosis, depression, and leukopenia	Bone mineral densitometry at lumbar spine and hip (preferably by dual energy X-ray absorptiometry)
Aromatase Inhibitors (AIs, 3rd generation)	Anastrozole Letrozole Exemestane	Inhibition of enzyme Aromatase	First line adjuvant therapy in postmenopausal women with HR+ early and locally advanced breast cancer. Primary hormone therapy in low-risk asymptomatic MBC (in premenopausal women along with ovarian function suppression)	Osteoporosis, bone, and joints pain. Less commonly—hot flushes, thromboembolic events, depression, cardiotoxicity, and arrhythmias	Bone mineral densitometry at lumbar spine and hip (preferably by dual energy X-ray absorptiometry)

(CVS: cardiovascular system; CDK: cyclin-dependent kinase; DCIS: ductal carcinoma *in situ*; ER: estrogen receptor; HR+: hormone receptor positive; IDC: invasive ductal carcinoma; MBC: metastatic breast cancer; USG: ultrasonography) thrombo-embolic events, and menopausal symptoms. Monitoring with transvaginal ultrasonography for monitoring the endometrial thickness is required during the therapy. Tamoxifen needs to be activated to an active molecule by the cytochrome P450 (CYP450) enzyme. Various SERMs are fraught with cross-resistance unlike SERDs.[15]

The SERDs are steroidal molecules, bind with great affinity with ER, block dimerization, and degrade the receptors thus resulting in greater and lasting anti-estrogenic effect than SERMs. These do not carry risk of endometrial cancer and thrombo-embolic events but result in increased menopausal symptoms, depression, myalgias, and osteoporosis.

The AIs are the inhibitors of the enzyme aromatase (estrogen synthetase) that normally catalyze various steps in the conversion of the circulating androgens into estrogens by aromatization, mainly in the peripheral adipose tissue, which is the major source of estrogens in postmenopausal women. Three generations of AIs have been investigated for use in breast cancer, and currently the third generation AIs are being used. The first generation AIs are aminoglutethimide, which is a non-selective inhibitor and prevents adrenal steroid production. The second generation AIs include formestane, while the third generation AIs include anastrozole, letrozole (both non-steroidal AIs), and exemestane (steroidal and irreversible AI). All the three third generation AIs are currently in common use, and there is no definite evidence to suggest which of them is superior to the rest.

The LHRH agonists namely leuprolide and goserelin act by inhibiting pituitary production of LHRH. Initially, they upregulate LH and follicle stimulating hormone (FSH) by flare effect (cyclical or intermittent action), which is then followed by a down-regulation (via continuous action) through hypothalamus-pituitary and ovary axis. They cause temporary, incomplete, and reversible ovarian suppression.

COMMON SCENARIOS IN WHICH ENDOCRINE THERAPY IS USED IN BREAST CANCER PATIENTS

Hormone manipulations have been shown to be of benefit in all stages of breast cancers. Majority of patients with early stage cancers treated with curative intent who express ER and/or PR in the breast tumors are treated with adjuvant HT in form of tamoxifen or one of the AIs. These have been shown to be of great benefit in prolonging overall survival, which has been a consistent finding of numerous large trials. Patients with MBCs too benefit from HT. The role of HT in pre-operative or neoadjuvant systemic treatment is evolving, and this strategy seems to be of some promise for elderly HR+ breast cancer patients with locally advanced cancers, who are poor candidates for neoadjuvant chemotherapy.

Adjuvant Hormonal Therapy in Non-metastatic Breast Cancer

The main utility of HT is in adjuvant setting. According to 2014 ASCO update, patients with HR+ tumors of all stages irrespective of menopausal status need to be offered HT as a standard of care. St Gallen consensus statement too endorses the same view, and identifies age less than or equal to 35 years and/or involvement of 4 or more lymph nodes (LNs) as factors based on which ovarian function suppression (OFS) too should be advised. Tablet tamoxifen given in dosage of 20 mg once a day is the drug of choice in premenopausal women. In 1990s, tamoxifen was approved for adjuvant therapy after the landmark meta-analysis by EBCTCG (1988), which had shown that addition of tamoxifen for 5 years significantly reduces the risk of local and distant recurrence, risk of contralateral breast cancer, and improves disease free and overall survival. Adjuvant Tamoxifen usage results in 50% reduction in risk of local recurrence in the first 5 years and 30% in next 5 years compared to controls. The risk of death due to breast cancer is 30% lesser in tamoxifen group even after 15 years. This benefit is irrespective of the use of chemotherapy, age, menopausal status, and axillary LN status. A study published in 2017 reporting 20 years follow-up of patients treated with 5-years adjuvant Tamoxifen has shown that the risk of recurrence and death due to breast cancer persists even after 5 years and are strongly dependent on the initial nodal status. The risk of recurrence steadily increased over 20-year period, while the risk of death due to breast cancer was low in first 5 years and increased thereafter. Young age at diagnosis, initial Ki-67 index, grade, and HER2 status had influenced outcomes only in the first 5 years.

While the standard duration of adjuvant tamoxifen treatment remains 5 years in low risk cancers, the results of ATLAS (Adjuvant Tamoxifen: Longer Against Shorter) and AttoM (adjuvant Tamoxifen—To offer more?) trials have shown that the breast cancer recurrence rates were lower, albeit only marginally so, in 10 year treatment arm than 5 years of tamoxifen. However, NSABP B-14 and few other trials have not shown any significant benefit in the recurrence rates or overall survival with extended adjuvant Tamoxifen therapy. Based on these, it is now recommended that duration of HT may be extended to up to 10 years in patients with intermediate and high-risk, HR+ breast cancers.

Though tamoxifen has been in use in post-menopausal women with HR+ disease for many decades now, the AIs have become the standard of care after they were proven to be more efficacious than tamoxifen in either sequentially or as a primary therapy in the ATAC (Arimidex, Tamoxifen, Alone or in Combination) and BIG 1-98 (breast international group) trials. The AIs decrease recurrence rates by 30%, compared to 5 years of tamoxifen (EBCTCG 15) irrespective of nodal status. The combination therapy of tamoxifen and AIs has intolerable side-effects without any additional benefits, compared to the individual or sequential therapy. The time to recurrence (TTR) increased over 10 years follow-up and the recurrence rates remained low in AIs group after treatment completion, compared to tamoxifen group. AIs should not be used in premenopausal patients unless used along with ovarian suppression therapy. The BIG 1-98 trial also showed that AIs significantly increase the disease-free survival (DFS). Combined analysis of both trials showed decreased recurrence rates with statistically in-significant improvement in survival with AIs. The extended use of AIs more than 5 years is not proven to be beneficial in terms overall survival though there was improvement in DFS (MA.17R), or breast cancer free interval and distant recurrence rate (NSABP B-42) than 5 years of use. There has been no proven superiority of one AI over the other so far. The ASCO guidelines on adjuvant endocrine therapy for women with ER+ breast cancer recommend incorporating AI therapy at some point during adjuvant treatment, while recognizing that the optimal timing and duration of therapy remain unresolved questions. Also, postmenopausal women receiving AI should be evaluated with bone mineral density and should be advised to receive with calcium and vitamin D supplementation, and bisphosphonate use, if deemed necessary. The duration of AIs treatment should not exceed 5 years, except in setting of a clinical trial.

As per the results of meta-analysis of trials evaluating the switching from tamoxifen to AIs compared with tamoxifen alone [Intergroup Exemestane Study (IES), Austrian Breast and Colorectal Cancer Study Group (ABCSG 8), Arimidex-Nolvadex (ARNO 95) and Italian Tamoxifen Anastrozole (ITA) studies], switching to anastrozole resulted in a statistically significant improvement in DFS (HR 0.59, $p < 0.0001$), and reduction in breast cancer mortality and death from any cause (HR 0.71, $p = 0.037$). This may be relevant as there is known resistance to tamoxifen on long-term therapy in addition to its adverse effects after prolonged usage. Switching from tamoxifen to AIs, compared with upfront AI has been evaluated in BIG 1-98 and TEAM (Tamoxifen Exemestane Adjuvant Multinational) trials. There was no significant difference in disease-free recurrence, overall survival or time to distant recurrence between the switch or monotherapy arms. However, there were early relapses in letrozole alone compared with the switch arm especially among node-positive patients at 5 years. Meta-analysis has failed to identify the specific factors, which may help choose patients for switch or monotherapy, but the absolute levels of ER, PR, and HER 2 expression are being considered to base upon. So, clinicians should consider patient and tumor factors, the side-effects of individual treatment to decide optimal strategy in individual patients.

Ovarian Function Suppression in Premenopausal Women

Ovarian function suppression (OFS) either by LHRH agonists, surgery, or by radiation has been reviewed by EBCTCG. These results document decreased recurrence and mortality with ovarian suppression usage. The benefits of ovarian suppression is more evident in young pre-menopausal patients who have not been treated with chemotherapy. Results of SOFT (Suppression of Ovarian Function Trial) and TEXT (Tamoxifen and Exemestane Trial) trials have shown that ovarian suppression along with tamoxifen has better disease free survival than tamoxifen alone at 8 years of follow-up in premenopausal women. However, ovarian suppression with exemestane is still better than ovarian suppression with tamoxifen in terms of survival, though at the cost of increased adverse effects.[16] Combination therapy is no better than single-agent therapy (ATAC trial). Based on evidence from these trials, ASCO 2016 update has recommended use of OFS in premenopausal women with HR+ disease along with tamoxifen or AIs in stage II and III patients who are candidates for chemotherapy and higher risk patients, but not in lower risk ones of stage I cancers which do not warrant chemotherapy. It was found beneficial in patients younger than 35 years of age on subset analysis.

Another major change in practice for adjuvant systemic treatment of early stage breast cancer in recent years has come as a result of being able to individualize or tailor the treatment according to the genomic risk profile established by multigene expression profiling, such as Oncotype-Dx. We are now able to classify the tumors based on ER, PR, HER 2 and Ki-67 index or gene-expression profiling into luminal A and B, and further risk-group them based on recurrence score using Oncotype-Dx, thus trying to select patients to do away with adjuvant chemotherapy. The results of 21 gene recurrence score study [Trial Assigning IndividuaLized Options for Treatment Rx (TAILORx) study] using Oncotype Dx in HR+, node-negative patients suggest that if recurrence score is less than or equal to 10, hormone treatment alone is sufficient and if the recurrence score is more than 25, chemotherapy and HT both are recommended.

Hormone Therapy for Metastatic Breast Cancer

Metastatic breast cancers are treated with palliative intent by and large, with some exceptions in low-risk oligometastatic patients. A Cochrane review by Wilcken N, et al. in 2011 of randomized trials comparing HT and chemotherapy in MBC yielded inconclusive data. The choice of therapy should depend on, besides the HR status of the tumor, on the site of metastasis, burden of disease, and performance status or general condition of the patient. Primary intention is to have effective symptom palliation and maintenance or improvement in quality of life, besides achieving a reasonable control of disease progression where ever possible. Though there is no strong evidence to back it, there is a trend in HR+ MBC patients having relatively longer survival.

First-line therapy: recommended for HR+ MBC patients who are asymptomatic, and are not in visceral crisis is tamoxifen or a III generation nonsteroidal (letrozole and Anastrozole) or steroidal (exemestane) AIs. Tamoxifen was the preferred drug in the past due to its proven benefits over other drugs (high dose estrogens, progesterones, first generation AIs, toremifene, and LHRH analogs (goserelin), in terms of better side-effect profile with similar overall response rate and survival.[17] Third-generation AIs—both the nonsteroidal (Anastrozole and letrozole) and steroidal (exemestane)—have been shown to be more effective compared to tamoxifen in terms of clinical benefit, time to progression (TTP 10.7 vs 6.4 in tamoxifen group),[18] but overall survival benefit was seen with Anastrozole in only one randomized controlled trial (RCT) [17.4 months vs 16 months (HR 0.64, 95% CI 0.47-0.86, p = 0.003)].[19] Of course, premenopausal MBC patients planned to be treated with AIs will need to be on OFS too. Metanalyses have shown improved overall survival with third generation AIs as first-line therapy in MBC compared to other HT.[20] Studies comparing fulvestrant at 500 mg per month with tamoxifen showed non-inferiority of fulvestrant and no differences in OS between both.[21] A phase III RCT comparing fulvestrant with Anastrozole (FALCON-fulvestrant and anastrozole compared in hormone therapy naive advanced breast cancer) showed survival benefit- with fulvestrant.

Second-line therapy in patients who have failed or have progressed on first-line HT is based on the fact that there is no cross-resistance between AIs. AIs as first-line followed by tamoxifen as second-line on progression is proven to have longer TTP than *vice-versa*, in the TARGET (Tamoxifen or Arimidex randomized group efficacy and tolerability) trial.[22,23] Fulvestrant as a second line has been shown to be non-inferior to III generation AIs in the EFECT (Evaluation of Faslodex versus Exemestane clinical trial) trial. In short, if a third generation AI was being used as the first-line HT in a patient who now has a HR+ MBC, tamoxifen, or another AI can be used as a second-line as long as possible. Fulvestrant can be added to, or can replace AIs, if a patient has progressive, yet non-visceral metastatic disease.

Neoadjuvant Hormone Therapy

A large proportion of patients with large operable and locally advanced breast cancers are treated with neoadjuvant or pre-operative systemic treatment to reduce the volume of the disease in breast and axilla, to make an inoperable cancer operable, and to render a non-conservable breast conservable. The neoadjuvant systemic therapy strategy is now being extended to a large proportion of early stage cancers too (mostly T2/ N0-2), in an effort to reduce the extent of breast (lower volume excision) and axillary [sentinel lymph node (SLN) rather than axillary lymph node dissection (ALND)] surgery. A meta-analysis[24] by Leal, et al. concluded that neoadjuvant chemotherapy (NACT) in inoperable breast cancer patients is better than neoadjuvant HT (NAHT) in premenopausal women in achieving overall response rate. Accordingly,

NACT is preferable in fit premenopausal patients for the lack of evidence for the benefits of NAHT. However, NAHT may be equivalent to NACT in postmenopausal, especially elderly patients with multiple comorbidities. AIs are preferred over tamoxifen due to better clinical response rates (CRR), and a combination of AIs and tamoxifen is no better than AIs alone [Immediate pre-operative anastrozole, tamoxifen, or combined with tamoxifen (IMPACT) trial]. The pathological complete response (pCR)-is low with any form of HT in HR+ tumors. A meta-analyses[25] in 2016 by LM Spring, et al. revealed that there is no difference between NACT and NAHT (using AIs) in clinical, radiological response rate (RRR), and breast conservation rates, with better toxicity profile in NAHT in post-menopausal HR+ elderly breast cancer patients. There is no difference among the AIs in terms of RRR.

Dual therapy using NAHT with additional agents like everolimus, celecoxib, zoledronic acid, and gefitinib has shown no difference in CRR, however, inconsistent better RRR has been reported. Against the classical notion that HT cannot be combined with chemotherapy, a trial has shown better CRR and pCR with addition of HT to NACT. Given the therapeutic success seen in the metastatic setting with the combination of endocrine therapy and cyclin-dependent kinase (CDK) 4/6 inhibition, it is also being investigated as a neoadjuvant therapy (LORELEI and PALLET trials). There is insufficient data on criteria for selection of appropriate patients for NAHT. Few studies have used Ki-67 index assessment during the NAHT to switch over to NACT [Alliance for Clinical Trials in Oncology cooperative group has designed a phase III neoadjuvant clinical (ALTERNATE)]. The current indications for use of NAHT are postmenopausal women, especially medically frail, and even the fit women with strongly ER or PR positive; HER-2 neu negative tumors, lobular carcinomas, either large operable breast cancers or locally advanced breast cancers or otherwise unfit for primary surgery. The duration of therapy, though somewhat arbitrarily is usually for 3-4 months or up to 6 months after a combined decision is made by a multidisciplinary team in discussion with the patient.

RESISTANCE TO HORMONAL THERAPY

Breast tumors show heterogeneity in expression of ER within different areas of tumors as well as circulating tumor cells showing positivity and negativity for ER staining.[13] So, Allred score uses percentage and intensity of staining of ER to give the final score. The response of HR+ tumors to the HT may vary over a period of time, owing to resistance to the drug. The pathways of resistance can be multiple, and include those that result in either decreased expression of HRs or by overexpression of cell cycle regulators like cyclin or CDK or PI3K or AKT or mammalian target of rapamycin (mTOR) or other growth factor receptor pathways.[26] For example, increased expression of amplified in breast cancer 1 (AIB1) protein correlates with tamoxifen resistance as this protein expression contributes to the agonistic activity of tamoxifen (rather than antagonism). Metabolites of tamoxifen are its physiologically active form, and have higher potency than tamoxifen itself. Alteration in CYP450 enzymes may result in failure or reduced tamoxifen metabolism, thus decreasing the efficacy of tamoxifen.[27,28] Few investigators claim that by studying fluorescence resonance energy transfer (FRET) analysis,[29] by directly monitoring conformational changes of ER(alpha) upon antiestrogen binding, the mechanisms of developing resistance by the antiestrogens can be known and thus may help in selection of a type of antiestrogen in a given patient. Recent studies have shown the prevalence of recurrent ESR1 mutations by next-generation sequencing which may play an important role in acquired endocrine therapy resistance.[30] Addition of certain other therapeutic molecules may help circumvent some of such problems.

OTHER STRATEGIES OF MANAGING HR+ BREAST CANCERS—CDK 4/6 INHIBITORS

As the resistance to HT may alter other cell cycle pathways, therapy directed against downstream cell cycle pathways and proteins may help to circumvent this problem. This was addressed in the PALOMA 3 [Palbociclib (PD-0332991) Combined With Fulvestrant In Hormone Receptor+ HER2-Negative Metastatic Breast Cancer After Endocrine Failure)—a phase III, prospective, randomized, double-blind, and placebo-controlled trial done in postmenopausal, treatment naïve HR+, HER2 negative MBC patients who had progressed on previous endocrine therapy, of fulvestrant with or without palbociclib (a CDK 4/6 inhibitor) plus or minus goserelin (required for premenopausal or perimenopausal participants). PALOMA-3 results revealed that the combination of palbociclib with HT improves the progression free survival significantly in these patients, irrespective of the type of endocrine therapy previously used in these patients.[31] The US Food and Drug Administration (FDA) approved palbociclib for use in combination with letrozole. The ASCO guidelines 2016 incorporated use of fulvestrant as a second-line therapy with or without palbociclib in these patients. Similarly, MONALEESA 2 [Mammary Oncology Assessment of LEE011's (Ribociclib's) Efficacy and Safety] trial assessed use of another CDK4/6 inhibitor-ribociclib, and found improved progression free survival in combination with letrozole than letrozole monotherapy.[32] The CDK 4/6 inhibitors are reasonably well tolerated, with neutropenia, QT prolongation being their important adverse effects. Abemaciclib is another molecule under investigation in phase I or II trials at present. How to choose a patient who can safely be started on AIs alone or in combination with CDK 4/6 inhibitors is matter of research. These are used in metastatic disease mainly to bones or if at all limited visceral disease.

EMERGING HORMONE THERAPIES

Newer, more efficacious hormone therapeutic agents with greater safety profile compared to the currently in-use drugs are an attractive area of active current research. Newer SERDs, such as the investigational molecule GDC-0810 are under evaluation to circumvent the need to administer fulvestrant deep intramuscular and its poor bioavailability. Combination therapies of AIs with molecules like bevacizumab, newer molecules like phosphoinositide 3-kinase inhibitors (e.g. buparlisib), strategies like combining anti-androgens with anti-estrogens are underway in phase I or II trials.

SUMMARY

Hormonal therapy in breast cancer is an extremely useful option that can improve outcomes in HR expressing breast cancer patients with relatively milder adverse effect profile. The indications for HT include its use in the adjuvant, metastatic, and neoadjuvant settings. The importance of HT is ever-increasing, with more acceptance of the fact that chemotherapy can be avoided in patients with suitable genomic risk profile, in whom HT alone may suffice. This is one area where the research has been able to de-escalate treatment rather than making it more and more intensive and toxic, as new information has emerged. Present time HT in HR+ breast cancer patients thus extends beyond the current standard of care tamoxifen, AIs, or ovarian function suppression, and incorporates strategies which utilize synergism of anti-estrogenic effects of these drugs with down-regulation of downstream cell cycle pathways, such as use of CDK4/6 inhibitors. Further research is underway to understand the resistance patterns, rescue therapies, and strategies for better adverse effect profile.

REFERENCES

1. Love RR, Philips J. Oophorectomy for breast cancer: history revisited. J Natl Cancer Inst. 2002;94(19):1433-4.
2. Moore DD. A Conversation with Elwood Jensen. Ann Rev Physiol. 2012;74(1):1-11.
3. Laudet V, Gronemeyer H. The Nuclear Receptor FactsBook [Internet]. London: Academic Press; 2002.
4. Dunnwald LK, Rossing MA, Li CI. Hormone receptor status, tumor characteristics, and prognosis: a prospective cohort of breast cancer patients. Breast Cancer Res. 2007;9(1):R6.

5. Althuis MD, Fergenbaum JH, Garcia-Closas M, et al. Etiology of hormone receptor-defined breast cancer: a systematic review of the literature. Cancer Epidemiol Biomarkers Prev. 2004;13(10):1558-68.
6. Ursin G, Henderson BE, Haile RW, et al. Does oral contraceptive use increase the risk of breast cancer in women with BRCA1/BRCA2 mutations more than in other women? Cancer Res. 1997;57(17):3678-81.
7. Hall JM, Couse JF, Korach KS. The multifaceted mechanisms of estradiol and estrogen receptor signaling. J Biol Chem. 2001;276(40):36869-72.
8. Williams C, Lin CY. Oestrogen receptors in breast cancer: basic mechanisms and clinical implications. Ecancermedicalscience. 2013;7:370.
9. Shaaban AM, O'Neill PA, Davies MPA, et al. Declining estrogen receptor-beta expression defines malignant progression of human breast neoplasia. Am J Surg Pathol. 2003;27(12):1502-12.
10. Yaşar P, Ayaz G, User SD, et al. Molecular mechanism of estrogen-estrogen receptor signaling. Reprod Med Biol. 2017;16(1):4-20.
11. Hammond MEH, Hayes DF, Wolff AC, et al. American Society of Clinical Oncology/College of American pathologists guideline recommendations for immunohistochemical testing of estrogen and progesterone receptors in breast cancer. J Oncol Pract. 2010;6(4):195-7.
12. Badve SS, Baehner FL, Gray RP, et al. Estrogen- and progesterone-receptor status in ECOG 2197: comparison of immunohistochemistry by local and central laboratories and quantitative reverse transcription polymerase chain reaction by central laboratory. J Clin Oncol. 2008;26(15):2473-81.
13. Clarke R, Tyson JJ, Dixon JM. Endocrine resistance in breast cancer: an overview and update. Molecular and Cellular Endocrinology. 2015;418(Pt 3): 220-34.
14. Van Asten K, Slembrouck L, Olbrecht S, et al. Prognostic value of the progesterone receptor by subtype in patients with estrogen receptor-positive, HER-2 negative breast cancer. Oncologist. 2018; pii:theoncologist.2018-0176.
15. Patel HK, Bihani T. Selective estrogen receptor modulators (SERMs) and selective estrogen receptor degraders (SERDs) in cancer treatment. Pharmacol Ther. 2018;186:1-24.
16. Francis PA, Pagani O, Fleming GF, et al. Tailoring adjuvant endocrine therapy for premenopausal breast cancer. N Engl J Med. 2018;379(2):122-37.
17. Fossati R, Confalonieri C, Torri V, et al. Cytotoxic and hormonal treatment for metastatic breast cancer: a systematic review of published randomized trials involving 31,510 women. J Clin Oncol. 1998;16(10):3439-60.
18. Nabholtz JM, Buzdar A, Pollak M, et al. Anastrozole is superior to tamoxifen as first-line therapy for advanced breast cancer in postmenopausal women: results of a North American multicenter randomized trial. Arimidex Study Group. J Clin Oncol. 2000;18(22):3758-67.
19. Milla-Santos A, Milla L, Portella J, et al. Anastrozole versus tamoxifen as first-line therapy in postmenopausal patients with hormone-dependent advanced breast cancer: a prospective, randomized, phase III study. Am J Clin Oncol. 2003;26(3):317-22.

20. Gibson L, Lawrence D, Dawson C, et al. Aromatase inhibitors for treatment of advanced breast cancer in postmenopausal women. Cochrane Database Syst Rev. 2009;(4):CD003370.
21. Howell A, Robertson JFR, Abram P, et al. Comparison of Fulvestrant Versus Tamoxifen for the Treatment of Advanced Breast Cancer in Postmenopausal Women Previously Untreated With Endocrine Therapy: A Multinational, Double-Blind, Randomized Trial. J Clin Oncol. 2004;22(9):1605-13.
22. Thürlimann B, Hess D, Köberle D, et al. Anastrozole ('Arimidex') versus tamoxifen as first-line therapy in postmenopausal women with advanced breast cancer: Results of the double-blind cross-over SAKK trial 21/95: a sub-study of the TARGET (Tamoxifen or 'Arimidex' Randomized Group Efficacy and Tolerability) trial. Breast Cancer Res Treat. 2004;85(3):247-54.
23. Bertelli G, Garrone O, Merlano M, et al. Sequential treatment with exemestane and non-steroidal aromatase inhibitors in advanced breast cancer. Oncology. 2005;69(6):471-7.
24. Leal F, Liutti VT, Antunes dos Santos VC, et al. Neoadjuvant endocrine therapy for resectable breast cancer: A systematic review and meta-analysis. Breast. 2015;24(4):406-12.
25. Spring LM, Gupta A, Reynolds KL, et al. Neoadjuvant Endocrine Therapy for Estrogen Receptor-Positive Breast Cancer: A Systematic Review and Meta-analysis. JAMA Oncol. 2016;2(11):1477-86.
26. Hayes EL, Lewis-Wambi JS. Mechanisms of endocrine resistance in breast cancer: an overview of the proposed roles of noncoding RNA. Breast Cancer Res. 2015;17:40.
27. Mittal B, Tulsyan S, Kumar S, et al. Cytochrome P450 in Cancer susceptibility and treatment. Adv Clin Chem. 2015;71:77-139.
28. Agarwal G, Tulsyan S, Lal P, et al. Generalized Multifactor dimensionality reduction (GMDR) analysis of drug-metabolizing enzyme-encoding gene polymorphisms may predict treatment outcomes in Indian breast cancer patients. World J Surg. 2016;40(7):1600-10.
29. Zwart W, Griekspoor A, Rondaij M, et al. Classification of antiestrogens according to intramolecular FRET effects on phospho-mutants of estrogen receptor α. Mol Cancer Ther. 2007;6(5):1526-30.
30. Alluri PG, Speers C, Chinnaiyan AM. Estrogen receptor mutations and their role in breast cancer progression. Breast Cancer Res. 2014;16(6):494.
31. Cristofanilli M, Turner NC, Bondarenko I, et al. Fulvestrant plus palbociclib versus fulvestrant plus placebo for treatment of hormone-receptor-positive, HER2-negative metastatic breast cancer that progressed on previous endocrine therapy (PALOMA-3): final analysis of the multicentre, double-blind, phase 3 randomised controlled trial. Lancet Oncol. 2016;17(4):425-39.
32. Hortobagyi GN, Stemmer SM, Burris HA, et al. Ribociclib as first-line therapy for HR-positive, advanced breast cancer. N Eng J Med. 2016;375(18):1738-48.

Index

Page numbers followed by *b* refer to box, *f* refer to figure,
fc refer to flowchart, and *t* refer to table.

A

Abdomen
  plain X-ray 93
  regions 223
  reveals encapsulation 171
  ultrasonography of 94
Abdominal
  carcinomatosis, treatment of 231
  compartment syndrome 56
  distension 91
  lymphadenopathy 179
  pain 91, 172
  tuberculosis 97, 165
Abemaciclib 292
Ablation
  techniques 38
  therapies 38, 207
Acetic acid 114
Acid-fast bacilli 172
Acquired immunodeficiency syndrome 172
Actinomycin D 241
Adenocarcinoma 109, 193
  risk of 116
Adenosine
  deaminase 179
  triphosphate 240
Adrenal gland
  ipsilateral 204, 205
  removal of 205
Adriamycin 5-fluorouracil 273
Agarose gel electrophoresis 175
Alkylating agents 220
American College of Chest Physicians 146
American College of Gastroenterology 116
American Diabetes Association 179
American Joint Committee on Cancer 202
American Society of Clinical Oncology 76, 245, 283
American Society of Colon and Rectal Surgeons 76
Americas Hepato-Pancreato-Biliary Association 30
Amikacin 182
Amyloidosis 199
Anastomotic stricture 90
Anastrozole 286, 288, 290
Anemia 199
Angioembolization 204, 210
  bone of 210
  role of 208
Angiogenesis 37, 249, 274, 275
Angiosarcoma 246
Anomalous pancreaticobiliary ductal junction 57
Anthracyclines 241, 273, 274
Antiangiogenic agent 245
Antibiogram 53
Anti-epidermal growth factor receptor, case of 244
Antiestrogen
  drug 281
  type of 292
Antiproliferative activity 274
Antireflux surgery 118
Anti-resorptive action 284
Antiretroviral therapy 182
Antitubercular
  drugs 181
  treatment 169
Apoptosis 23
Appendiceal mucinous neoplasm 221
Appendiceal origin 219, 233
Appendix 8

Argon
    beam coagulator 13
    plasma coagulation 119, 121
    pumped dye laser 20
Arimidex-nolvadex 288
Aromatic amino acids 115
Aromatization 286
Arterial
    hemorrhage 54
    oxygen, partial pressure of 48
Arteriovenous fistula 263
Arteriovenous malformation 249, 253, 255, 256
    clinical staging system for 254t
    rapid progression of 254
    therapy of 263
Ascariasis 90
    obstruction due to 98
Ascites
    high density 177
    malignant 230
Ascitic fluid 172
    analysis 179
Aspergilloma, cases of complex 152
Aspirin 123
Atezolizumab 275
Atlanta classification 48
Atrial flutter, recurrent 22
Atrial tachycardia 22
    multifocal 22
Austrian Breast and Colorectal Cancer Study Group 288
Autofluorescence 115
Autosonix system 16
Axillary lymph node 272
    dissection 290
Axitinib 213

B

Bacillus Calmette-Guérin vaccination 173
Back pain, chronic lower 22
Bacteria, mucosal translocation of 92
Bacterial translocation 172
Balloon-diffusing fibers 122
Bannayan-Rilay-Ruvalcaba syndrome 256
Barium meal 169f
Barium studies 176b
Barrett's esophagus 108

advanced imaging for 114
clinical features 110
diagnosis 110
endoscopic image of 111f
epidemiology 108
histological diagnosis 111
management 116
natural history of disease 109
risk factors 109
role of biomarkers 113
screening guidelines for 116
therapy of 117
treatment of 120t
trials 113, 114
Vienna classification for 112t
Basal-like breast cancer 270
Bedaquiline 186
Belmont hyperthermia pump 228f
Bevacizumab 37, 38, 75, 212, 274, 275, 293
Biophysics 5
Bipolar current, effects red area 12f
Bipolar electrosurgery 11
    modified 15
Birt-Hogg-Dubé syndrome 194
Bladder catheter 57
Blebectomy for pneumothorax 149
Bleomycin 210, 262
Blood brain barrier 241
Blue rubber bleb nevus syndrome 251, 259
Body and tail lesions 133
Body mass index 109, 116
Bone tumors 24
Bowel
    decompression, role of 96
    edema 91, 94
    hypoperfusion 93
    ischemia ensues 91
    large 93
    obstruction: small and large, clinical features of 92t
    small 93
Brachiocephalic vein 156
Brachytherapy 75
BRCA mutant tumors 276
Breast cancer
    free interval 288
    hormone therapy for 280
        antiestrogen therapy in 282

emerging 293
endocrine therapy, used in 286
estrogen exposure as a risk-factor 282
evolution of 281
hormone receptor positivit 283
modalities of 284
resistance to 291
CDK 4/6 inhibitors 292
large proportion of 280
major molecular subtypes of 269*t*
mammographic diagnosis of 271
molecular classification of 268
progesterone receptors in 283
quadruple-negative 276
resistance protein 241
TNM staging 269
triple-negative 268-276
concept of 276
imaging studies 271
immunotherapy 275
natural history of 271
prevalence of 270
prognosis of 272
radiotherapy in 275
surgery in 272
synonymous with basal-like breast cancer 270
targeted therapy in 273
treatment in 272
Breast conserving surgery 272
Breast tumors 281
British Society of Gastroenterology 111
British Thoracic Society 182
Bronchial blocker 150
Bronchogenic cyst 149
Bullectomy 149

C

Cabozantinib 213
Cachexia 199
Cancer
Care Ontario 76
related intestinal obstruction, management of 101
specific mortality 205
specific survival 210
stem cells 244
war on 246
Candida species 53

Capacitive coupling 6
Capecitabine 74, 274, 276
plus oxaliplatin 38
Capillary
arteriovenous malformation 255
lymphatic-arteriovenous malformation 255
lymphaticovenous malformation 255
malformation 249, 252, 254, 255, 256
therapy of 262
Capsule endoscopy 178
Carbohydrate antigen 19-9 130
Carbon dioxide, partial pressure of 46
Carboplatin 242, 273, 274
versus docetaxel 273
Carcinoembryonic antigen 28, 65, 77
Cardiac defibrillation 3
Cardiac-specific mortality 206
Cardiovascular system 284, 285
Cavitational
fragmentation 17
ultrasonic aspirating device 17
Cecal, management of 100
Cecostomy 104
Cecum, head of 67
Celiac plexus neurolysis 141
Cell adhesion-mediated drug resistance 243
Cell death 24
receptor-ligand-1 244
Central caseous necrosis 180
Central nervous system, metastases 268
Cerebral cavernous malformation 251
Certain familial syndromes 192
Cetuximab 37, 38, 76
multidisciplinary concept 37
Chemical photosensitizer 262
Chemoprevention 123
agents, role of 124
Chemoradiotherapy
after initial chemotherapy 140
neoadjuvant 135, 136, 290
Chemoresistant
cancers, treatment of 246
cells 244
clones 244
Chemotherapy 36
adjuvant intraperitoneal and systemic 229

by killing chemosensitive clones 244
early postoperative intraperitoneal
    229
intraoperative HIPEC plus
    intravenous 229
neoadjuvant intraperitoneal plus
    intravenous 228
pharmacokinetic properties of 239
Chest wall invasion 150
Chicken intestine 176
Cholangitis 135
    incidence of 141
Cholecystectomy 57, 226
Chorioretinopathy 253
Chromoendoscopy 114
Cisplatin 241, 242, 273, 274
Cisplatinum 210, 273
Clinical Outcomes of Surgical Therapy
    trial 77
Clinical risk score 36
Clonal evolution 244
Clots, removal of 97
Cold spray anesthetics 24
Colectomies 226
Collagen, presence of 115
College of American Pathologists 283
Colo Rectal Endoscopic Stenting trial 73
Colon cancer
    adjuvant and neoadjuvant therapy
        74
    approach to patients with metastatic
        disease 73
    computed tomography of chest 64
    differences between right-and left-
        sided 63t
    disseminated to ovaries 229
    epidemiology, changing trends 62
    involving adjacent organs 229
    low anastomotic leak rate in right 71
    management of 62
    ongoing research impact future
        practice 78
    open versus laparoscopic surgery for
        69
    preoperative
        investigations 63
        management 65
    role for
        positron emission tomography 64
        radiation therapy in 75
    surgery for 66
    surveillance 76
    use of monoclonal antibodies 76
Colon head, ascending of 67
Colonic
    decompression 104
    lesions 171
    obstruction 90
    resection 74
    stenting 101
Colonography 63
Colonoscopic 179
    decompression 104
Colonoscopy 223
    versus computed tomography
        colonography 63
Colorectal
    cancer 27
        investigation to detect 63
        metastatic 27
        screening down 62
    liver metastases 64
        defining resectability 30
        factors influencing the treatment
            strategy 30
        lesions 28
        majority of 27
        management of 27
        MRI 29f
        surgical management of 30
    malignancy 90
    surgery 98
Compensatory anti-inflammatory
    response syndrome 46
Confocal laser endomicroscopy 114
    probe-based 115
Conglomerate mass 172
Constipation 92
Contrast-enhanced computed
    tomography 28, 43
Coregulators 282
Corneal burn 21
Cough 199
Coupling
    capacitive 9, 10f, 11
    direct 9, 9f
C-reactive protein 151
Crohn's disease 90, 97, 102, 169, 178,
    183
Cryoablation 119, 207

Cryotherapy 23, 24, 121
    uses of 24
Crystal violet 114
Current density 4
Cyclic vomiting syndrome 47
Cyclin-dependent kinase 285, 291
Cyclophosphamide 273
Cystic masses 200
Cystitis 184
Cystoduodenostomy 50
Cystogastrostomy 50
Cytochrome P450 enzymes 241
Cytokeratin 223
Cytoreductive nephrectomy 209, 210
Cytoreductive surgery 220, 223, 225
Cytoreductive surgery and HIPEC
    complications of 230
    contraindications to 230
    indications for the combined
        treatment 229
    role of 231
Cytosponge: trefoil factor-3 113

D

Debulking
    procedure 73
    surgery 219
Deep vein thromboembolism 66
Dehydrated alcohol 141
Demodulated currents 7
Deoxyribonucleic acid 242
    damage repair 242
Depression 286
Diaphragmatic
    pinch 110
    plication 149
Diatrizoate meglumine 94
Diatrizoate sodium 94
Diffusion weighted images 221
Dihydropyrimidine dehydrogenase 78
Dilated small bowel loops 175
Disease-free survival 288
    benefit 74
Disease-specific survival 36
Distal gastrectomy 226
Distal pancreatectomy 138
    pancreaticoduodenectomy 54
Diverticulitis 90
DNA crosslinking agents 276
Docetaxel 274

Double balloon enteroscopic 103, 178
Double wall sign 93
Doxorubicin 211, 225, 240, 242, 262
Drug delivery system 78
Drug-eluting beads preloaded with
        irinotecan 38
Drug resistance
    in cancer 239
        chemotherapy sensitivity 245
        different mechanisms of 240
        looking into future 246
        mechanisms of 240f
        overcoming resistance:
            challenging present dogmas
            245
        principles of 239
        reaching the moon 246
        tumor microenvironment 243
    strains 186
    tumor subpopulation 240
Drug sensitivity test 173
Ductal carcinoma in situ 285
Duodenal mobilization 100
Duodenojejunostomy 100
Duodenum, head of 67
Dysfunctional apoptosis 240, 243
Dyspepsia, symptoms of 168
Dysphagia detect 116
Dysplasia 111
    high-grade 118
    indefinite for 119
    low-grade 112f, 118
Dyspnea 199

E

Early Breast Cancer Trialists'
        Collaborative Group 281
Eastern Cooperative Oncology Group
        139
Efavirenz 182
Elective colonic resection 72
Electrocautery 3
Electrolyte imbalance 92
Electrosurgery 2
    in laparoscopic applications, use of
        13
    recent technological advances in 13
    use of 7
Electrosurgical
    device 9, 17

generator units 4
pencil works 3
Embolization technique 263
Embolotherapy 263
Emesis 91
Emphysema and lung volume reduction surgery 158
Empyema, early stage 152
Enchondroma 256
Endobronchial suction 150
Endocytosis 240
Endogenous biological substances 115
Endometrial carcinoma, risk of 284
Endopelvic fascia 66
Endoprosthesis 22
Endoscopic
  ablative therapies 119
  biopsy 169
  diagnosis 110
  mucosal resection 122
  resection 122-123
  retrograde pancreatography 134
  submucosal dissection 122-123
  transgastric and transduodenal drainage 50
  ultrasonography 52, 131
  ultrasound- fine-needle aspiration 179
Endoscopy 178, 223
  findings surveillance 120
Endosuturing 159
Endotracheal intubation, introduction of 149
Endotracheal tube 150
Endovascular treatment 263
Endovenous
  laser ablation 260
  radiofrequency ablation 260
Energy sources, different 17f
Enhanced recovery after surgery protocols 65
Enteral stents for colonic obstruction 73
Enterobacteriaceae 53
Enterococcus 53
Enterocutaneous fistula 181, 183
Enteroliths 90
Enterovesical fistula 184
Enzyme aromatase, inhibitors of 286
Epidermal growth factor receptor 37, 76, 283

Epigastric pain 110, 130
Epilepsy 255
Epipodophyllotoxins 241
Epirubicin 273
Epithelial
  appendix cancer 233
  mesenchymal transition to 243
  ovarian cancer 234
Epithelioid 233
  tubercles 166
  variants 234
Eribulin 276
Erlotinib 140, 241, 244
Erythrocyte sedimentation rate 199
Erythropoietin 212
Esophageal
  leiomyoma enucleation 149
  premalignant lesion 24
Esophagectomies 159
Esophagectomy 117, 149
  in esophageal cancer 153
Esophagus 146, 149
Estrogen receptor-mediated
  membrane signaling 283
  mitochondrial 283
  nuclear signaling 283
Estrogen response elements 282
Estrogen synthetase 286
Ethambutol 165, 181, 182
Ethanols 263
Ethylene-vinyl-alcohol-copolymer 263
European Institute of Oncology 269
European Organisation for Research and Treatment of Cancer 37
Everolimus 214, 275
Excimer laser, uses of 21
Exemestane trial 289
Extracellular stroma 243
Extraintestinal structures, obstruction of 55

F

Familial leiomyomatosis 194
Fecal
  impaction 90
  tagging, use of 64
Fecaluria 184
Fibrin degradation product 47
Fimbrial 8
Finney's strictureplasty 183

Fistulography 184
Flank mass 199
Fludeoxyglucose 131
Fluid resuscitation 95
Fluorescence
   in-situ hybridization 175
   resonance energy transfer 292
Fluorescent nanoparticles 78
Fluorodeoxyglucose 29*f*
   positron emission tomography 65
Fluorophores 115
   differential amounts of 115
Fluoroquinolones 182
Folinic acid plus either irinotecan 36
Follicle stimulating hormone 286
Football sign 93
Forced vital capacity 151
Foreign material 97
Fraction of inspired oxygen 48
Fuhrman's grading 198, 214
Fulguration 5
   maximum pause in 5
Fulminant hepatitis 182
Fulvestrant 290
Fundoplication partial 118

G

Gallstone ileus 90
Galvanic current 3
Ganglia 141
Gastric
   cancer, recurrent 219
   emptying 66
   folds, proximal margin of 110
   outlet obstruction 168
Gastroduodenal artery 137
Gastroesophageal junction 108
Gastroesophageal reflux disease 108, 116
Gastrointestinal
   obstruction 47, 55
   tract, mucosal layer of 166
   tuberculosis, cases of 180
Gastrojejunostomy 100, 135
Gastroparesis 66
Gefitinib 241, 244
Gelatinous ascites 233
Gemcitabine 134, 135, 140, 210, 211, 273
   monotherapy 139
Gene expression pattern 269

Germline mutations 109
Gerota's fascia 204, 205
Gland, tail of 49
Glaucoma 255
Glissonian capsule removal 226
Glomuvenous malformation 251
Glutathione S-transferase 242
Gonadotropin releasing hormone 284
Goose neck deformity 176
Gorham stout syndrome 256
Goserelin 286, 290
Granulomatous ailment, chronic 165
Granulomatous inflammation 166, 177, 180
Greater omentum 220
Ground pad failures 6
Growth factor receptor pathways 291

H

Harmonic scalpel 16
Hartmann's procedure 71, 100, 101
Heineke-Mikulicz technique 183
Hemangioendothelioma 250
Hemangioma 250
Hemangiopericytoma 250
Hematemesis 110
Hematogenous
   dissemination 166
   spread to lungs 198
Hematoporphyrin derivative 20
Hemidiaphragm
   left 226
   right 226
Hemiparesis, form of 255
Hemodialysis 192
Hemodynamic instability 183
Hemoptysis 199
Hemorrhagic shock, acute 54
Hemostasis 6, 14
Hepatic parenchyma, sparing partial hepatectomy 32
Hepatic resection, technical aspects of 32
Hepatocellular carcinoma 24
Hepatoduodenal ligament, involvement of 226
Hepatosplenomegaly 177
Hereditary lymphedema, primary 253
Hereditary type papillary 194

Hernia
   internal, management of 97
   obstructed 96
Holmium laser 20
Holmium:Yag laser 21
Homeobox transcription factor 223
Homogeneous collection 49
Hormone
   receptor positive 280, 285
   replacement therapy 282
   therapeutic agents and clinical usage 285t
   therapy
      adjuvant 287
      neoadjuvant 290
Host immune components 211
Hounsfield units 200
Hour-glass stenosis 176
Human epidermal growth factor receptor 2 268, 284
Human immunodeficiency virus 165
Hyaluronate carboxymethylcellulose 98
Hydro-dissection 21
Hydrophilic nontoxic metabolite conjugates 242
Hydroxy-progesterone caproate 284
Hyperbaric oxygen therapy 97
Hypercalcemia 199
Hyperglycemia 48, 214
Hyperhidrosis 158
Hypersegmentation of barium column 176
Hypertension 192, 199
Hyperthermia 225
   induced tissue changes 1
Hyperthermic
   intraperitoneal chemotherapy 220, 223
      rationale of 225
      various techniques of 226
   solution 226
Hypertrichosis-lymphedema-telangiectasia 253
Hypocalcemia 48
Hypodense
   areas in around organ 177
   lesions on portvenous phase 28
Hypofractionated 210
Hypokalemia 92
Hypophosphatemia 214
Hypoplastic deep veins 255

I

Iatrogenic factors 192
Ileocecal 182
   region 176, 183
Ileorectal anastomosis 101
Ileostomy 71
Ileotransverse bypass is reserved 71
Imatinib resistance mutation analysis 245
Immune system 244
Immunoglobulin G4 57
Immunohistochemical staining 221, 283
Immunohistochemistry 193
Immunological factors 211
Immunomodulatory properties 211
Immunotherapy 210, 277
   strategies, newer 211
Indigo carmine 114
Indocyanine green 159
Infected pancreatic necrosis 52
Inflammation, acute 97
Inflammatory bowel disease 90, 102, 179
Infraclavicular nodes 272
Infrared: near, advantages of 78
Infundibulopelvic 8
Iniparib 274, 275
Insulation failure 7
Insulin-like growth factor 1 283
Intensive care unit 47, 151
Interaortocaval lymph nodes 198
Interferon-gamma release assay 173
Interferons 211
Intergroup Exemestane Study 288
Interleukin-2 211
International Society for the Study of Vascular Anomalies classification 250t
International Society of Urological Pathology 198
International Study Group of Pancreatic Surgery 135
International Union for Cancer Control 202
Interstitial edematous pancreatitis 43
Intestinal
   metaplasia 121
   obstruction 89, 181
      accuracy of diagnosis of 93

causes of 90*t*
choice of surgical procedures 101
classification of 89
clinical manifestations 91
diagnosis 92
large 92
management of 89, 95
pathophysiology 91
role of laparoscopy in
management of 102
signs of 92
small 92
tuberculosis 175
ulcers 181
Intestine
non-viable 97
viable 97
Intra-abdominal adhesions
common causes of 97
grades of 90*t*
Intra-abdominal free fluid 178
Intracranial components 255
Intractable diarrhea 138
Intramucosal cancer 108, 112, 116
Intraperitoneal chemotherapy
regimens, types of 228
role of 220
use of 220
Intraperitoneal viscera 219
Intratumoral signal intensity 272
Intussusception 90
Invasive ductal carcinoma 285
Inverted umbrella sign 176
Irinotecan 36
Ironoxide nanocrystal contrast agent in MRI 78
Ischemia 23, 24
presence of 92
Isolated and grounded generator system 4
Isoniazid 165, 181, 182
Italian Tamoxifen Anastrozole 88
Ixabepilone 273

J

Japanese Society for Cancer of the Colon and Rectum 67
Jaundice 199
obstructive 134
Jejunal obstruction 55

K

Kinase receptor inhibitor 213
Kirsten rat sarcoma wild-type 38
Klebsiella 53
Klippel-Trenaunay syndrome 255, 256, 259
K-ras 73
Krukenberg tumor 230

L

Lactate dehydrogenase 93, 200
Laparoscopic
necrosectomy 54
procedures 15
surgery 6, 9, 24
oncological safety of 70, 79
use in 5
versus open colon cancer surgery 77
versus robotic surgery 70
Large intestine 10
Laser 18
beam, methods of release of 19
biophysical, principles of 19
generation, method of 18
properties of commonly used 9*t*
therapy 262
tissue interaction 20
unique properties of 18
Laxatives overuse 103
Letrozole 286, 288, 290
Leucovorin 36, 74
Leukemia 241
Leuprolide 286
Ligasure
instruments 15
vessel sealing system 15
Light Amplification through Stimulated Emission of Radiation 18
Liposomal 273
Liquefactive necrosis 166
Liver
abscess 184
first approach, systemic chemotherapy 32
function test 182
metastases 29*f*
approach to patient with synchronous 31
oncosurgery management of 32

synchronous *versus* metachronous 27
synchronously detected 34*fc*
unresectable, treatment options for 38
parenchyma 38
resection 38
Lobectomy 146, 149, 157, 159
Lobular carcinomas 291
Locoregional therapy 38
Loop colostomy 72
Low-molecular-weight heparins 141, 259
Luminal tumors 273
Lung 149
and breast cancers 241
and diaphragm 146
cancer
early stage 149
resection for 153
video-assisted thoracic surgery 153
volume reduction surgery 149
Lymph node 150
dissection 153, 209
involvement 178
tuberculosis 177
Lymphadenopathy 177
Lymphatic malformation 249, 252, 255, 256, 262
classification of 253*b*
therapy of 261
Lymphaticovenous malformation 255
Lymphedema 253
choanal atresia 253
distichiasis 253
Lympho-adipose tissue 67, 69
Lymphocyte 151*t*
Lymphoma 241
Lymphovascular invasion 77, 276

M

Macrocephaly 256
Macrocystic, treatment of 262
Maffucci syndrome 256
Magnetic resonance angiography 253
Malignancies, primary 231
Malignancy 178
spreads 223
Malignant peritoneal mesothelioma 233

Malnourished patients 99
Mantoux test 173
Marshall scoring system, modified 47, 48*t*
Maryland dissector 9*f*
Mediastinal biopsies 158
Mediastinal space for thymic surgery 156
Mediastinal tumors, posterior 149, 159
Mediastinum 146, 149
Megestrol acetate 284
Melted extracellular water 1
Memorial Sloan Kettering Cancer Center 36
Menopausal symptoms 286
Mental retardation syndrome 253
Mesenchymal components 249
Mesenteric artery syndrome, superior 90, 99, 130, 132
precipitating factors for 99
radiological criteria for diagnosing 99
surgical procedures 100
Mesenteric ischemia 91
Mesenteric lymph nodes 166
Mesenteric tubercles, multiple 180
Mesenteric vein, superior 67, 130, 137
Mesocolic excision
complete 68*f*
main component of 67
Mesorectal excision 66
Metabolic complications 48
Metachronous cancer, detect 76
Metachronous lesions 74
Metal
cannula system 12
stent, self-expanding 71, 135
Metaplastic mucosa causes 110
Metastasectomy 204
Metastatic breast cancer 280, 285
hormone therapy for 289
Metastatic colorectal tumor 76
Metastatic lesions 199
Methylation 242
Methylene blue 114
Microarray-based technology 268
Microsatellite instability 74
Microsomal enzymes metabolize 241
Microtubule stabilizer 273
Microvascular invasion 214

Microwave ablation 22
Minimal access retroperitoneal
          pancreatic necrosectomy 54
Minimally invasive technique 183
Minimally invasive thoracic surgery
          146-159
    benefits of 151, 151*b*
    benign indications for 152
    contraindications 150
    future prospects in 156
    indications for 149
    indications for diagnostic 149
    indications for therapeutic 149
    oncological aspect of 153, 155
    principles of 150
    technological advances in 158
    thymoma for 155
Mitochondria 21
Mitomycin C 225, 228
Molecular
    genetics 193
    methods 173
    subtype 269
Monoclonal
    antibodies 212
    antibody bevacizumab 76
Monopolar electrosurgery 11
Mucinous tumors 226
Mucosal integrity, loss of 91
Multidrug resistance 239
    emergence of 165
Muscle strength 66
Mutation
    detected 245
    in the signaling pathway 76
    of exon 2 76
Myalgias 286
Myasthenia gravis 155
    thymectomy for 149
Mycobacteria detection, culture and
          drug sensitivity 174*t*
Mycobacterial culture 173
Mycobacterium tuberculosis 172
Myeloid leukemia, chronic 244
Myeloma cell 243
Myeloma upregulate 241

N

Nab-paclitaxel 134, 274
Nanotechnology 78

Nasogastric tube 91
National Comprehensive Cancer
          Network 28, 64, 76, 129, 146
National Surgical Adjuvant Breast and
          Bowel Project 281
Necrotic collection 52*f*
    acute 50
Neodymium-doped:yttrium aluminum
          garnet 260
Neostigmine 104
Nephron-sparing
    kidney cancers prostate cancer 24
    surgery *versus* radical nephrectomy
          206
Neuroblastoma RAS 73
Nicotinamide adenine dinucleotide
          hydrate 115
Nitroimidazole-oxazine PA-824 185, 186
Nonhomologous end joining pathway
          242
Nonmetastatic hepatic dysfunction 199
Nonne-Milroy syndrome 253
Non-nucleoside reverse transcriptase
          inhibitor 182
Nonsteroidal anti-inflammatory drugs
          110
Nuclear pleomorphism 268
Nuclear scintigraphy 200, 202
Nucleic acid amplification tests 173
Nucleotide excision repair 242
    pathway 242

O

Obesity 192
Obstructed colonic cancer, management
          of 70
Odynophagia 110
Olaparib 274, 275
Oligometastatic disease 210
    presence of 138
Oncotype-Dx 289
Ophthalmologic lasers, hallmark of 18
Oral contraceptive pills 282
Organ dysfunction syndrome, multiple
          46, 47
    risk of 46
Organ failure
    assessment, sequential 47
    multiple 44
    persistent 46, 47
    transient 46, 47

Orthopedic surgery 22
Osteolytic metastatic bone 199
Osteoporosis 286
Ovarian
　cancer, recurrent 230
　function suppression 287, 288
　ligaments 8
　tumors 101
Oxaliplatin 36, 75, 228, 273

P

Paclitaxel 274, 275
Pain 199
Pain and infection 252
Palbociclib 292
Palliative
　care 140
　interventions 204
　measures, specific 140
Pancreas
　divisum interfering 57
　head of 49, 67
　protocol 130
Pancreatic
　abscess 47, 52
　ascites 56
　cancer, advanced 129
　cancer, borderline resectable 129-141
　　definitions 131
　　evaluation and workup 130
　　principles of management 134
　　prognosis 142
　cancer, locally advanced 132f, 138, 139
　cancer, surgical techniques for 138
　fistula 138
　necrosis 51f
　parenchymal necrosis, presence of 44
　pleural effusion 56
　pseudocyst 49, 50f
　resection 54
　sphincterotomy 57
　stump 138
　tests 57
Pancreaticoduodenal arteries 54
Pancreaticoduodenectomy 138, 172
　specimen 137f

Pancreatitis, acute 43
　classification of 45fc
　complications of 43, 46, 47t
　phases of 45
　recurrent 57
　　causes of 57
　severity, classification of 44
　severity, grades of 44t
　systemic complications of 47
　types of 43
Pancreatitis edematous 44
Pancreatitis, mild acute 44
Pancreatitis, moderately severe acute 44
Pancreatitis necrotizing 43
Pancreatitis, severe acute 44
Pancreatoduodenectomy 138
Panitumumab 37, 38, 76
Para-aminosalicylic acid 165
Paracolic gutters, left and right 226
Paraneoplastic
　phenomenon 199
　syndromes 199
Parathyroid hormone-like peptides 199
Parenchymal
　dissection 21
　organs 21
Parkes Weber syndrome 256
Partial nephrectomy 206, 207
Paustian's criteria 181
Pazopanib 213
Peak hepatic enhancement 130
Pegylated variety 273
Pembrolizumab 275
Peptide growth factor mediated 283
Percutaneous
　catheter drainage 53
　microwave ablation 23
　sclerotherapy 264
Perianal fistulae 181, 184
Pericardium 233
Periduodenal lymph nodes 168
Perinephric
　tissues 204
　fat 205
Peripancreatic
　arteries 130
　collection 55f
　fluid collection, acute 48, 49
　necrotic 51
Perirenal hematomas 199

Peritoneal
  adhesion 89
  carcinomatosis 219
    assessment of 224f
    cases with mucinous 223
    colorectal cancer 231
    detection 221, 222t
    diagnosis 220
    gastric cancer 232
    management of 223
    ovarian cancer of 234
    prevent of 232
    staging, disease burden 223
  cavity 57, 99
  epithelial implants, multifocal 233
  malignant mesothelioma, treatment choice for 234
  mesothelioma 229, 233, 234
  metastasis 74, 220
  mucinous carcinomatosis 233
  pseudomyxoma 229
  sarcomatosis 230
Peritoneum 166, 233
Peritonitis 97
Peritumoral inflammation 72
Phenothiazines 103
Phosphoinositide 3-kinase inhibitors 293
Photoablative 19
Photochemical 20
Photodynamic therapy 119, 122, 262
Photokeratitis 21
Photothermal 20
Picibanil 262
Pinocytosis 240
Platelet-derived growth factor 212, 274
Platinum-based primary intraperitoneal chemotherapy 234
Pleura 149
  serosal layer of 233
Pleural
  biopsy 149
  effusion 56, 158
Pleurodesis 149
Pneumaturia 184
Pneumonectomy 149
Pneumonitis 214
Poly (ADP-ribose) polymerase inhibitors 274

Poly-adenosine diphosphate 243
Polycythemia 199
  account of 199
Polymerase chain reaction 175, 179
Porfimer sodium 122
Porphyrins 115
Portal fashion 147
Portal vein 130, 132, 133, 137
Portal venous phase 28, 130
Port-wine stains 254
Positron-emission tomography 77, 131, 222
  role of 202
Postmenopausal
  obesity, case of 282
  women 288
Potassium 183
  titanyl phosphate lasers 262
Potent multikinase inhibitor 274
Pouch of Douglas 226
Power cutting 17
Premenopausal women 288
Procarbazine 242
Progestins 284
  like medroxy-progesterone acetate 284
Progressive disease, supportive care for 140
Prostaglandins 199
Prosurvival signals, external 240
Protective stoma, use of 71
Protein
  calorie malnutrition 48
  correlates 292
  denaturation 15
Proteus syndrome 256, 261
Proton pump inhibitors, use of 109
Pseudoaneurysm-associated bleeding 54
Pseudocapsule 193
Pseudocysts 49, 50
  contents of 52
  pancreatic 54
  reports of 56
Pseudomyxoma peritonei 219, 227f, 233
Pseudo-obstruction 103
  causes of 103
  old age 90

Pulmonary
    aspergilloma 152
    biopsies 158
    fibrosis 262
    nodules, resection of 158
Pulse mode 18
Pulsed current 3
Pure coagulation current 6
Purified protein derivative 173
Purse-string stenosis 176
Purtscher's retinopathy resulting 57
Purulent form 172
Pyogenic granuloma 250
Pyrazinamide 181, 182
Pyrexia 199

R

Radiation
    in neoadjuvant setting 136
    proctitis 90
    therapy, intensity modulated 75
Radical nephrectomy 204, 206, 206f, 210
    part of 205
    procedure 205
Radical total pancreaticosplenectomy 137f
Radioembolization 28
Radiofrequency
    ablation 22, 38, 119, 207, 208
    current 2
    output 14
Radioisotope renogram 202
Radiotherapy 139
Radiotherapy, conventional 210
    versus stereotactic 136
Ranson's criteria 43
Rapamycin 275
    mammalian target of 213, 274, 275, 291
    mechanistic target of 259
Rectal cancer 29f
Regional lymphadenopathy 200
Renal
    cell carcinoma 190, 206, 209f
        bilateral 201f
        clinical features 198
            computed tomography 200
            imaging 200
            investigations 202
            laboratory findings 200
        magnetic resonance imaging 201
        physical examination 199
    epidemiology 191
    etiology 191
    familial subtypes 194t
    grading systems 198t
    histological, subtypes of 196t
    immunotherapy 211
    management 204
    pathology 193
    pulmonary metastases in 203f
    recent advances in 190
    role of genetic factors 192
    staging 202
    systemic therapy for advanced/metastatic 210
    targeted therapies 212
    TNM staging 203
    treatment of
        advanced 208, 209
        localized 205
    disease, end-stage 192
    failure, acute 47
    parenchyma 193
    tumors 200
    vein 204
Retinal damage 21
Retinoblastoma 24
Retrograde transvenous embolization technique 263
Retroperitoneal
    hematoma 54, 103
    lymph nodes 172
Retroperitoneoscopic approaches 207
Retroperitoneum 54, 57
Rhabdoid morphology 198
Ribociclib's 292
Ribose polymerase 243
Rifampicin 165, 181, 182
    resistance 175
Rigler's sign 93
Robotic thoracic surgery 159
Roux-en-Y cystojejunostomy 50

S

Sarcomatoid
    components 211
    elements 214
    variants 210

Schobinger classification 263
Sclerotherapy 259, 262
　　principle of 260
Segmentectomy 149, 157, 159
Selective ER
　　degraders 284
　　modulators 284
Semiclosed technique 226
Sentinel lymph node 290
Seprafilm 98
Serosal surfaces 219
Sertraline 246
Serum amino transferases 130
Servelle-Martorell syndrome 256
Short bowel syndrome 183
Sigmoid colectomy, specimen of 32
Sigmoid lesion, synchronous resection
　　of 33
Sigmoid volvulus 100
Sigmoidopexy 100
Single strand DNA breast 274
Sinusoidal fashion 3
Sirolimus 261
　　role of 259
Skeletal pain 199
Skin
　　discoloration 252
　　malignancy 21
Small bowel
　　disease, extent of 225
　　feces sign 95
　　obstruction 89, 90
　　tuberculosis 182
Smart electrode technology 14
Smoking, cessation of 192
Sodium 183
Soft tissue densities 177
Sorafenib 212, 274, 275
Sparking and arcing 9
Spinal
　　deformity 99
　　metastatic sites 210
　　trauma 99
Spindle cell hemangioma 256
Splenectomy 55, 138, 226
Splenic
　　artery 54
　　artery embolization 55
　　vein thrombosis 54, 55
Spontaneous pneumothorax 158

Squamocolumnar junction 110
Staphylococcus aureus 53
Statins 123
Stauffer's syndrome 199
Stem cell transplantation 211
Stereotactic
　　body radiation therapy 38, 74, 140,
　　　　210
　　radiosurgery 210
Sternotomy, median 156
Steroid hormone 17-beta-estradiol 281
Stierlin sign 176
Stoma related complications 76
Stromal
　　cells 243
　　elements 282
Sturge-Weber syndrome 254, 256
Submucosa
　　cancer 112
　　lymphoid tissue 166
Subtotal colectomy
　　limitations with 72
　　versus segmental colectomy 72
Succinate dehydrogenase 194
Suck cut technique 122
Sulfotransferases 242
Sunitinib 213, 241, 274, 275
Supraclavicular
　　lymphadenopathy 200
　　tachycardia 22
Surgery
　　anterior mediastinal masses for 149
　　locally advanced pancreatic cancer
　　　　for 140
　　sexual problems, after 76
Surgical
　　glove injury 6
　　practice, energy sources in 1
　　technique, good 97
Systemic chemotherapy 38
Systemic inflammatory response
　　syndrome 45, 46*b*, 47
Systemic platinum-taxanes
　　chemotherapy 234

T

Talc pleurodesis 158
Tamoxifen 281, 286, 287, 288, 289, 290,
　　292
Taxane-anthracycline combination 277

Taxanes 273
Temozolamide 242, 274
Temsirolimus 214
Testicular cancer 192
Thermal
　injury 8
　tissue effects 1
Thioridazine 246
Thoracolaparoscopic esophagectomy 153
Thoracoscopic
　instruments 148
　pericardial window 149
　surgery 147
　　and video-assisted thoracic surgery, difference 147
　　equipment for 148
　　equipment required for 148
　　multiportal 157
　　ports for 147*f*
　sympathectomy for hyperhidrosis 149
　thymectomy 155
Thoracotomy
　group 154
　procedures 151
Thrombocytopenia 214
Thromboembolism 259
Thrombophlebitis, recurrent 255
Thymectomy 159
　for thymoma 153
　in myasthenic patients 158
Thymic horns 156
Thymidine phosphorylase 78, 242
Thymoma 149
　early stage 156
Tissue
　changes, temperature determined 2
　injury 7
　　distal site 8*f*
　　during adhesionolysis 8*f*
　management system 14
Tobacco consumption 192
Toldt's fascia, lifting of 68*f*
Topoisomerase II inhibitors 242
Topotecan 274
Total pancreatectomy 138
Transabdominal ultrasonography 43, 130
Transarterial chemoembolization 38

Transcriptase-polymerase chain reaction 283
Transmembrane domain exists 241
Transmembrane proteins 282
Transoral endoscopy 110
Trastuzumab monoclonal antibody therapy 272
Trefoil factor-3 113
Tricyclic antidepressants 103
Trocar cannula units 148
Tubercular ascitis 179
Tuberculin test 173
Tuberculosis 102, 165
　abdominal 97, 165-185
　　clinical presentation of 167*t*
　　criteria for diagnosis of 181
　　from Crohn's disease 170*t*
　　histopathology in 180
　　laboratory diagnosis 172
　　management of 181
　　pathophysiology of 166
　　role of
　　　diagnostic laparoscopy 180
　　　surgery 182
　　sites involvement of 166
　colorectal 170
　current diagnostic methods for 174*t*
　esophageal 168
　extrapulmonary 175
　　risk of 166
　gastroduodenal 168, 182
　in Asia and Africa 90
　jejunal and ileocecal 168
　lymph node 172
　new modalities in management of 185*t*
　peritoneal 171
　solid organs of 172, 177
Tuberous sclerosis 192
Tubule formation 268
Tufted angioma 250
Tumor
　borderline resectable 132, 133
　cells 225
　　with sarcomatoid 198
　central 38
　derived 1,25-dihydroxycholecalciferol 199
　detecting synchronous 65
　extends 204

giant cells 198
heterogeneity 240, 244
locally advanced 138
marker 130, 221
microenvironment 244
non-metastatic 131
polyps 65
primary 31, 32
resection of 22
rupture primary resection 230
small 65
thrombus 198
unresectable 131
venous thrombus 200
Tunica vaginalis testi 233
Tyrosine kinase 275, 277
Tyrosine kinase inhibitor 213, 244, 274

U

UK Special Interest Group in Gastrointestinal and Abdominal Radiology 63
Ulcerohypertrophic variety 169
Ultracision, high power system 16
Ultracold liquid causes 23
Ultrasonic
 cutting 16
 dissectors 15
 energy 15
Ultrasound, physics of 15
Ultrasurgical hook 16
Ureteral obstruction 199
Ureters 55
Urethral sling, mid 37
Uridine 5'-diphospho glucuronosyltransferases 242
US Food and Drug Administration 292
Uterosacral 8

V

Vagal-sparing esophagectomy 119
Vaginal prolapse repair 37
Valvulae conniventes 93
Vapor pulse coagulation 14
Vascular endothelial growth factor 76, 273
 development of 212
 pathway antagonists 212

Vascular malformation 249, 250, 251f, 264
 associated with other anomalies 256b
 chest wall involvement in 258f
 classification of 250, 251b
 combined therapy 255, 255b
 diagnosis tool 256, 257
 extensive involvement of trunk 251f
 major vessels of 255
 therapy of fast-flow 263
 treatment 258
  endovenous intervention 260
  laser excision 260
  medical management 259
  sclerotherapy 259
  surgical excision 260
Vascular organ 172
Vascular tumor 249, 250
Vasculogenesis 249
Veliparib 274, 275
Vena cava, inferior 55, 198, 199, 202, 209
Vena cavography, inferior 202
Venous
 malformation 249, 250, 255, 256
  elbow region of 261
  therapy of 258
 phase contrast-enhanced CT 28f
 thromboembolism 141
 tumor thrombus management of 208
Ventricular arrhythmias, types of 22
Video-assisted
 fistula therapy 184
 retroperitoneal debridement 54
 thoracic surgery 146, 148
  augmented reality in 159
  instruments 148f
  limitations of 151
  ports 148f
  three-dimensional 158
  two-dimensional 158
  uniportal 156
  versus open thoracotomy, benefits of 150
Vienna classification 111
Vinblastine 210, 240
Vinca alkaloids 241
Vinorelbine 276

Virgin abdomen 96
Visceral organ tuberculosis 184
Voltage waveform 12
Volumetric laser endomicroscopy 115
Volvulus 90
Vomiting 91
von Hippel-Lindau disease 192-194, 212

W

Walled-off necrosis 52
Water jet dissection, high-velocity 21
Whirl sign 95

Wilms tumor 191, 192
World Health Organization 155, 165, 193
Wound protector 148*f*

X

Xpert *M. tuberculosis* 175

Y

Yttrium-90
    microspheres 75
    selective internal radiotherapy 38

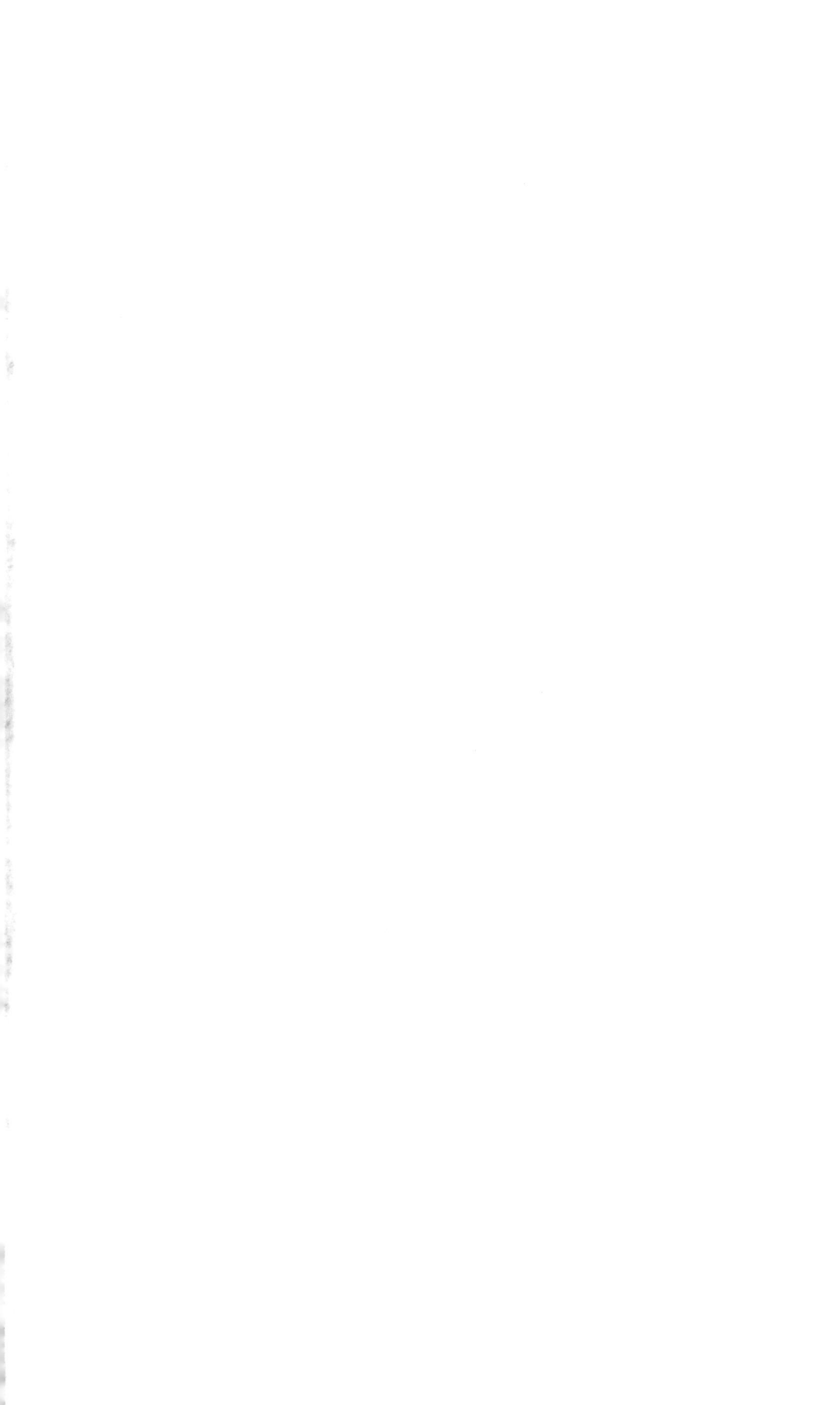

EU GSPR Authorised Reprsentative
Logos Europe, 9 rue Nicolas Poussin
1700, La Rochelle, France
Phone: +33 (0) 6 67 93 73 78
E-mail: contact@logoseurope.eu

www.ingramcontent.com/pod-product-compliance
Ingram Content Group UK Ltd.
Pitfield, Milton Keynes, MK11 3LW, UK
UKHW050428150426
5217IPUK00019B/1284